Hematology *for the* Medical Student

Hematology *for the* Medical Student

Alvin H. Schmaier, MD
Professor of Internal Medicine and Pathology
Director, Coagulation Laboratory
University of Michigan
Ann Arbor, Michigan

Lilli M. Petruzzelli, MD, PhD
Associate Professor, Internal Medicine-Hematology/Oncology
University of Michigan
Ann Arbor, Michigan

 LIPPINCOTT WILLIAMS & WILKINS
A **Wolters Kluwer** Company
Philadelphia · Baltimore · New York · London
Buenos Aires · Hong Kong · Sydney · Tokyo

Editor: Neil Marquardt
Managing Editor: Anjou K. Dargar
Marketing Manager: Scott Lavine
Project Editor: Paula C. Williams
Designer: Risa Clow
Compositor: Peirce Graphic Services, Inc.

351 West Camden Street
Baltimore, Maryland 21201-2436 USA

530 Walnut Street
Philadelphia, Pennsylvania 19106-3621 USA

Printed in the United States

Library of Congress Cataloging-in-Publication Data

Schmaier, Alvin H.
    Hematology for the medical student / Alvin H. Schmaier and Lilli Petruzzelli.
        p. cm.
    Includes bibliographical references and index.

    ISBN-13: 978-0-7817-3120-1
    ISBN-10: 0-7817-3120-8

    1. Blood—Diseases. 2. Hematology. I. Petruzzelli, Lilli. II. Title.

RC633.S365 2003
616.1'5—dc21   2003040115

To purchase additional copies of this book call our customer service department at **(800) 638-3030** or fax orders to **(301) 824-7390**. International customers should call **(301) 714-2324**.

Visit Lippincott Williams & Wilkins on the Internet:: **http://www.lww.com**. Lippincott Williams & Wilkins customer service representatives are available from 8:30 am to 6:00 pm, EST, Monday through Friday, for telephone access.

8 9 10

Dedications

I would like to thank Drs. Harold M. Mauer and Robert Colman for introducing me to the exciting and challenging field of hematology/hemostasis and Linda and Alec Schmaier whose presence and support make endeavors like this worthwhile.

—Alvin Schmaier

I would like to dedicate this book to my parents, Gloria and Anthony Petruzzelli, whose approach to life has been inspiring.

—Lilli Petruzzelli

Preface

The idea for this volume arose from the need to redesign the hematology course for second-year medical students at the University of Michigan. In preparing for this core sequence in the second year of the medical school curriculum, the hematology faculty realized that there was no current comprehensive, concise, multiauthor textbook that could serve as a reference for our second-year medical students. Furthermore, the need for such a volume was made clear by many students who sought a quality text that they could use as a supplement to lectures and course notes. Thus we have designed a multiauthor textbook highlighting the important basic concepts and diseases in red cells, white cells, and platelets. In particular, this text focuses on the approach to the patient with anemia, the approach to the bleeding patient, and the approach to the patient with thrombosis. Further, the hematologic malignancies are covered at the appropriate level for the practicing non-hematologist. Basic concepts of hematopoiesis, hemostasis, and bone marrow transplantation are also examined at the level of the practicing physician. Blood banking and transfusion practices are reviewed. Last, a special note is made on the distinctive hematologic features seen in pediatrics. Since this book is intended to be the student's first text in hematology, the entire volume has the goal to provide an introductory chapter on each of the many topics and to guide the student through the many diverse paths of this fundamental area in medical science. Because most students will never practice this area of medicine, this text is also intended to be a concise reference to the field for the nonexpert.

Acknowledgments

We would like to thank Dr. Will Finn for his aid in assembling the color atlas. We would also like to thank Sonja Girouard for her tireless efforts to help complete any task related to this volume.

Contributors

Paula L. Bockenstedt, M.D.
Clinical Associate Professor, Internal Medicine-Hematology/Oncology
Director, Adult Coagulation Disorder Program
University of Michigan
5301 MSRB III
1150 W. Medical Center Drive
Ann Arbor, MI 48109-0640

Robertson D. Davenport, M.D.
Associate Professor of Pathology
Medical Director, Blood Bank & Transfusion Services
University of Michigan
2G332 Agh
Ann Arbor, MI 48109-0054

Harry P. Erba, M.D., Ph.D.
Clinical Assistant Professor, Internal Medicine-Hematology/Oncology
University of Michigan
1355 CCGC
Ann Arbor, MI 48109-0922

James L. M. Ferrara, M.D.
Professor of Internal Medicine/Pediatrics & Communicable Diseases
Director of Bone Marrow Transplantation
University of Michigan
6308 CCGC
Ann Arbor, MI 48109-0942

William G. Finn, M.D.
Clinical Associate Professor of Pathology
Director of Hematopathology
University of Michigan
M5242 Medical Science Building I
Ann Arbor, MI 48109-0602

Scott D. Gitlin, M.D.
Assistant Professor of Internal Medicine-Hematology/Oncology
Director, Hematology/Oncology Fellowship Program
University of Michigan
5301 MSRB III
1150 W. Medical Center Drive
Ann Arbor, MI 48109-0640

Andrzej J. Jakubowiak, M.D., Ph.D.
Clinical Assistant Professor, Internal Medicine-Hematology/Oncology
University of Michigan
1353 CCGC
Ann Arbor, MI 48109-0922

Mark S. Kaminski, M.D.
Professor, Internal Medicine-Hematology/Oncology
Co-Director, Leukemia, Lymphoma and Bone Marrow Transplantation Program,
University of Michigan
4316 CCGC
Ann Arbor, MI 48109-0936

Kevin McDonagh, M.D.
Associate Professor, Internal Medicine-Hematology/Oncology
University of Michigan
5301 MSRB III
1150 W. Medical Center Drive
Ann Arbor, MI 48109-0640

Lilli M. Petruzzelli, M.D., Ph.D.
Associate Professor, Internal Medicine-Hematology/Oncology
University of Michigan
5301 MSRB III
1150 W. Medical Center Drive
Ann Arbor, MI 48109-0640

Samuel M. Silver, M.D., Ph.D.
Clinical Professor of Internal Medicine-Hematology/Oncology
Director, University of Michigan Care Center Network
University of Michigan
Bone Marrow Transplant
B1-207 CCGC
Ann Arbor, MI 48109-0914

Alvin H. Schmaier, M.D.
Professor of Internal Medicine and Pathology
Director, Coagulation Laboratory
University of Michigan
5301 MSRB III
1150 W. Medical Center Dr.
Ann Arbor, MI 48109-0640

Lloyd M. Stoolman, M.D.
Associate Professor of Pathology
Co-director Flow Cytometry Laboratory
University of Michigan
4224 Medical Science Building I
Ann Arbor, MI 48109-0602

Joseph Uberti, M.D., Ph.D.
Associate Professor of Internal Medicine-Hematology/Oncology
Clinical Director, Adult BMT
University of Michigan
Bone Marrow Transplant
B1-207 CCGC
Ann Arbor, MI 48109-0914

Gregory Yanik, M.D.
Clinical Associate Professor of Pediatrics-Hematology/Oncology
University of Michigan
Bone Marrow Transplant
B1-207 CCGC
Ann Arbor, MI 48109-0914

Contents

Introduction to Hematology

- ALVIN H. SCHMAIER AND LILLI M. PETRUZZELLI

I. INTRODUCTION

A. **Definition.** Hematology is the study of the normal and pathologic aspects of blood and blood elements.

B. **Hematopoietic system.** The hematopoietic system is characterized by turnover and replenishment throughout life. The pluripotent hematopoietic stem cell (HSC) is the progenitor of the cells in blood.

1. The cellular elements that arise from the HSC and normally circulate in blood include red blood cells (RBCs), white blood cells (WBCs), and platelets. WBCs include neutrophils, monocytes, lymphocytes, eosinophils, and basophils.

2. Because the HSC also gives rise to cells of the lymphoid system, hematology has traditionally included the lymph nodes and lymph tissue.

3. No specific organ is associated with hematologic disorders; diseases can arise in the bone marrow, lymph nodes, or intravascular compartment. The intravascular compartment, where blood cells and platelets circulate, includes the endothelial cell lining of blood vessels and the proteins in the blood plasma.

C. **Overview of this text.** This text introduces the medical student to hematology. Although most medical students do not become hematologists, all medical students must learn certain essential items about this area of medicine. After reading this text, the student will:

1. Learn the physician's approach to anemia and RBC disorders

2. Be able to fully evaluate a complete blood count

3. Understand screening tests for bleeding disorders as they apply to the classification of an individual with a protein or cellular defect that is associated with bleeding

4. Learn the clinical, protein, and genetic risk factors that contribute to thrombosis

5. Distinguish the WBC disorders that are recognized by nonhematologists from those that require consultation with a hematologist

II. ORIGINS OF HEMATOPOIETIC CELLS

A. **Embryogenesis.** Hematopoiesis begins early in embryonic development.

1. The cells that constitute the blood are derived from a common precursor cell, the HSC.

2. HSCs and the endothelial cells lining the blood vessels are thought to be derived from the same precursor cell in the aorta–mesonephros–gonad (AGM) region—the hemangioblast.

3. HSCs are present in small numbers and retain their ability to differentiate into blood cells of all origins as well as proliferate. During the earliest stages of embryogenesis, these cells circulate through the embryo to supply oxygen and deliver nutrients.

4. The HSCs that arise from the AGM system later in embryogenesis give rise to the blood system that seeds the liver and then the bone marrow.

5. Under the influence of specific growth and transcription factors, cells become committed to specific lineages.

B. **The myeloid system.** Cells of this group arise in the central marrow cavity (i.e., the medullary cavity). Myeloid lineage blood cells arising elsewhere in the body are designated as extramedullary in origin. The myeloid system consists of RBCs (erythrocytes), WBCs (neutrophils, monocytes, eosinophils, basophils), and platelets (thrombocytes). Neutrophils, eosinophils, and basophils are collectively called granulocytes because their function is defined by the presence and nature of their cytoplasmic granules. However, when physicians use the term granulocytes, they are often referring to just neutrophils.

1. **Erythrocytes** (RBCs) are specialized, nonnucleated cells that package hemoglobin, the protein that carries oxygen to and carbon dioxide from tissues.

   a. Erythrocytes undergo erythropoiesis, whereby they mature from a myeloid progenitor cell to a nonnucleated biconcave disk. Erythropoiesis is regulated by the growth factor erythropoietin and takes 4 days. The mature erythrocyte enters the circulation with residual RNA in its cytoplasm.

   b. A new RBC in the circulation is slightly bigger than older cells. Old RBCs lose their energy-producing capacity, develop stiff membranes, and are removed from circulation by the macrophages of the mononuclear phagocyte system of the spleen. The iron is normally retained in the reticuloendothelial system.

   c. The reticulocyte count reflects the percentage of early RBCs in the total number of RBCs in the circulation. RBC RNA remains in the erythrocyte about 1 day, so a normal reticulocyte count is less than 2%.

   d. The RBC lifespan is 120 days. Normally, there are about 5 million RBCs/μL of whole blood in adult men and 4.5 million RBCs/μL of whole blood in adult women.

2. **Neutrophils** (also called polymorphonuclear neutrophils, segmented neutrophils, or granulocytes) contain a nucleus that is usually a 3- or 4-lobed structure and stains a bluish color with Wright-Giemsa stain. An early form of a neutrophil is a band that shows an unsegmented nucleus. Neutrophils phagocytize and digest bacteria, cellular debris, and dead tissue.

   a. A neutrophil normally takes 12–13 days to be produced in bone marrow. Its lifespan in the circulation is about 12 hours, and it can live in tissues for several days. The marrow pool of mature neutrophils is 30–40 times that seen in the circulation. In the circulation, half are marginated (i.e., adherent to the endothelial cells) and half flow in the bloodstream.

   b. Only half of the neutrophils that are circulating are reflected in the WBC count. In the adult, neutrophils constitute 50%–80% of the total WBC counted (i.e., 4000–10,000/μL).

   c. Neutrophils exit the circulation via diapedesis to the tissues in response to chemotactic stimuli.

3. **Monocytes** are large, mononuclear cells with an indented (kidney shaped) nucleus. They form the circulating component of the mononuclear phagocyte sys-

tem. The nucleolus in mature monocytes circulating in the peripheral circulation is usually not identified on blood by light microscopy. Their role in host defense against organisms while in the circulation is similar to that of neutrophils.

    a. Monocytes spend 1–3 days in bone marrow and 8–72 hours in the peripheral blood.

    b. Once they traverse into tissues, they can differentiate into **macrophages,** which can survive in tissues for long periods (up to 80 days). Macrophages are characterized by and named for their tissue origin (e.g., alveolar macrophages in the lungs, Kupffer cells in the liver, splenic macrophages, and oligodendrocytes or glial cells in the brain). Macrophages phagocytize pathogens, cellular debris, and dead tissue.

  4. **Eosinophils** are characterized by prominent reddish orange granules seen with Wright-Giemsa stain. They usually have bilobed nuclei.

    a. Eosinophils increase in reaction to foreign protein; thus, they are seen in parasitic infections (especially larva of roundworms, helminths), allergic conditions, cancer, and certain drugs.

    b. The granules contain several proteins, most notably major basic protein.

    c. Normally, eosinophils constitute 0%–2% of the WBC count.

  5. **Basophils** are colorful cells with very dark bluish prominent granules on Wright-Giemsa stain.

    a. The granules contain histamine, heparin, and hyaluronic acid. Histamine release (basophil degranulation) is part of allergic reactions.

    b. Normally, basophils constitute up to 1% of the WBC count. The counts are often higher in patients with chronic myelogenous leukemia and other myeloproliferative disorders.

    c. Mast cells, which may have a common origin to basophils, contain histamine, have prominent granules, and play a role in host defenses against parasites.

  6. **Platelets** (thrombocytes) are nonnucleated cell fragments that contain remnant messenger RNA. Platelets are derived from the cytoplasm of the bone marrow megakaryocytes. Megakaryocyte growth and platelet development is regulated by thrombopoietin.

    a. Platelets have an 8–10 day lifespan. Their first 1–2 days are spent in the spleen. However, platelets can be entrapped by an enlarged spleen, as seen in congestive and inflammatory disorders.

    b. Platelets play a central role in hemostasis because they contain many hemostatic cofactors and inhibitors in their granules. At the megakaryocyte level, plasma proteins can be adsorbed and packaged into platelet granules. Platelets also contain many growth factors.

C. **Mononuclear phagocyte system** (also called the reticuloendothelial system). The mononuclear phagocyte system consists of circulating monocytes that are derived from myeloid progenitor cells in the bone marrow. The monocytes migrate from the circulation into tissues and differentiate into macrophages. Macrophages are found in the bone marrow, thymus, lymph nodes, spleen, serosal surfaces, adrenal cortex, Peyer patches, and Waldeyer throat ring. They function as a cleanup system for circulating debris; microorganisms; and aged, defective, or antibody-coated RBCs.

III. THE PHYSICAL STATES OF BLOOD

A. Blood is a **suspension** of cells in a solute of water, water-soluble proteins, and electrolytes.

   B. The **viscosity** of blood is equal to 1.1–1.2 centipoise. The viscosity of blood is highly influenced by RBC and protein concentration. Increased viscosity can occur from an elevation in cellular components (e.g., polycythemia) or protein (e.g., multiple myeloma [elevated immunoglobulin G levels], Waldenström macroglobulinemia [elevated immunoglobulin M levels]). Viscosity is also influenced by RBC size (smaller size increases viscosity) and the speed of blood flow in a given vessel (viscosity in the aorta is much less than in a small arteriole).
   C. **Blood volume** averages 70 mL/kg of body weight. The blood volume of an individual (e.g., man, dog) is approximately 7% of the total body weight. Using these two guidelines, a 70-kg person will have a blood volume of about 5 L.
   D. **Cellular composition** of blood averages 38%–42% in women and 40%–44% in men. The percent volume contributed by RBCs is called the **hematocrit** or packed cell volume.
   E. **Plasma** is anticoagulated blood from which the cellular components (RBCs, WBCs, and platelets) have been removed by centrifugation. It contains the coagulation proteins. **Serum** is the liquid in blood that has been collected without an anticoagulant. The coagulation proteins have clotted and formed a precipitate along with the cellular components of the blood. Plasma coagulation studies can be performed only on a sample collected with an anticoagulant and separated from the blood cells.

IV.   SUMMARY

Hematology consists of the study of normal and abnormal cellular components of blood: red blood cells, white blood cells, platelets, and the proteins in plasma that participate in coagulation, anticoagulation, and fibrinolytic reactions.

Hematopoiesis

- LILLI M. PETRUZZELLI

I. INTRODUCTION

A. **Definition.** Hematopoiesis is development of the hematopoietic elements, that is, the cells and other formed elements of blood.

B. **The hematopoietic system.** The hematopoietic system is composed of the blood elements, the protein components, and the supporting structures (i.e., stroma) that are necessary for blood development. In addition, the hematopoietic system includes a series of organs that serve as sites of hematopoiesis; these sites vary throughout development.

C. **Blood cells.** Blood cells perform a variety of functions, including delivery of oxygen by erythrocytes, formation of blood clots by platelets, host defense against infectious organisms by members of the myeloid series, and immune regulation by lymphocytes. Despite the wide functional diversity of blood cells, it appears that they originate from a common precursor cell. Research into development of the hematopoietic cells has yielded information not only on how blood cells develop but also on stem cells and how they relate to organ development.

II. HEMATOPOIESIS IN THE DEVELOPING HUMAN (FIG. 2–1)

A. During the first 8 weeks of embryonic development, nutrients and oxygen are delivered to the embryo by cells that arise in the extraembryonic yolk sac. The cells formed in the yolk sac contain a nucleus and use globin protein chains that are different from those used in adults to form the oxygen-carrying molecule.

B. Once the liver develops, it becomes the major site of hematopoiesis. The spleen also functions as a hematopoietic organ during this stage.

C. Later in fetal development, the bone marrow becomes the exclusive site of production of blood cells.

D. Throughout life, the bone marrow of the axial skeleton functions as a site of hematopoiesis; before age 20 years, the long bones also contribute significantly to blood cell production.

III. THE HEMATOPOIETIC STEM CELL (HSC)

A. **Overview**

1. Throughout life, hematopoietic cells age, are destroyed, and are replenished to maintain nearly constant levels in the normal host. In addition, blood cells increase in number in response to wound healing, blood loss, and infection.

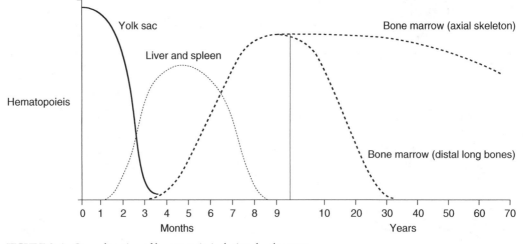

FIGURE 2–1. Organ location of hematopoiesis during development.

The hematopoietic system relies on the ability to replenish a pool of cells that can establish all blood elements. The HSC is defined by its ability to maintain this proliferation and differentiation.

2. HSCs are present in small numbers at any one time. Under the influence of growth factors and cytokines, HSCs develop or become committed to develop into a particular class of hematologic elements.

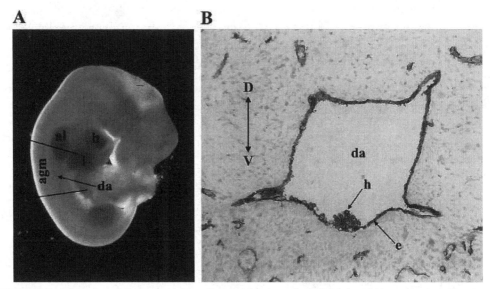

FIGURE 2–2. Generation of the hemangioblast during embryogenesis. A. A 34-day-old human embryo showing the heart (*h*), liver (*l*), and anterior limb bud (*al*). The aorta–gonad–mesonephros (*agm*) region extends from the umbilicus to the anterior limb bud and contains the dorsal aorta (*da*). B. Transverse section through the *agm* region indicated in A showing the dorsal aorta (*da*) and surrounding mesenchyme, which is stained with a monoclonal antibody to the membrane glycoprotein CD34 (*brown cells*). A cluster of CD34$^+$ hematopoietic cells (*h*) are associated with the ventral floor of the aorta in this region and are in contact with the endothelial cells (*e*) lining the wall of the aorta, which also express CD34. (Original magnification 39×.) (Reprinted with permission from Marshall CJ, Thrasher AJ: The Embryonic Origins of Human Haematopoiesis. *Br J Haematol*, 112:838–850.)

3. Although the HSC has been confirmed in mice, it has not yet been isolated in humans. The HSC is generated during embryonic development. In humans, HSCs are thought to arise from hemangioblasts, which are progenitor cells in the aorta–mesonephros–gonad (AGM) region of the embryo, at 30–37 days of gestation (Fig. 2–2).

4. The shared expression of a number of cell surface glycoproteins, transcription factors, and growth factor receptors with endothelial cells has led to the hypothesis that the hemangioblast is the precursor for endothelial cells as well as HSCs.

B. **Factors that influence hematopoietic stem cell development**

1. **Overview.** HSC development and lineage commitment depend on the activity of a number of transcription factors. These transcription factors establish gene expression programs that are specific for each hematopoietic cell lineage. Growth factors, such as erythropoietin and granulocyte–macrophage colony–stimulating factor (GM-CSF), and cytokines, such as interleukin (IL) 3 and IL-6 create an environment that sustains hematopoiesis by permitting viability or preventing cell death. The expression and concentration of a given transcription factor influences what lineage the HSC will develop. In HSC development, there is interplay between positive and negative regulatory transcription factors.

2. **Role of specific transcriptional regulators**

a. A single transcription factor responsible for turning a cell from the AGM region into an HSC or committed cell has not been defined, and development of blood cells is likely to involve the interplay of a number of transcription factors.

b. As a cell becomes committed (i.e., more restricted in its ability to develop into other cell types), there is a regulatory balance between the transcription factors that firmly establish the lineage to which the cell will develop. Both the cell-specific expression of certain transcription factors and the relative levels influence the development of specific cell lineages. Other factors are likely to function as either activators or repressors of specific panels of genes, so that as blood cells differentiate, certain genes are transcribed and others are turned off, depending on the cell line in which they are expressed.

3. **Potential for cells to exhibit lineage-specific development.** The HSC gives rise to all of the progenitors of blood cells (Fig. 2–3).

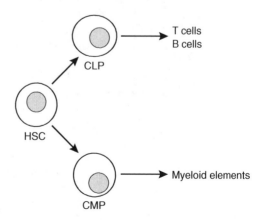

FIGURE 2–3. Hematopoietic stem cell differentiation into early progenitor cells. The hematopoietic stem cell (*HSC*) retains the potential to develop into common lymphoid progenitor (*CLP*) or common myeloid progenitor (*CMP*). The CLP generates both T and B cells, and the CMP differentiates into erythrocytes, neutrophils, monocytes, basophils, eosinophils, mast cells, and megakaryocytes.

    a. The earliest separation occurs at the level of the HSC when it becomes committed to give rise to the common lymphoid progenitor (CLP) or common myeloid progenitor (CMP).

    b. The use of transplantation models and cell culture has advanced the understanding of the capacity of cells to establish hematopoiesis.

      (1) The transplantation model is designed to introduce cells from a donor into mice whose own blood cells have been destroyed. This model has been used to characterize the developmental potential of a given population of blood cells. Using this model, it is now established in mice that there is a cell capable of repopulating all hematopoietic elements.

      (2) Cell culture techniques have been used to assess the developmental potential of isolated hematopoietic cells. Burst-forming units (BFUs) retain the ability to proliferate; however, they do not establish the entire hematopoietic compartment (see Figs. 2–4 to 2–7). BFUs take longer than colony-forming units (CFUs) to repopulate each cell lineage but establish a wider range of hematopoietic elements. BFUs are earlier cells.

    c. Flow cytometry is used to identify specific molecules on or in the cell using antibodies and fluorescent tagging. It has refined the analysis of cell lineages and the developmental hierarchy, particularly in cells that cannot be identified by morphology.

IV. ERYTHROPOIESIS

    A. Overview. The earliest separation of blood cell components in myeloid cell differentiation occurs at the development of the myeloid and lymphoid cells (Fig. 2–3). The myeloid-committed progenitor cell differentiates into cells that establish the granulocyte, erythroid, and megakaryocyte lineages. As each branch point is reached, cells become more restricted in their ability to form blood cells and divide. Most blood cell development occurs in the bone marrow; lymphoid development is established in the lymphoid tissue.

    B. Development of the erythroid lineage (Fig. 2–4)

    1. The earliest erythroid cells appear as nucleated red blood cells early in the embryonic development of humans. These cells do not lose their nuclei and are thought to be derived from a cell that is distinct from the HSC that gives rise to definitive hematopoiesis.

    2. Erythropoiesis begins when the multipotent CMP becomes committed to a burst-forming unit, erythrocyte (BFU-E). This unit is defined from culture techniques as a cell that gives rise in 14–16 days to erythroid colonies in humans. IL-3 is required for its growth. Other factors (e.g., GM-CSF, thrombopoietin, stem cell factor-1) influence its ability to proliferate.

    a. The BFU-E is a progenitor to the colony-forming unit, erythrocyte (CFU-E), which can generate erythroid colonies in culture in 6–7 days. The CFU-E undergoes approximately three to five divisions.

    b. Dependence on erythropoietin for development of the mature erythrocyte begins at the end of the BFU-E stage and remains a critical factor in subsequent stages of erythroid development.

    3. Characterization of the initial erythroid precursors relies on the ability to form colonies in a culture system. As the red cell matures, its development can be tracked by morphologic changes.

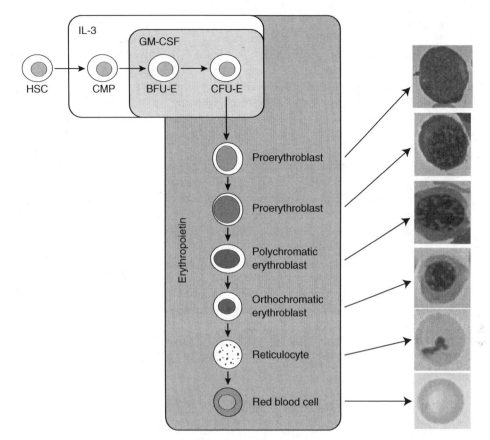

FIGURE 2–4. Erythropoiesis. Erythropoiesis begins with the HSC. Interleukin-3 (IL-3) and granulocyte–macrophage colony–stimulating factor (GM-CSF) are required to maintain viability of the earliest progenitors. Erythropoietin is required for maintenance of the erythroid lineage. Cells that require erythropoietin for viability are indicated by the *dark shaded area*. The stages when the cells are visible morphologically are indicated in the photographs to the right. *BFU-E,* burst-forming unit, erythrocyte; *CFU-E,* colony-forming unit, erythrocyte; *CMP,* common myeloid progenitor.

 a. The proerythroblast is the first visibly recognizable erythroid precursor. The proerythroblast is thought to retain its ability to divide and undergoes another three to five cell divisions. Only small amounts of hemoglobin are present at the proerythroblast stage.

 b. During the basophilic erythroblast stage, condensation of the chromatin begins. The ribosomes that are active in synthesizing hemoglobin reach their peak at this stage.

 c. During the polychromatic erythroblast stage, hemoglobin in the cytoplasm can be noted, and there is no further cell division. The chromatin continues to condense, and mitochondria in the cell are reduced.

 d. The full complement of hemoglobin is coincident with the appearance of the orthochromatic erythroblast. During this stage the nucleus begins to condense.

 e. The next species that is noted after extrusion of the nucleus is the reticulocyte. It contains ribosomes, mitochondria, and the Golgi apparatus. Methyl alcohol fixative enables visualization of the reticulin deposits in the cell. After several days in the circulation, the reticulocyte matures and the biconcave red blood cell becomes evident.

C. Hemoglobin synthesis

1. Most of the erythrocyte is composed of hemoglobin, and synthesis of hemoglobin is closely associated with the development of the erythrocyte. Production of hemoglobin involves the synthesis of the globin chains, the synthesis of protoporphyrin (heme), and the incorporation of iron into the heme moiety.

2. Tissue oxygen levels and the resultant elaboration of the glycosylated protein hormone erythropoietin by the kidney influence the maintenance of normal levels of hemoglobin. Erythropoietin interacts with a specific cell surface receptor on erythroid precursors. The cell between the CFU-E and proerythroblast is most sensitive to erythropoietin, and erythroid cells are critically dependent on the secretion of erythropoietin to maintain viability.

3. There are five globin genes, α, β, γ, δ, and ε. There are two pairs of α (chromosome 16), two different pairs of γ, and one pair of genes for β (chromosome 11) and δ. The genes are coordinately regulated and expressed at restricted periods in development (Fig. 2–5).

   a. The α cluster produces two types of globin, α-globin and ζ-globin. ζ-Globin is produced during the first 8 weeks in the human embryo. As α- and γ-globin appear, several hemoglobin pairings are seen (Fig. 2–5).

   b. From 2 months until birth, hemoglobin F is the major hemoglobin species responsible for oxygen delivery.

   c. At the end of gestation, under normal conditions, the β-subunit is synthesized and the hemoglobin F concentration begins to fall.

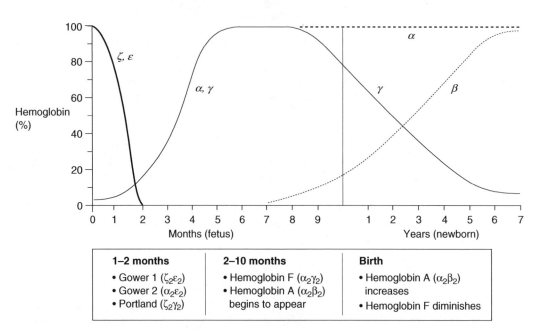

1–2 months	2–10 months	Birth
• Gower 1 ($\zeta_2\varepsilon_2$) • Gower 2 ($\alpha_2\varepsilon_2$) • Portland ($\zeta_2\gamma_2$)	• Hemoglobin F ($\alpha_2\gamma_2$) • Hemoglobin A ($\alpha_2\beta_2$) begins to appear	• Hemoglobin A ($\alpha_2\beta_2$) increases • Hemoglobin F diminishes

FIGURE 2–5. Hemoglobin synthesis in the developing organism. There are two main loci of globin genes: those containing the α cluster (ζ is part of this cluster) and a β cluster containing the ε-, γ-, δ-, and β-chains. Hemoglobin genes are synthesized from two groups or clusters of genes, the α and β clusters. During development, the genes are transcribed from the α cluster (ζ, α) and the β cluster (ε, γ, δ, β) and the pattern during development is indicated in the figure. As the fetus develops, some genes are turned off and others are turned on. However, the net result is the formation of a protein that is composed of two protein chains from the α-locus and two from the β-locus to form a four-chain heterodimer.

d. After birth, hemoglobin A continues to rise, and 30 weeks after delivery, hemoglobin F levels fall below 10% of the hemoglobin concentration.

V. DEVELOPMENT OF NEUTROPHILS

A. Overview. Similar to basophils and eosinophils, neutrophils are white blood cells that express granules. They share a precursor cell with monocytes, but all are originally derived from the CMP (Fig. 2–6).

B. The neutrophil before birth. The neutrophil is not required for host defense in utero; however, its establishment before birth is critical for extrauterine survival.

  1. The colony-forming unit, granulocyte monocyte (CFU-GM) appears as early as 5–6 weeks of gestation; however, there is no evidence of maturation at this stage.

  2. The first mature neutrophil is thought to appear as early as 15–16 weeks of gestation. At this stage in the developing fetus, mature neutrophils are found in the liver, spleen, and bone marrow.

  3. The neutrophil at birth is not functionally mature.

C. Maturation of the neutrophil in the normal host. The appearance of the granules that are critical to neutrophil function characterize the developmental stages of the neutrophil.

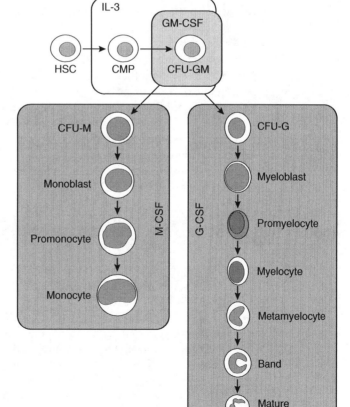

FIGURE 2–6. Granulopoiesis and monocytopoiesis. The colony-forming unit granulocyte macrophage (*CFU-GM*) gives rise to both the monocytic and granulocytic (neutrophil) lineages. It is derived from the common myeloid progenitor (*CMP*). IL-3 and granulocyte–macrophage colony–stimulating factor (*GM-CSF*) are required for production of these cells. Two distinct growth factors, granulocyte colony-stimulating factor (*G-CSF*) and macrophage colony-stimulating factor (*M-CSF*), support neutrophil and monocyte differentiation, respectively. *CFU-G*, colony-forming unit, granulocyte; CFU-M, colony-forming unit, monocyte; HSC, hematopoietic stem cell.

1. The CFU-GM is the common precursor to the monocyte and neutrophil. IL-3 and GM-CSF are required for the development of the CFU-GM.
2. The myeloblast, the first recognizable member of this family, is found primarily in the bone marrow. Primary granules that contain lysozyme in addition to other bactericidal proteins are found at this stage. Cell division occurs during this stage and is characteristic of cells in this series until the myelocyte stage.
3. Development of the promyelocyte is characterized by the appearance of azurophilic granules.
4. The myelocyte stage is characterized by the appearance of secondary granules that contain lysozyme, alkaline phosphatase, and other bactericidal proteins.
5. Cell division is no longer evident at the metamyelocyte stage, and the nucleus begins to indent. The cytoplasm also takes on the hue of the mature neutrophil on staining.
6. The band form is characterized by condensation of the nuclear chromatin and constriction of the nucleus. Tertiary granules containing gelatinase appear at this stage.
7. As the nucleus divides into two or more lobes separated by a thin filamentous strip, the cell enters the polymorphonuclear (i.e., neutrophil) stage. The absence of granulocyte colony–stimulating factor (G-CSF) results in a marked reduction in neutrophils.

VI.   MONOCYTOPOIESIS

A. **Overview.** The CFU-GM also forms the precursor cell to the monoblast, which forms mature monocytes in culture but is difficult to identify visually (Fig. 2–6).
B. **Developmental stages**
   1. The promonocyte is the earliest recognizable member of this family.
   2. Monocytes represent the mature blood-bound form of this lineage. These cells are capable of opsonizing or phagocytizing bacteria and contain granules that aid in bacterial killing. Although peroxidase production stops at this stage, it is present in the granules and helps the cells phagocytize and kill bacteria. Macrophage colony–stimulating factor (M-CSF) influences the survival and differentiation of the monocyte.
   3. Macrophages represent the tissue-bound form of monocytes that have differentiated in response to local factors.

VII.   DEVELOPMENT OF EOSINOPHILS, BASOPHILS, AND MAST CELLS

A. **Overview.** The members of this family are all derived from the common HSC, the CMP. Although basophils and mast cells are characterized by dense basophilic granules, basophils are not tissue-bound; they circulate similarly to monocytes.
B. **Mast cells.** The mast cell develops from the HSC and undergoes differentiation from a pre–mast cell to an early, intermediate, and then mature mast cell.
C. **Eosinophils and basophils.** The eosinophil and the basophil are derived from a common precursor cell that differentiates into mature eosinophils and basophils. Because of their small numbers, morphologic recognition of early precursors is limited. The early stages of eosinophil and basophil development require the presence of GM-CSF and IL-3. IL-5 is required for both eosinophil and basophil growth and differentiation.

VIII. MEGAKARYOCYTOPOIESIS

A. **Overview.** Thrombopoiesis (or megakaryocytopoiesis) results in the generation of circulating blood platelets (Fig. 2–7). The CMP is the earliest identified progenitor cell. It differentiates into the BFU of the megakaryocyte (BFU-MK), which becomes more restricted in development and becomes the CFU of the megakaryocyte (CFU-MK). The BFU-MK forms colonies in culture in 21 days, whereas the CFU-MK gives rise to colonies in 10–12 days. When proliferation ceases, the progenitors are committed to become megakaryocytes. The promegakaryoblast is the first cell to exhibit platelet-specific markers. None of these precursor cells can be distinguished by eye.

B. **Developmental stages.** The megakaryocyte is the first identifiable species in the pathway to platelet production. It is characterized by the ability to undergo endomitosis or nuclear division in the absence of cytoplasmic division. It is believed that the entire DNA content is replicated each time there is a round of division. The megakaryocyte can be identified by eye when there is 4N DNA content. Cytoplasmic maturation begins at the time of endomitosis and continues after DNA replication is complete. The megakaryocyte can be characterized in four stages based on the quality and quantity of the cytoplasm, size, and nuclear lobulation.

1. The megakaryoblast is the earliest megakaryocyte and constitutes approximately 20% of the megakaryocyte pool. Its nucleus is round; however, it can be lobulated or indented.

2. The promegakaryocyte is the next stage. It contains a lobulated nucleus and more abundant cytoplasm. The final DNA ploidy is achieved by this stage.

3. The megakaryocyte undergoes its final maturation, which is characterized by two morphologic forms.

   a. The earlier mature megakaryocyte (approximately 50% of the megakaryo-

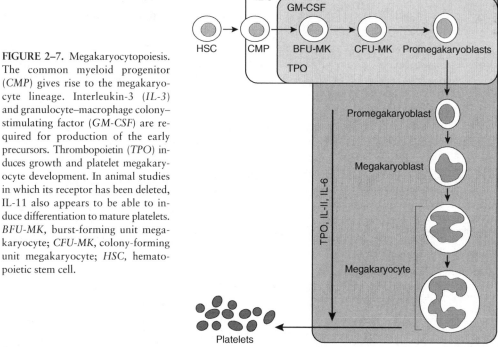

FIGURE 2–7. Megakaryocytopoiesis. The common myeloid progenitor (*CMP*) gives rise to the megakaryocyte lineage. Interleukin-3 (*IL-3*) and granulocyte–macrophage colony–stimulating factor (*GM-CSF*) are required for production of the early precursors. Thrombopoietin (*TPO*) induces growth and platelet megakaryocyte development. In animal studies in which its receptor has been deleted, IL-11 also appears to be able to induce differentiation to mature platelets. *BFU-MK*, burst-forming unit megakaryocyte; *CFU-MK*, colony-forming unit megakaryocyte; *HSC*, hematopoietic stem cell.

cytes at any one time) is characterized by a low ratio of nuclear to cytoplasmic matter and a loss of basophilic staining of the cytoplasm. The membrane system in the cell is well demarcated and the nucleus is pushed to one side.

b. The latter or second stage involves the formation of mature platelets. During this morphologic phase, the cytoplasm becomes irregular, and large platelets are shed. Cells with 8N DNA content or greater are generally involved in platelet production. The mechanism by which the platelets are shed from the cytoplasm and the nucleus is left behind is not known.

C. **Regulation of thrombopoiesis.** Thrombopoiesis is well regulated and is under the influence of a range of cytokines and growth factors.

1. Thrombopoietin stimulates the proliferation of progenitor cells such as BFU-MK and CFU-MK. It also supports differentiation of the megakaryocyte.

2. Like other hematopoietic elements, IL-3 is needed to support development of the BFU-MK and CFU-MK.

3. IL-6 acts in synergy with thrombopoietin to increase megakaryocyte numbers.

4. IL-11 stimulates platelet production and is elevated in response to low platelets in the circulating blood (thrombocytopenia). It is thought to act both on the early progenitor cells and in development of the megakaryocytes.

IX. LYMPHOPOIESIS

A. **Overview.** The development of lymphocytes begins as the earliest branch point from the HSC. Lymphocytes are a diverse set of cells that originate from the CLP in the bone marrow. However, in an emerging model some stem cells possess T lymphocyte–myeloid activity or B lymphocyte–myeloid activity. Development is different for each of the subclasses of lymphocytes.

B. **B-cell development**

1. B cells originate in the bone marrow.

2. Development is modulated by the cytokines elaborated by the bone marrow stromal cells and by cell–cell interactions (Fig. 2–8). The expression of immunoglobulin (Ig) on the cell surface is critical to its function and begins at the pro–B cell stage.

a. IL-7 plays a central role in B-cell development from the pro–B cell to the pre–B cell stage by directly stimulating proliferation. This is the period when a repertoire of B cells are generated; there are approximately eight cell divisions at this stage.

b. The movement of the B cell through maturation, eventually to reach the pre–B cell stage, is associated with the appearance of increasingly mature Ig on the cell surface. The first is IgM, followed by IgD and later IgG or IgA. Maturation is also associated with a change in density of less mature Ig.

3. Terminal differentiation of B cells occurs in the peripheral lymph organs (e.g., lymph nodes).

4. The life of the mature B cell is characterized by circulation from the tissue into the blood and back into the tissue.

5. Finally, B cells differentiate into plasma cells that are capable of antibody production.

C. **T-cell development**

1. Development of T cells also occurs in several stages.

a. The duration of interaction of the lymphocyte with the stroma is critical for development of T-cells in the thymus. Stem cells migrate to the thymus and begin maturing at the subcapsular cortex (Fig. 2–9).

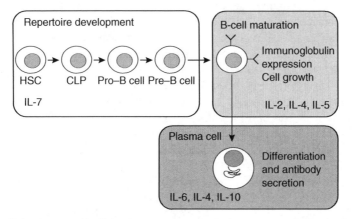

FIGURE 2–8. B-cell development. B-cell development occurs in the bone marrow during the early stages; however, final maturation of the B cell occurs in the peripheral lymph organs. The common lymphoid progenitor (*CLP*) gives rise to lymphocytes, and the hallmark of cell development is the rearrangement of the VDJ regions of the immunoglobulin chains to establish the lymphocyte repertoire. Rearrangement of the immunoglobulin begins in the pro–B cell stage and continues in the B cell. Immunoglobulin is expressed on the cell surface, and antigen promotes expression of the B cell. The indicated factors also stimulate the B cell to grow. The plasma cell is the terminally differentiated B cell. *HSC*, hematopoietic stem cell; *IL*, interleukin.

FIGURE 2–9. T-cell development. T-cell development begins with the common lymphoid progenitor (*CLP*) and depends on migration of the precursor cell to the thymus. T-cell development is associated with movement of the T cell through the cortex and medullary regions of the thymus. Cell surface markers identified by antibodies directed against cluster of differentiation (CD) antigens characterize each step of development and are indicated by the numbers associated with each T cell. The T-cell receptor expressed on the cell surface also varies with the developmental program; it can be the α β or γ δ form. The combination of the T-cell receptor expressed on the cell surface and the different CD molecules has established the developmental order in T cells. Most T-cell development occurs in the thymus, but the final stages that result in the cytotoxic or helper T cells occur in the peripheral blood. *TdT*, terminal deoxynucleotidyltransferase.

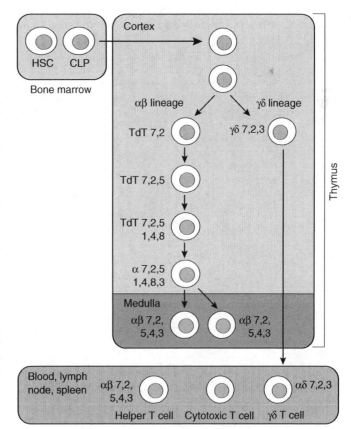

     b. As T-cells mature, they migrate toward the medulla. The developmental stages are marked by the appearance of specific cell surface proteins and by the T-cell receptor generated on the cell surface.

     c. Ultimately, the CLP develops into the terminal cells that function as either cytotoxic T or helper T cells.

  2. As T cells progress through development, identification is aided by a panel of antibodies that recognize cell surface molecules on leukocytes.

     a. The cluster of differentiation (CD) antigens are numbered; however, many of the molecules have now been identified at the molecular level. Figure 2–9 demonstrates their expression on major identifiable cells during T-cell development.

     b. In addition, the T-cell receptor subunits (α, β, γ, δ) are important in distinguishing T-cell receptor subsets.

  3. Like B-cell development, T-cell development depends on IL-7. IL-1, IL-2, and IL-4 have also been shown to play a role in differentiation. Specific adhesive interactions also contribute to differentiation and migration of the T cell through the thymus.

X.   SUMMARY

Hematopoiesis is a well-regulated process that encompasses the development of the blood cells. The cells originate from a common hematopoietic stem cell, and under the influence of transcription factors and growth factors, they become committed to developing into distinct compartments of the blood system. The molecular details outlined here present a scheme that continues to evolve as we learn more about the specific components involved in the process.

SUGGESTED READING

Bondurant MC, Koury MJ. Origin and development of blood cells. In: Lee GR, Foerster J, Lukens J, et al. *Wintrobe's Clinical Hematology.* 10th ed. Baltimore: Lippincott Williams & Wilkins, 1999:145–168.

Marshall CJ, Thrasher AJ. The embryonic origins of human haematopoiesis. *Br J Haematol* 2001;112:838–850.

Orkin SH. Diversification of haematopoietic stem cells to specific lineages. *Nat Rev Genet* 2000;1:57–63.

CHAPTER 3

Red Blood Cell Biochemistry and Physiology

- KEVIN MCDONAGH

I. INTRODUCTION

Understanding the factors that regulate RBC growth and development and the genetic and biochemical basis of RBC physiology is critical for an informed approach to the diagnosis and treatment of anemia.

II. RED BLOOD CELL DEVELOPMENT (ERYTHROPOIESIS)

A. Early development. Red blood cells (RBCs) are normally produced in the **bone marrow.** RBCs are derived from **pluripotent hematopoietic stem cells (HSCs)** and share a common precursor (or **progenitor cell**) with other **myeloid lineage cells,** including megakaryocytes, granulocytes, monocytes, macrophages, eosinophils, and basophils. Thus, inherited or acquired abnormalities in HSCs or myeloid progenitor cells may be associated with functional or quantitative defects in multiple types of blood cells.

B. Regulation of growth. The growth and maturation of RBCs from the HSC and myeloid progenitor cells is regulated by a complex interplay between specific genetically defined developmental programs and external signals generated by remote and neighboring cells.

1. **Growth factors** are an important class of external signals used to regulate hematopoiesis. Multiple hematopoietic growth factors have been identified and characterized.

2. **Erythropoietin (EPO)** is the single most important growth factor regulating erythropoiesis.

   a. EPO is produced in the **kidneys** by peritubular cells that sense tissue oxygen content. When oxygen delivery to the kidneys falls because of anemia, hypoxemia, or other cause, these renal peritubular cells rapidly increase synthesis and release of EPO.

   (1) The normal rise in EPO associated with anemia may be blunted or absent in patients with renal disease.

   (2) As a result, renal disease is frequently associated with anemia and is a common indication for treatment with recombinant EPO.

   b. In response to EPO, erythroid precursors in the bone marrow are stimulated to proliferate and mature, resulting in increased production and release of RBCs.

   c. There is normally an **inverse relationship** between the hematocrit and plasma EPO levels (Fig. 3–1). In individuals with a normal hematocrit, EPO levels are low or undetectable. As the hematocrit declines, EPO levels increase **logarithmically.**

C. **Stages of development**

   1. The development stages of red blood cells are presented in Chapter 2 (see Fig. 2–4).

   2. At the time of release from the bone marrow, the erythrocyte has not assumed the normal biconcave disk shape of the mature RBC. This young erythrocyte is anucleate but is larger than a mature RBC and has a spherical shape characterized by the absence of central pallor.

      a. On a Wright-stained peripheral blood smear, these cells have a faint bluish coloration in the cytoplasm (**polychromatophilia**) that reflects staining of the last remnants of the synthesis of hemoglobin by messenger RNA.

      b. When stained with a supravital dye, such as new methylene blue, the RNA and polyribosomes in these cells aggregate and are identified as **reticulocytes.**

   3. Reticulocytes differentiate into fully mature RBCs (smaller cells with central pallor and no polychromatophilia) within 1–2 days after release into the circulation from the bone marrow. Thus, reticulocytes are the youngest erythrocytes normally identified in the peripheral blood. An elevation in the number of reticulocytes in the circulation is an indication that RBC production is increased, usually in response to the loss of RBCs from bleeding or hemolysis (i.e., shortened RBC survival).

III.   HEMOGLOBIN: STRUCTURE AND FUNCTION

A. **Structure**

   1. Hemoglobin is the major protein in mature RBCs. A hemoglobin molecule is composed of four **globin** chains. Each globin chain is bound to a **heme** moiety containing **iron**. Two of the globin chains are derived from the **α-globin** locus on chromosome 16, and the remaining two globin chains are derived from the **β-globin** locus on chromosome 11 (Fig. 3–2).

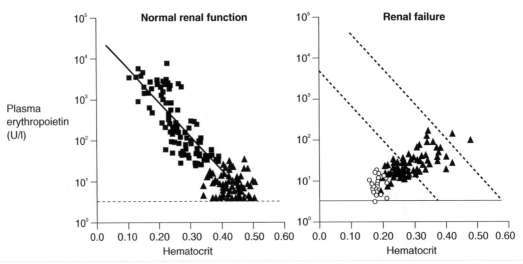

FIGURE 3–1. Relationship between hematocrit and erythropoietin levels in normal individuals and patients with renal failure. (Reprinted with permission from Erslev AJ, Erythropoietin. *N Engl J Med* 1991;324: 1339–1344.)

2. Different globin chains are expressed during the embryonic, fetal, and post-natal (adult) stages of development. Hemoglobin molecules containing different globin chains can be distinguished from one another by electrophoresis or liquid chromatography.

   a. **Fetal hemoglobin** contains two α-globin chains and two γ-globin chains ($\alpha_2 \gamma_2$). Fetal hemoglobin is the major hemoglobin during the later stages of fetal development (Fig. 2–5).

   b. Around the time of birth, expression of γ-globin is suppressed.

   c. β-Globin is the major β-like globin chain expressed after birth and in adults, although small amounts of γ-globin and δ-globin are also produced.

   d. **Hemoglobin A,** which is composed of two α-globin chains and two β-globin chains ($\alpha_2 \beta_2$), normally represents more than 95% of the hemoglobin in adult RBCs.

   e. Hemoglobin A_2 ($\alpha_2 \delta_2$) and fetal hemoglobin $\alpha_2 \gamma_2$) are also normally found at low levels in adult RBCs.

3. Genetic mutations in the α-globin or β-globin locus may result in the expression of an abnormal hemoglobin (**hemoglobinopathy**) with a different amino acid composition and aberrant migration pattern on electrophoresis. Although the variant hemoglobin may be functionally normal, it may have physical or physiologic properties that differ from those of a normal hemoglobin molecule.

4. A second category of genetic mutations in the globin loci (**thalassemia**) is characterized by a quantitative reduction in the synthesis of α-globin or β-globin chains and a net reduction in the formation of hemoglobin.

B. Function

1. The major physiologic role of hemoglobin is transport of oxygen from the lungs to the tissues. Oxygen binds to hemoglobin with high affinity in the oxygen-rich environment of the alveolar capillary bed and dissociates from hemoglobin in the relatively oxygen-poor environment of the tissue capillary bed. The loading and unloading of oxygen from hemoglobin is facilitated by conformational changes in the hemoglobin molecule that alter its affinity for oxygen (**cooperativity**).

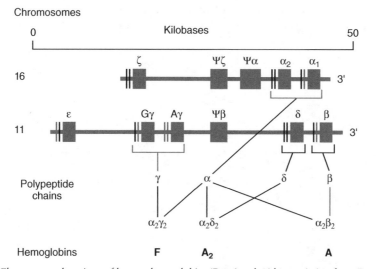

FIGURE 3–2. Chromosome locations of human hemoglobin. (Reprinted with permission from Benz EJ. *Hemoglobinopathies.* Fig. 106–1. Harrison's online.)

2. Hemoglobin oxygenation is classically depicted by an **oxyhemoglobin dissociation curve,** which is based on the oxygen saturation of hemoglobin measured as a function of the partial pressure of oxygen (Fig. 3–3). A convenient measure of the oxygen affinity of hemoglobin is the partial pressure of oxygen when hemoglobin is 50% saturated (P_{50}). The P_{50} of hemoglobin varies as a function of temperature, pH, and the concentration of 2,3-diphosphoglycerate (2,3-DPG).

   a. Acidosis (low pH) and elevations in RBC 2,3-DPG content stabilize the deoxyhemoglobin conformation, resulting in decreased affinity for oxygen, an increase in the P_{50}, and a right shift in the oxyhemoglobin dissociation curve.

   b. Physiologic changes in the oxyhemoglobin dissociation curve occur as adaptive responses to anemia or hypoxia. Levels of 2,3-DPG within the erythrocyte are increased in individuals with chronic hypoxia or anemia and in individuals living at high altitudes. These changes in RBC 2,3-DPG levels result in a right shift of the oxyhemoglobin dissociation curve and the release of a greater proportion of hemoglobin-bound oxygen in tissue capillary beds.

IV. RED BLOOD CELL MEMBRANE

A. A mature RBC assumes the shape of a **biconcave disk.** When viewed from above on a peripheral blood smear, it shows an area of central pallor that corresponds to the region where the upper and lower membrane surfaces of the RBC are in closest proximity. The unique morphology of the RBC is adapted for transit through extremely narrow capillary beds and splenic sinusoids.

   1. Young, healthy RBCs are highly deformable yet rapidly return to their native shape after exiting a capillary bed.

   2. RBCs become more rigid and less deformable as they age, which contributes to their senescence and elimination from the circulation in the spleen. The average life span of an RBC is 120 days.

B. The skeleton of the RBC is formed by a complex network of structural proteins that tether the membrane lipid bilayer to the cell (Fig. 3–4). Key structural proteins in the RBC cytoskeleton include **spectrin, ankyrin,** and **band 3.** Congenital deficiencies in the function or quantity of these proteins are associated with abnormalities in RBC shape (**spherocytosis** or **elliptocytosis**) and shortened RBC survival (**hemolysis**).

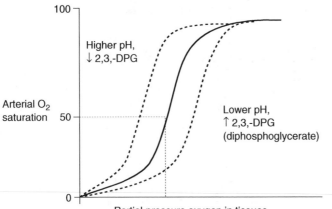

FIGURE 3–3. Red blood cell oxyhemoglobin dissociation curve. *DPG,* diphosphoglycerate.

C. The volume and ionic content of the RBC are actively regulated by energy-dependent pumps that traverse the membrane. These pumps depend on a constant source of **adenosine triphosphate (ATP)**, which is generated by **glycolysis** in the RBC. Defects in the production of ATP are associated with loss of cell volume, increased RBC rigidity, and decreased RBC survival.

V.   METABOLIC PATHWAYS IN RED BLOOD CELLS

The RBC has a relatively simple pattern of metabolic pathways (Fig. 3–5).

A. **Embden-Meyerhof pathway (anaerobic glycolysis).** The anaerobic glycolytic pathway is the major source of ATP production in the RBC. It generates the ATP necessary to power the ionic pumps that regulate cellular ion content and hydration status. Congenital defects in the glycolytic pathway, which are rare, are associated with a wide range of clinical disorders (e.g. myopathy, mental retardation, neuropsychiatric abnormalities, hemolysis of variable severity).

1. The hemolysis associated with defects in glycolysis is referred to as **congenital nonspherocytic hemolytic anemia** because the RBC morphology is minimally altered. The common biochemical consequence for the RBC is **ATP deficiency** leading to abnormalities in sodium, potassium, calcium, and water homeostasis. RBCs are typically more rigid than normal cells and are susceptible to retention and destruction in the spleen.

2. A subset of glycolytic enzyme defects (**Rapaport-Luebering pathway**) may also lead to reduction in RBC 2,3-DPG concentrations, causing a left shift in the hemoglobin-oxygen affinity curve (increased affinity) and further impairing oxygen delivery to the tissues.

B. **Hexose monophosphate shunt.** A small portion of glucose metabolism proceeds through the hexose monophosphate shunt. The RBC is designed to transport high concentrations of oxygen, an extremely reactive molecule with the potential to do chemical damage to vital components of the RBC. The RBC has elaborate defense mechanisms to protect itself from **oxidative damage. Glutathione** is a critical molecule necessary to detoxify **hydrogen peroxide,** the primary chemical intermediate in oxidative damage. Glutathione is maintained in a reduced state by the hexose monophosphate shunt. This pathway can also indirectly contribute to glycolysis and ATP production.

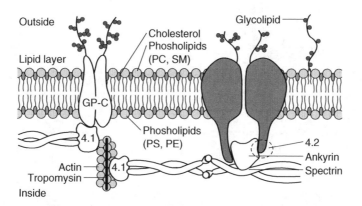

FIGURE 3–4. The red blood cell cytoskeleton. *GP-C*, glycophorin C; *PC*, phosphatidylcholine; *PE*, phosphatidylethanolamine; *PS*, phosphatidylserine; *SM*, sphingomyelin. (Reprinted with permission from Bunn HF, Rosse W. *Hemolytic Anemias and Acute Blood Loss.* Chapter 108. Harrison's online, 1999.)

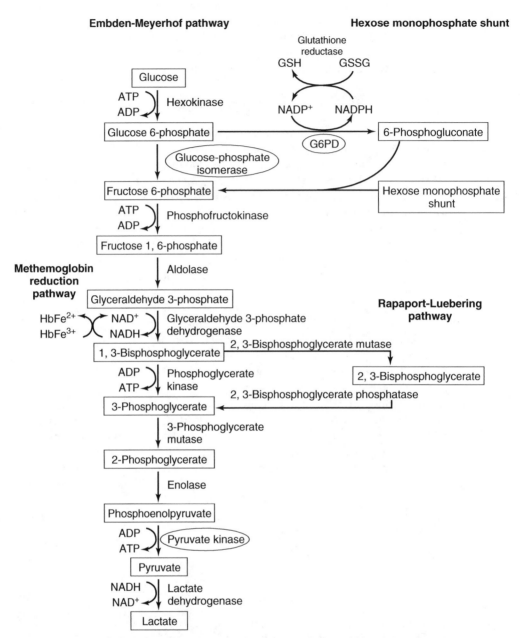

FIGURE 3–5. Red blood cell glucose metabolic pathways. *ADP,* adenosine diphosphate; *ATP,* adenosine triphosphate; *G6PD,* glucose-6-phosphate dehydrogenase; *GSH,* glutathione; *GSSG,* oxidized glutathione; *HbFe²⁺,* ferrous hemoglobin; *HbFe³⁺,* ferric hemoglobin; *NAD,* nicotinamide adenine dinucleotide; *NADH,* reduced nicotinamide adenine dinucleotide; *NADP,* nicotinamide adenine dinucleotide phosphate; *NADPH,* reduced nicotinamide adenine dinucleotide phosphate. (Reprinted with permission from Bunn HF, Rosse W. *Hemolytic Anemias and Acute Blood Loss.* Figure 103. Harrison's online, 2002.)

C. **Methemoglobin reduction pathway.** The methemoglobin reduction pathway maintains hemoglobin iron in the ferrous (Fe^{2+}) state, and defects in the pathway lead to hemolytic disorders due to unstable hemoglobins.

VI.   SUMMARY

Red blood cells are derived from precursor cells in the bone marrow. The major physiologic function of RBC is oxygen transport. Oxygen status has important direct effects on RBC production by the bone marrow and the biochemical properties of hemoglobin. The metabolic pathways of the RBC are streamlined to provide a simple, reliable source of ATP from glycolysis and maintain a steady pool of reducing substrates to protect RBC components from oxidative damage.

Evaluation and Classification of Anemia

• KEVIN MCDONAGH

I.   INTRODUCTION

Anemia is an extremely common medical condition that all physicians must address in clinical practice. The diagnostic approach to anemia is based on an understanding of the disease mechanisms that lead to it. Important clues to the cause of anemia may be obtained from the patient's history, laboratory studies, and an examination of the peripheral blood smear.

II.   CLINICAL DEFINITION OF ANEMIA

A. Anemia is best defined and monitored by measurement of the **hemoglobin (Hb) concentration.** The **normal range** for Hb is established by measuring the values from a large sample of healthy individuals and varies as a function of age and gender (Table 4–1).
   1. Males and females have equivalent Hb values until **puberty.**
   2. The increase in Hb that occurs in men is largely attributed to the effect of **androgens** on the release of erythropoietin (EPO) and the responsiveness of red blood cell (RBC) precursors to EPO.
   3. The gender disparity in the normal range for Hb concentration is less significant in elderly individuals.
B. Anemia is defined as Hb concentration more than two standard deviations below the normal range for age and gender. Using this definition, there is less than a 5% chance that a Hb concentration below the normal range is a "normal" value for the individual. Worldwide, almost one-third of the population is anemic.

III.   CLINICAL MANIFESTATIONS OF ANEMIA

A. The symptoms of anemia are correlated with the following five factors:
   1. The degree of reduction in the oxygen-carrying capacity of the blood
   2. The extent of change in the whole blood volume
   3. The rate at which the reduction in oxygen-carrying capacity and change in whole blood volume developed
   4. The ability of the cardiopulmonary system to compensate for the reduced oxygen-carrying capacity of the blood (cardiopulmonary reserve)
   5. Manifestations of the underlying illness that caused the anemia

TABLE 4–1 • Mean and Lower Limit of Normal for Adults*

	Hb (g/dL)		Hct (%)		RBC (10^{12}/L)		MCV (fL)	
	Mean	−2 SD	Mean	−2 SD	Mean	−2 SD	Mean	−2 SD
Female	14.0	12.0	41	36	4.6	4.0	90	80
Male	15.5	13.5	47	41	5.2	4.5	90	80

Hb, hemoglobin; Hct, hematocrit; MCV, mean corpuscular volume; RBC, red blood cell; SD, standard deviation.
*These values are for individuals 18–49 years of age.

    B. The specific symptoms associated with anemia and their duration may provide important clues to the chronicity and underlying disease process.

        1. Symptoms of acute hemorrhage are largely related to **hypovolemia** (hypotension, orthostasis, syncope, shock).

        2. A reduction in the oxygen-carrying capacity of the blood results in **tissue hypoxia**. Symptoms attributed to tissue hypoxia include fatigue, dyspnea, light-headedness, cognitive abnormalities, and ischemic pain (e.g., angina, claudication).

        3. Cardiovascular manifestations of anemia include tachycardia, palpitations, and congestive heart failure.

    C. The Hb concentration alone does not determine the severity of anemic symptoms. In the absence of underlying cardiac, pulmonary, vascular, or other significant systemic disease, chronic anemia of gradual onset is generally well tolerated until the Hb declines to very low levels (≤8 g/dL). The body has a number of adaptive physiologic responses to anemia:

        1. Cardiac output rises due to an accelerated heart rate (mild to moderate anemia) and increased ventricular stroke volume (severe anemia).

        2. Acute blood loss and the concurrent hypovolemia trigger reflex vasoconstriction. In contrast, chronic anemia is associated with a decrease in vascular resistance.

        3. Cerebral blood flow is preserved, while renal blood flow is decreased.

        4. The kidneys retain salt and water, leading to expansion of intravascular volume. Therefore, **blood transfusion in an individual with well-compensated chronic anemia may cause acute volume overload and precipitate congestive heart failure.**

        5. The unloading of oxygen in tissues is enhanced by an increase in RBC levels of 2,3-diphosphoglycerate and a right shift in the oxyhemoglobin dissociation curve.

        6. Renal peritubular cells detect anemia by sensing tissue oxygen content. The peritubular cells respond with an increase in the production of EPO. As EPO levels rise, erythroid precursors in the bone marrow are stimulated to divide and mature, leading to increased RBC production.

IV.　MECHANISMS OF ANEMIA

The clinical approach to the diagnosis of anemia is guided by an understanding of the underlying mechanisms responsible for anemia. The clinical history and physical examination are an attempt to gather initial clues to the cause of anemia. This information is correlated with laboratory studies to establish the underlying cause of the anemia.

A. **Hemorrhage.** The loss of RBCs through bleeding should always be the **initial focus** in any patient with anemia and should prompt an evaluation of the **hemostatic system.** Bleeding may be secondary to trauma, surgery, or an underlying disease. The **gastrointestinal tract** is a common location for clinically significant bleeding. **Menstruation** is an important source of blood loss in women of reproductive age. Chronic blood loss may be associated with concurrent iron deficiency and impaired ability of the bone marrow to generate replacement RBCs.

B. **Hemolysis.** Hemolysis is defined as a shortened RBC survival time not explained by bleeding. The average survival time of an RBC after leaving the bone marrow is 120 days.

1. Hemolysis is associated with changes in serum and urine **chemistry** values that reflect accelerated metabolism of RBC components and serve as important clues to the presence of a hemolytic process (Table 4–2). These biochemical changes may vary as a function of the anatomic location of RBC destruction (i.e., **intravascular** versus **extravascular**).

   a. RBCs contain a rich supply of **lactate dehydrogenase,** which is liberated from RBCs into the plasma with hemolysis.

   b. Hb released from RBCs is bound by a plasma carrier protein called **haptoglobin,** resulting in decreased levels of plasma haptoglobin. If RBCs are destroyed in the intravascular space, free **plasma Hb** may be present after all available haptoglobin has been bound and cleared and may spill into the urine.

   c. **Bilirubin** is a metabolic byproduct of hemoglobin. Unconjugated (**indirect**) bilirubin is frequently elevated in hemolysis, manifested clinically as **jaundice.**

   d. Chronic longstanding hemolysis is associated with increased excretion of bile pigments through the biliary system, which may result in the formation of **pigment gallstones.**

2. **Morphologic changes** in RBCs may provide important clues to the underlying cause of hemolysis (Table 4–3).

3. Hemolysis can be subclassified according to the **anatomic site** of RBC destruction.

TABLE 4–2 • Laboratory Evaluation of Hemolytic Anemia

	Extravascular Hemolysis	Intravascular Hemolysis
Hematologic studies		
Routine blood film	Polychromatophilia	Polychromatophilia
Reticulocyte count	↑	↑
Bone marrow examination	Erythroid hyperplasia	Erythroid hyperplasia
Plasma or serum		
Bilirubin	↑ unconjugated	↑ unconjugated
Haptoglobin	↓, absent	Absent
Plasma hemoglobin	N-↑	↑↑
Lactate dehydrogenase	↑ (variable)	↑↑ (variable)
Urine		
Bilirubin	0	0
Hemosiderin	0	+
Hemoglobin	0	+ (severe cases)

Reprinted with permission from Bunn HF, Rosse W, Hemolytic anemias and acute blood loss, Chapter 108, Table 108–1, Harrison's online 2002.

TABLE 4–3 • RBC Morphology Associated with Hemolytic Anemia

Morphology	Cause	Disorders
Spherocytes (or micro-spherocytes)	Loss of membrane	Hereditary spherocytosis, auto-immune hemolytic anemia
Target cells	Increased ratio of RBC surface area to volume	Hemoglobin disorders (thalassemias, Hb S disease, Hb C disease, liver disease
Schistocytes	Traumatic disruption of membrane	Microangiopathy, intravascular prostheses (artificial heart valves), Intravascular fibrin deposits (DIC, TTP), metastatic cancer
Sickled cells	Polymerization of Hb S	Sickle cell disease
Acanthocytes	Abnormal ratio of membrane lipids	Severe liver disease (spur cell anemias), abetalipoproteinemia
Agglutinated cells	Presence of IgM antibody	Cold agglutinin disease
Bite cells	Precipitated Hb (Heinz bodies)	Unstable Hb, oxidant stress

DIC, disseminated intravascular coagulation; Hb, hemoglobin; IgM, immunoglobulin M; RBC, red blood cell; TTP, thrombotic thrombocytopenic purpura.
Reprinted with permission from Bunn HF, Rosse W, Hemolytic Anemias and acute blood loss, Chapter 108, Table 108–2, Harrison's Online, 2002.

    a. **Intravascular hemolysis** (i.e., destruction of RBCs within blood vessels) is associated with the following conditions:

        (1) **Mechanical damage:** artificial heart valve, vascular anomalies (arterial dissection, arteriovenous malformation)

        (2) **Vascular damage:** microangiopathic hemolytic processes (disseminated intravascular coagulation, thrombotic thrombocytopenic purpura, hemolytic uremic syndrome, metastatic cancer) (see Chapter 7)

        (3) **Immune-mediated damage:** ABO incompatibility, paroxysmal cold hemoglobinuria

        (4) **RBC defect:** sickle cell anemia, paroxysmal nocturnal hemoglobinuria

    b. **Extravascular hemolysis** occurs when reticuloendothelial cells in the spleen destroy RBCs that are perceived as aberrant. This may be secondary to:

        (1) **Membrane-bound immunoglobulin G or complement:** autoimmune hemolytic anemia

        (2) **Damaged RBC membrane:** Heinz body anemia

        (3) **Loss of RBC membrane:** hereditary spherocytosis

  4. Hemolysis is also subclassified according to the **pathophysiologic cause.**

    a. In the case of an **intrinsic RBC defect,** RBC survival is shortened by a defect in the RBC. In most cases it is an inherited disorder, although acquired disorders exist. Possible causes include the following:

        (1) **Membrane disorder:** hereditary spherocytosis, paroxysmal nocturnal hemoglobinuria

        (2) **Enzymatic defect:** glucose-6-phosphate dehydrogenase deficiency

        (3) **Hb disorder:** sickle cell disease, Hb H disease

    b. In the case of an **extrinsic RBC defect,** the disease process is centered outside the RBC, which is a bystander or target of the disease. Most causes are acquired, although congenital disorders exist. Possible causes include the following:

        (1) **Mechanical or vascular disorders:** mechanical heart valve, arteriove-

nous malformation, arterial aneurysm, vasculitis, malignant hypertension

(2) **Immune disorders:** autoimmune hemolytic anemia (warm antibody and cold antibody type)

(3) **Drug-associated disorders:** drug-induced autoimmune hemolytic anemia, glucose-6-phosphate dehydrogenase deficiency

(4) **Metabolic disease:** abetalipoproteinemia, Wilson disease

C. **Decreased production of RBCs.** Deficient production of RBCs may result from a multitude of underlying causes.

1. Nutritional deficiencies of iron, vitamin B_{12}, or folic acid are common and readily correctable causes of hypoproliferative anemia.

2. Kidney disease may be associated with decreased production of EPO.

3. Nonhematologic systemic illness is often associated with anemia (e.g., anemia of chronic disease).

4. Anemia may result from a primary bone marrow disorder (e.g., myelodysplasia, leukemia, aplastic anemia).

V. LABORATORY EVALUATION OF ANEMIA: COMPLETE BLOOD COUNT

A. **Overview.** The complete blood count (CBC), or **automated blood count,** is a laboratory report of the cellular elements of the blood. The CBC is now routinely performed with an automated instrument. The CBC provides detailed information on RBCs, white blood cells, and platelets.

B. **Measured values.** Seven values relating to RBCs are reported on a CBC, including **Hb, RBC count, mean corpuscular volume (MCV), hematocrit (Hct), mean corpuscular hemoglobin (MCH), mean corpuscular hemoglobin concentration (MCHC), and red blood cell distribution width (RDW).** The Hb, Hct, and RBC count provide quantitative information about the RBC compartment. The MCV, MCH, MCHC, and RDW provide descriptive information about the RBC and are referred to collectively as **RBC indices.** Hb, RBC count, and MCV are measured directly, and Hct, MCH, MCHC, and RDW are calculated from the directly measured values.

1. The **Hb** is a direct measure of the **concentration** of Hb in grams per deciliter. Hb is the most accurate and reproducible value to describe and monitor anemia.

2. The **Hct** is the **volume** of RBCs expressed as a percentage of whole blood volume. The Hct reported by an automated blood count is a calculated value. The Hct can be directly measured by centrifugation of blood in a capillary tube, which is typically higher with anemic red blood cells than a calculated Hct because of plasma trapping during centrifugation.

3. The **RBC count** is a direct measure of the **number** of RBCs ($\times 10^{12}$ per liter).

4. The **MCV** is a direct measure of mean RBC volume in femtoliters (1 fL = 10^{-15} L). The MCV is obtained by dividing the Hct by the RBC count. For example, in a patient with an Hct of 45% and an RBC count of 5×10^{12} cells/L, the MCV equals:

$$\frac{0.45}{5 \times 10^{12}/L} = 90 \times 10^{-15}L = 90 \text{ fL}$$

The normal range for MCV is 80–100 fL.

5. The **MCH** is calculated by dividing the Hb by the RBC count and is expressed in picograms (pg). The normal range is 27–31 pg. The MCH is a calculated

value. It is linearly correlated with the MCV and provides little additional diagnostic information.

6. The **MCHC** is a value calculated by dividing the Hb by the Hct and is expressed in grams per deciliter. The normal range is 32–36 g/dL. Hypochromia is detectable when the MCHC is below 31 g/dL. MCHC may be increased in disorders characterized by membrane loss (e.g., hereditary spherocytosis) or cellular dehydration (e.g., Hb C disease). The MCHC is not usually clinically useful.

7. The **RDW** is a statistical value describing the coefficient of variation of the MCV, according to this formula:

$$RDW = \frac{\text{Standard deviation of MCV}}{\text{MCV}}$$

This value is calculated from the directly measured MCV. The RDW is especially useful in the subclassification of anemia when used in conjunction with the MCV.

VI. CLASSIFICATION OF ANEMIA BY THE ERYTHROPOIETIC RESPONSE

A. **Overview.** Measurement of the **reticulocyte count** provides a rapid method to differentiate between anemia due to defective production of RBCs and anemia due to decreased survival of RBCs from bleeding or hemolysis (Fig. 4–1).

1. Young erythrocytes just released from the bone marrow (**reticulocytes**) differ biochemically and morphologically from fully mature RBCs.

   a. Reticulocytes are larger than fully mature RBCs and more spherical.

   b. Reticulocytes are still in the process of synthesizing Hb. **Messenger RNA** is being translated into globin chains on **polyribosomes.** The staining characteristics of messenger RNA allow reticulocytes to be differentiated from older RBCs. Nucleic acid stains blue in a Wright stain. As a result, the cytoplasm of newly released RBCs will stain faint blue (**polychromatophilia** or **polychromasia**).

   c. The combination of increased size, spherical shape, and polychromasia, the hallmark of reticulocytes, differentiates them from other macrocytic RBCs. For example, in megaloblastic anemia due to vitamin B_{12} deficiency, large macroovalocytes are present in the peripheral blood smear but lack polychromasia.

   d. The polyribosomes in reticulocytes stain with supravital dye, such as new methylene blue or acridine orange.

2. Reticulocytes persist in the circulation for 1–2 days before they lose their RNA and undergo additional physical changes (e.g., loss of volume and membrane), becoming mature RBCs.

3. Reticulocytes are counted manually with a microscope or an automated fluorescent cell counter (**flow cytometer**). The reticulocyte count may be expressed as a percentage of total RBCs or as an absolute number of reticulocytes in a given volume of blood.

   a. In an anemic individual, the reticulocyte percentage must be corrected for the severity of the anemia. The **corrected reticulocyte count** is calculated by multiplying the reticulocyte percentage by a factor adjusting for the degree of anemia (i.e., actual Hct divided by ideal Hct).

   b. The **reticulocyte index** incorporates a second adjustment to account for the early release of reticulocytes from the marrow that occurs in anemia (Fig. 4–1).

   c. Early-released reticulocytes enter the circulation a day earlier than normal reticulocytes, and the corrected reticulocyte count is further multiplied by 0.5 to obtain the **reticulocyte production index** (RPI).

   (1) An RPI greater than 2% is consistent with preservation of the erythropoietic response and suggests that acute blood loss or hemolysis is responsible for the anemia.

   (2) An RPI less than 2% in the face of anemia is consistent with a bone marrow production defect.

   d. Modern automated measurements of reticulocytes by flow cytometry yield an **absolute reticulocyte count.**

   (1) An absolute reticulocyte count greater than 100×10^9/L is consistent with peripheral loss or destruction (shortened RBC survival).

   (2) An absolute reticulocyte count less than 75×10^9/L in the face of anemia is consistent with a production defect.

B. Elevated reticulocyte count. In an individual with normal bone marrow function, the reticulocyte count will be elevated in the presence of anemia. An elevated reticulocyte count suggests RBC loss (bleeding) or destruction (hemolysis) as the underlying cause of the anemia.

1. The RBC mass is maintained within the normal range by closely matching the rate of RBC production with the rate of RBC loss.

2. In normal conditions, approximately 0.8% of the circulating RBC mass must be replaced daily.

3. At maximum stimulation, the bone marrow is capable of increasing the production of new RBCs up to eightfold in response to anemia.

C. Normal or decreased reticulocyte count. If the reticulocyte count is not elevated in the face of anemia, the production of RBCs is defective. The following conditions should be considered as a cause of **hypoproliferative anemia.**

1. **Acute blood loss or destruction.** The bone marrow requires several days to a week to increase production of RBCs. Therefore, in the face of a precipitous drop in Hb, the reticulocyte count may not be elevated.

2. **Vitamin or mineral deficiency** (e.g., iron, vitamin B_{12}, folic acid)

3. **Bone marrow depression** (e.g., drugs, chronic infection, chronic inflammation, malignancy)

4. **Defective RBC production** (e.g., kidney disease, myelodysplastic syndrome, hereditary pure red cell aplasia (Diamond-Blackfan anemia), lead poisoning, alcoholism)

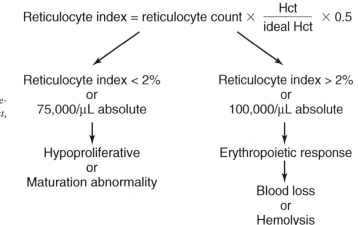

$$\text{Reticulocyte index} = \text{reticulocyte count} \times \frac{\text{Hct}}{\text{ideal Hct}} \times 0.5$$

Reticulocyte index < 2%
or
75,000/μL absolute

Reticulocyte index > 2%
or
100,000/μL absolute

Hypoproliferative
or
Maturation abnormality

Erythropoietic response

Blood loss
or
Hemolysis

FIGURE 4–1. Classification of anemia based on reticulocyte index. *Hct*, hematocrit.

5. **Destruction of marrow or erythroid precursors** (e.g., aplastic anemia, acquired pure red cell aplasia, parvovirus infection)
6. **Replacement of normal bone marrow** (e.g., leukemia, lymphoma, myeloma, carcinoma, granuloma, fibrosis)

VII.   CLASSIFICATION OF ANEMIA BY RED BLOOD CELL SIZE

A. **Overview.** The average size of the RBC (**MCV**) provides a convenient and informative framework to categorize the various types of anemia and their associated causes (Fig. 4–2). This classification system is commonly used by physicians in daily practice.

B. **Microcytic anemia**
1. Microcytosis is present when the MCV is less than 80 fL (Fig. 4–2).

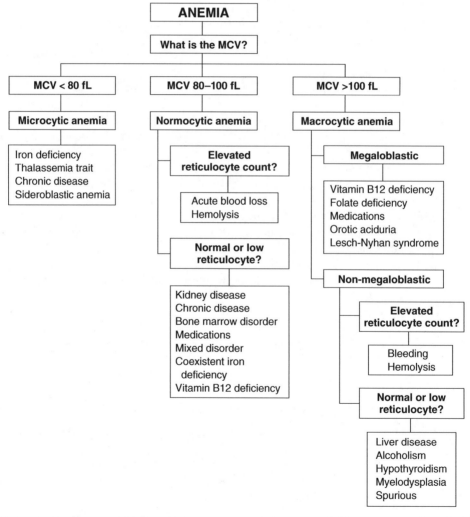

FIGURE 4–2. Classification and differential diagnosis of anemia based on red blood cell size. *MCV*, mean corpuscular volume.

2. Microcytic anemia generally reflects a deficiency in the synthesis of Hb. Defects in globin chain synthesis (thalassemia) or heme synthesis (iron deficiency, sideroblastic anemia) may be involved.
3. It is useful clinically to subdivide microcytic anemias into inherited and acquired causes.
   a. **Inherited** causes of microcytic anemia:
      (1) **α-Thalassemia** (deficiency in α-globin synthesis)
      (2) **β-Thalassemia** (deficiency in β-globin synthesis)
      (3) **Hb E disease** (a mild type of β-thalassemia)
      (4) Inherited sideroblastic anemia (defective heme synthesis)
   b. **Acquired** causes of microcytic anemia:
      (1) **Iron deficiency** (most common anemia overall in all populations)
      (2) **Anemia of chronic disease** (most common anemia in hospitalized patients)
      (3) **Lead poisoning**
      (4) **Medications** that interfere with heme synthesis (e.g., isoniazid)
C. **Macrocytic anemia**
   1. Macrocytosis is present when the MCV is greater than 100 fL.
   2. Macrocytic anemia can be divided into megaloblastic and nonmegaloblastic causes (Fig. 4–2).
      a. **Megaloblastic anemia** is caused by impaired DNA synthesis. Marked increases in MCV (> 110 fL) are generally associated with megaloblastic anemia.
      b. **Nonmegaloblastic anemia** is associated with a variety of causes (Fig. 4–2).
D. **Normocytic anemia**
   1. Normocytic anemias are characterized by an MCV that falls within the normal range (80–100 fL).
   2. In many respects, normocytic anemias present the greatest diagnostic challenge because they may reflect an underlying systemic illness (e.g., anemia of chronic disease) or a more complex presentation of a hematologic disorder (e.g., combined iron and vitamin B_{12} deficiency) (Fig. 4–2).
   3. Patients with hypoproliferative normocytic anemia (i.e., a low reticulocyte count) may require a bone marrow examination for an accurate diagnosis of the underlying problem.

VIII. CLASSIFICATION OF ANEMIA BY VARIABILITY IN RBC SIZE

A. The MCV represents an average of the RBC size. Subpopulations of RBCs of different sizes may be present within the total RBC pool but will not be identified by the MCV alone. The **RDW** is the coefficient of variation of the MCV:

$$RDW = \frac{\text{Standard deviation of MCV}}{\text{MCV}} \times 100$$

The RDW describes the heterogeneity in RBC size within a blood sample. The normal range is 11.5%–14.5%.
B. The information provided by the RDW can be qualitatively obtained by examination of the peripheral blood smear. **Anisocytosis** is the descriptive term for variation in RBC size observed on a peripheral blood smear. **Poikilocytosis** is the descriptive term for variation in RBC shape observed on a peripheral blood smear.
   1. A normal RDW indicates that the RBCs are relatively uniform in size.
   2. An elevated RDW indicates that the RBCs are heterogeneous in size and/or shape.

C. The RDW is used in conjunction with the MCV to subclassify the likely cause of anemia. For example, both thalassemia and iron deficiency are associated with microcytic anemia.
   1. The RDW is normal in thalassemia, an inherited disorder with a uniform deficiency in the synthesis of Hb.
   2. In contrast, the RDW is increased in iron deficiency, an acquired disorder with variable impairment in Hb synthesis from cell to cell.

IX. SUMMARY

The differential diagnosis of anemia is broad. The likely cause of anemia in an individual patient can be narrowed by a thorough and systematic evaluation. Critical information includes measurement of the erythropoietic response to anemia (reticulocyte count) and measurement of red blood cell size (MCV and RDW). These data provide a framework that guides the selection of more specific studies to establish the underlying diagnosis.

CHAPTER 5

Nutritional Anemias

- SCOTT D. GITLIN

I. INTRODUCTION

The term *nutritional anemia* refers to a decreased concentration of hemoglobin or a decreased number of red blood cells (RBCs) in the blood that results from the lack of a substance obtained and replenished by ingestion of foodstuffs (Table 5–1). Deficiencies of iron, vitamin B_{12}, and folic acid are the most commonly encountered clinical nutritional anemias.

II. IRON DEFICIENCY ANEMIA

A. **Total body iron content**
   1. The normal body iron content is 3–4 g for an adult. Typically, men have 50 mg/kg and women have 35 mg/kg of iron in their bodies.
   2. Less than 0.2% of the total body iron content is found in the plasma, where it is carried bound to a transport protein (transferrin). Approximately 70% of the total body iron content is found in heme compounds, with hemoglobin (67%) and myoglobin (3%) making up most of these compounds. Approximately 29% of the remaining iron (nonheme iron) is stored as ferritin and hemosiderin.
      a. **Ferritin,** the major storage form of iron, is sequestered in a nontoxic form and available for future use.
      b. **Hemosiderin** is a water-soluble form of iron.
      c. Heme-containing enzymes (e.g., cytochromes, catalase, peroxidase) and the iron transport compartment contain less than 1% of the total body iron.
   3. For reference purposes, packed RBCs contain 1 mg/mL of iron. Each unit of packed RBCs used for transfusion contains 200–223 mg of iron. Every gram of hemoglobin contains 3.3 mg of iron.
B. **Iron metabolism**
   1. **Overview**
      a. The metabolism of iron is dominated by its role in hemoglobin synthesis. In this process, iron is used over and over again; therefore, the internal movements of iron can be described as a cycle (Fig. 5–1).
         (1) Iron absorbed from the duodenum and proximal jejunum in the gastrointestinal (GI) tract or modified from iron stores in the liver enters the plasma, where it is bound to transferrin.
         (2) This circulating iron is transported from the plasma to cells that have the capacity to make hemoglobin (e.g., in the bone marrow).

TABLE 5–1 • Nutrients Required for Normal Erythropoiesis

Iron
Vitamin B_{12} (cobalamin)
Folic acid
Proteins, amino acids, calories
Vitamin B_6
Vitamin B_2 (riboflavin)
Nicotinic acid (niacin)
Vitamin C (ascorbic acid)
Vitamin A
Vitamin E
Copper
Cobalt

(3) The iron, now part of the hemoglobin in mature erythrocytes, is delivered to the circulation.

(4) At the end of an RBC's life span, the RBC is engulfed by macrophages of the reticuloendothelial system, primarily in the spleen, and the iron is extracted from the hemoglobin.

(5) Some of this iron may be stored in macrophages as ferritin or hemosiderin, but most is delivered to the plasma and bound to transferrin, completing the cycle.

b. Each day, approximately 30 mg (normal man) of iron completes the iron cycle. An additional small amount of iron (probably less than 2 mg/day)

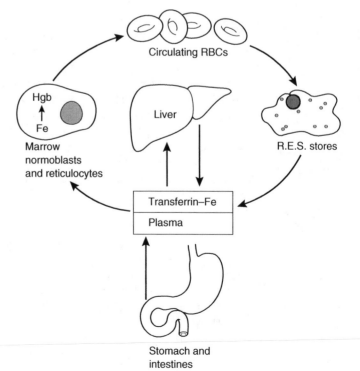

FIGURE 5–1. The metabolism of iron. Once absorbed into the body, iron is stored and recycled. The only normal loss of iron from the body is through the loss of cells. *Fe*, iron; *Hb*, hemoglobin; *RBCs*, red blood cells; *RES*, reticuloendothelial system. (Adapted with permission from Lee GR, Herbert V. Nutritional factors in the production and function of erythrocytes. In: Lee GR et al., eds. *Wintrobe's Clinical Hematology*. 10th ed. Baltimore: Williams & Wilkins, 1999:247.)

leaves the plasma to enter hepatic parenchymal cells and other tissues, where it is stored or used for synthesis of tissue heme proteins (e.g., myoglobin, cytochromes).

2. **Components of the iron cycle**
   a. **Iron absorption**
      (1) The average American diet contains 7 mg of iron per 1000 kcal (10–15 mg/day). Only 10% (1–2 mg) is typically absorbed.
         (a) Heme iron makes up 10%–15% of the nonvegetarian Western diet and is absorbed intact.
         (b) Nonheme iron absorption is affected by many factors, including reduction of ferric iron (Fe^{+3}) found in food to the ferrous form (Fe^{+2}), which is absorbed at the duodenum and proximal jejunum across the brush border. Nonheme iron absorption is also affected by foods that either inhibit (e.g., grains, tea, egg yolks) or enhance (e.g., vitamin C) absorption.
      (2) The extent of iron absorption depends on the amount of iron stored in the body. In other words, iron absorption increases with diminished body iron stores and with increased erythropoietic activity (and vice versa).
   b. **Iron transport: transferrin**
      (1) **Transferrin** (β_1-globulin) is the major physiologic **transport protein** for iron in blood. It transports iron to the cells.
      (2) Transferrin has the capacity to bind approximately 300 (250–450) μg Fe/dL. This value is known as the **total iron-binding capacity (TIBC)**.
      (3) **Transferrin saturation** is the proportion of available sites on transferrin for iron binding that are occupied by iron atoms, expressed as a percentage. Typically, only 33% (20%–50%) of transferrin is saturated (i.e., 100 μg Fe/dL).
      (4) A number of factors can affect serum transferrin levels and therefore the TIBC.
         (a) Iron deficiency, pregnancy, and estrogen therapy increase transferrin (TIBC) levels.
         (b) Inflammation, malignancy, liver disease, nephrotic syndrome, and malnutrition decrease transferrin (TIBC) levels.
   c. **Cellular iron use**
      (1) Transferrin-bound iron is delivered to RBCs by binding to specific transferrin receptors. Although transferrin receptors are found on all nucleated cells, erythroblasts, placental cells, and hepatocytes have more receptors than do other types of cells.
      (2) After transferrin binds to the transferrin receptor, transferrin–transferrin receptor complexes are endocytosed.
      (3) Once inside the cell, the iron is released into the cytosol and the transferrin is released back into the plasma.
         (a) Most (80%–90%) of the iron that enters an erythrocyte precursor is used to synthesize hemoglobin, myoglobin, and the cytochromes.
         (b) A small amount of the iron is used in the production of nonheme enzymes (e.g., ribonucleotide reductase).
         (c) Most of the remaining iron is stored in ferritin, which is found in all cells.
   d. **Iron excretion**
      (1) There is no physiologic mechanism for iron excretion. Iron is lost from

the body only when cells are lost, especially epithelial cells from the GI tract, skin, and renal tubules.

    (a) Normally, 1–2 mg of iron is lost each day.

    (b) Menstruating women lose an additional 0.006 mg/kg/day of iron (on average) prorated over the entire menstrual cycle.

    (c) Pregnant women lose iron at a rate approximately 3.5 times that of normal men.

  (2) Regulation of total body iron content depends primarily on control of absorption because there is little control on iron excretion.

C. **Etiology of iron deficiency anemia**

  1. A number of clinical situations can lead to iron deficiency, including the following:

    a. Increased iron requirements due to physiologic stresses (e.g., growth, pregnancy, lactation)

    b. Increased iron requirements due to pathologic causes (e.g., blood loss)

    c. Inadequate iron supply (e.g., consumption of foods low in iron, impaired absorption of iron, abnormal transferrin function)

  2. **Iron deficiency in an adult is almost always due to blood loss.** Dietary insufficiency and impaired absorption alone are rare causes of iron deficiency. Identification of the source of the blood loss should be the focus of the physician's attention.

D. **Clinical presentation of iron deficiency anemia**

  1. Patients may be asymptomatic or may present with signs and symptoms of anemia, including fatigue, weakness, pallor, palpitations, headaches, tinnitus, exertional dyspnea, and light-headedness.

  2. Some patients have signs and symptoms associated with the underlying cause of iron deficiency, such as GI symptoms (e.g., ulcers, gastritis, malignancy) or bleeding (e.g., menorrhagia, melena, hematochezia, hemoptysis, hematemesis, hematuria).

  3. History and physical examination may reveal signs and symptoms that reflect the effects of iron deficiency on nonhematopoietic tissues, such as:

    a. Glossitis (a red, smooth, waxy-appearing tongue with atrophy of the papillae)

    b. Angular cheilitis (ulcerations or fissures at the corners of the mouth)

    c. Esophageal webs and strictures (a web of mucosa that forms at the juncture between the hypopharynx and the esophagus and often leads to dysphagia)

    d. Koilonychia (concave or spoon-shaped nails)

    e. Blue sclerae

    f. Gastric atrophy

    g. Pica (obsessive consumption of substances with no nutritional value such as ice, clay, starch, dirt, or paper)

E. **Laboratory evaluation of iron deficiency anemia** (Fig. 5–2)

  1. **Complete blood count**

    a. A decrease in hemoglobin and hematocrit are the last events to occur in the progressive depletion of body iron stores. Small (microcytic), pale (hypochromic) RBCs are produced during iron-deficient erythropoiesis. However, this microscopic appearance of the RBCs is not specific for iron deficiency (Table 5–2).

    b. The earliest sign of iron deficiency erythropoiesis in the complete blood count (CBC) is an elevated red cell distribution width (RDW), which is the standard deviation of the mean corpuscular volume (MCV).

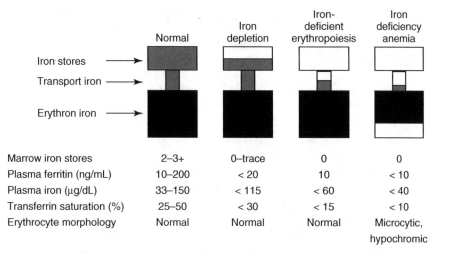

	Normal	Iron depletion	Iron-deficient erythropoiesis	Iron deficiency anemia
Marrow iron stores	2–3+	0–trace	0	0
Plasma ferritin (ng/mL)	10–200	< 20	10	< 10
Plasma iron (µg/dL)	33–150	< 115	< 60	< 40
Transferrin saturation (%)	25–50	< 30	< 15	< 10
Erythrocyte morphology	Normal	Normal	Normal	Microcytic, hypochromic

FIGURE 5–2. The location and level of iron in various states. Shading in each compartment indicates the level of iron; white indicates lack of iron. Also listed are the expected ranges of various measures of iron in the body. Marrow iron stores are rated as 0 (absent) to 3+ (maximum normal amount). (Adapted with permission from Brittenham GM. Disorders of iron metabolism: iron deficiency and overload. In: Hoffman R et al., eds. *Hematology: Basic Principles and Practice.* 3rd ed. New York: Churchill Livingstone, 2000:410.)

TABLE 5–2 • Differential Diagnosis of Microcytic, Hypochromic Anemia

Disorders of iron metabolism
  Iron deficiency
  Anemia of chronic disease[a]
  Atransferrinemia
  Familial microcytic anemia (impaired absorption and metabolism of iron)
  Antibodies to the transferrin receptor
  Gallium administration
  Aluminum intoxication
Disorders of globin synthesis
  Thalassemias (α and β)[b]
  Some hemoglobinopathies (e.g., hemoglobin E, hemoglobin C, unstable hemoglobins)
Disorders of porphyrin and heme synthesis
Disorders of heme biosynthesis (sideroblastic anemias)
  Inherited (usually X-linked)
  Acquired
    Alcohol
    Lead poisoning
    Drugs (e.g., isoniazid)
    Myelodysplastic disorders
    Vitamin B_6 deficiency

---

[a]Anemia of chronic disease is thought to be due to the blockade of iron release from the reticuloendothelial system to the developing erythron by cytokines.
[b]A high normal RBC count in the setting of low hematocrit and hemoglobin suggests thalassemia trait. The RBC distribution width tends to be normal, and the mean corpuscular volume is often much lower than expected for the level of anemia.

      c. Eventually, the MCV and mean corpuscular hemoglobin fall as older (normal) RBCs are removed from the circulation and hypochromic microcytes continue to be produced.

    2. Serum iron, TIBC, and percent transferrin saturation

      a. Serum iron levels decrease and TIBC increases **after** storage iron is depleted.

      b. A transferrin saturation of less than 10% with an elevated TIBC is diagnostic of iron deficiency in an otherwise healthy person.

      c. Serum iron levels and TIBC are both reduced by inflammation, infection, and malignancy. Therefore, reduced transferrin saturation alone is not specific for iron deficiency.

    3. Serum ferritin

      a. The serum ferritin level reflects the total body iron stores.

      b. A serum ferritin level less than 12 μg/L is diagnostic of iron deficiency.

      c. However, because ferritin levels may be elevated in patients with inflammation, infection, malignancy, hemolysis, and other clinical entities, a serum ferritin level greater than 12 μg/L does not eliminate the possibility of iron deficiency.

    4. Bone marrow aspiration

      a. This test is the gold standard for evaluating bone marrow iron stores and is the most sensitive indicator of iron deficiency.

      b. The diagnosis of iron deficiency requires the complete absence of intracellular iron deposits in an adequate bone marrow specimen.

F. Treatment of iron deficiency anemia

    1. Treatment of iron deficiency anemia is directed at the underlying associated condition (e.g., blood loss).

    2. Oral iron replacement is the therapy of choice (e.g., ferrous sulfate, other iron salts or preparations).

    3. Parenteral iron (e.g., iron dextran, iron gluconate) can be administered, but because of the associated risks and toxicities (e.g., allergic reactions, anaphylaxis), it should be reserved for specific clinical situations (e.g., unable to absorb iron from GI tract, unable to tolerate oral iron).

III.   MEGALOBLASTIC ANEMIA

A. General features

    1. The term *megaloblastic anemia* is used to describe a group of disorders characterized by a distinct morphologic pattern in the hematopoietic cells. These cells have a common biochemical feature, a defect in DNA synthesis. There are typically only minor defects in the synthesis of RNA and proteins.

    2. Overall, the result is unbalanced cell growth and impaired cell division characterized by cells with an immature-appearing nucleus, mature-appearing cytoplasm, and cell volume that is above normal.

    3. Vitamin B_{12} (cobalamin) and folic acid deficiency are the two most common causes of megaloblastosis.

B. Clinical presentation of megaloblastic anemia

    1. Megaloblastic hematopoiesis typically presents as anemia.

    2. A number of nonhematologic manifestations of vitamin B_{12} and folic acid deficiency may appear clinically. These include effects on epithelial tissues, such as the characteristic beefy, red, smooth tongue (vitamin B_{12} and folic acid deficiency), and neuropsychiatric manifestations (vitamin B_{12} deficiency only).

      a. The neuropsychiatric manifestations of vitamin B_{12} deficiency are thought to be due to the requirement for vitamin B_{12} in myelin synthesis and may include the clinical signs and symptoms associated with the following:

        (1) Peripheral neuropathies (e.g., paresthesia, numbness, hyporeflexia)

        (2) Dorsal column involvement (e.g., loss of position and vibratory sense, ataxia)

        (3) Subacute combined degeneration of the spinal cord

        (4) Optic atrophy

        (5) Psychiatric symptoms (e.g., dementia, psychosis, personality change)

      b. The neuropsychiatric manifestations induced by vitamin B_{12} deficiency may be present in the absence of anemia and other hematologic abnormalities. These clinical manifestations are reversible if the vitamin B_{12} deficiency is treated early.

C. Hematologic manifestations of megaloblastic anemia

    1. CBC and peripheral blood smear examination

      a. The morphologic appearance of the peripheral blood is the same whether the deficiency causing megaloblastic anemia is of vitamin B_{12} or folic acid. In both cases, the erythrocytes demonstrate an increased MCV with anisocytosis (elevated RDW) and poikilocytosis.

      b. Polymorphonuclear neutrophils (PMNs) may demonstrate nuclear hypersegmentation, defined as 5% of PMNs with five lobes or one PMN with six lobes. A finding of three or more PMNs with five lobes is highly suggestive of vitamin B_{12} or folic acid deficiency.

      c. Mild to moderate leukopenia and thrombocytopenia may be present.

    2. Bone marrow aspiration

      a. Bone marrow aspirate typically reveals hypercellularity with hyperplasia of all three major hematopoietic cell lines and abnormal appearance of the hematopoietic cells.

      b. The hematopoietic cell abnormalities in the bone marrow are often confused with those of acute erythroblastic leukemia.

D. Differential diagnosis of macrocytic anemia

    1. RBCs that are larger than normal (elevated MCV) are called macrocytic. A number of clinical situations can lead to macrocytic anemias, including the causes of both megaloblastic anemias and other macrocytic anemias (Table 5–3). Differentiation between megaloblastic and nonmegaloblastic causes of macrocytic anemia is important for identifying underlying diseases and determining appropriate treatment.

    2. In addition to vitamin B_{12} and folic acid deficiency, a number of other disorders can also present with megaloblastosis (Table 5–3).

    3. Artifactual macrocytosis can occur in the presence of cold agglutinins or marked hyperglycemia.

IV. COBALAMIN (B_{12}) DEFICIENCY

A. Cobalamin metabolism

    1. Overview

      a. Cobalamin is an essential cofactor for two enzymatic reactions: the conversion of methylmalonyl-coenzyme A (CoA) to succinyl-CoA and the conversion of homocysteine to methionine. The latter reaction generates tetrahydrofolate, which is required for DNA synthesis.

      b. Cobalamin is produced in nature only by microorganisms (bacteria and

TABLE 5–3 • Differential Diagnosis of Macrocytic Anemias

Clinical Condition	Differential Diagnoses
Megaloblastosis	Inherited disorders of DNA synthesis
	Orotic aciduria
	Lesch-Nyhan syndrome
	Thiamine-responsive megaloblastic anemia
	Deficiency of enzymes required for folate metabolism
	TCII deficiency or abnormalities
	Homocystinuria and methylmalonic aciduria
	Congenital dyserythropoietic anemias
	Erythroleukemia
	Drugs and toxins that interfere with DNA synthesis
	Chemotherapy drugs (e.g., antimetabolites, alkylating agents, hydroxyurea)
	Antiviral drugs (e.g., zidovudine)
	Antibiotics (e.g., trimethoprim)
	Oral contraceptives
	Anticonvulsants (e.g., phenytoin)
	Arsenic
	Herbicides, pesticides (e.g., chlordane)
	Nutritional anemias
	Vitamin B_{12} (cobalamin) deficiency
	Folic acid deficiency
Other macrocytic anemias	Reticulocytosis
	Hepatic disease
	Postsplenectomy
	Aplastic anemia
	Alcoholism
	Hypothyroidism
	COPD
	Benign familial macrocytosis
Artifactual macrocytosis	Cold agglutinins
	Marked hyperglycemia

COPD, chronic obstructive pulmonary disease; TCII, transcobalamin II.

fungi). Humans obtain cobalamin solely from the diet, particularly plants (legumes) that carry cobalamin-producing bacteria and animal muscular and parenchymal organs. The cobalamin produced by the bacteria that colonize the large intestine of humans is too distal for physiologic absorption.

  c. The average Western diet contains 5–7 μg of cobalamin per day. Cobalamin is stored in tissues in its coenzyme forms. The total body content in an adult is 2–5 mg, of which approximately 1 mg is stored in the liver. It takes 3–4 years to deplete cobalamin stores if absorption suddenly ceases.

2. Steps in cobalamin metabolism

  a. Cobalamin in food is usually nonspecifically protein bound in coenzyme form (Fig. 5–3).

  b. Peptic digestion at low pH in the stomach is required for release of cobalamin from food protein.

  c. Released cobalamin binds to R protein in saliva and gastric juice.

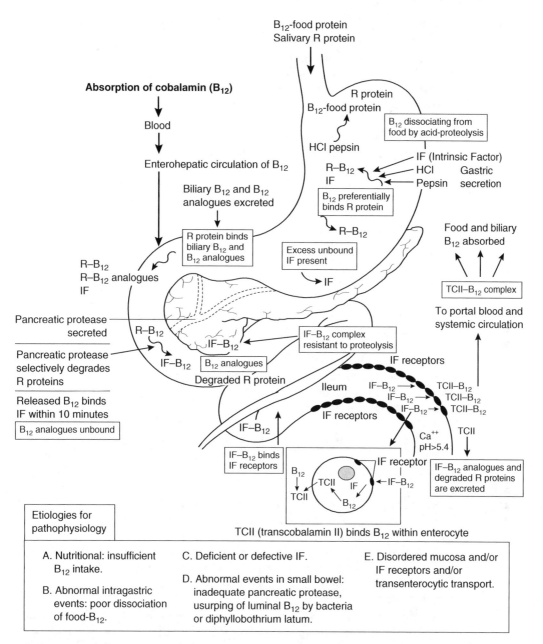

FIGURE 5–3. Cobalamin (B_{12}) metabolism through the gastrointestinal tract. *Cbl*, cobalamin; *HCl*, hydrochloric acid; *IF*, intrinsic factor; *TCII*, transcobalamin II. (Reprinted with permission from Antony AC. Megaloblastic anemias. In: Hoffman R, et al, eds. *Hematology: Basic Principles and Practice*. 3rd ed. New York: Churchill Livingstone, 2000:450.)

   d. Pancreatic proteases degrade R protein in the second part of the duodenum, where cobalamin can bind to intrinsic factor (IF), which is produced in the fundus and cardia of the stomach.
   e. The IF–cobalamin complex binds to specific membrane-associated IF–cobalamin receptors on microvilli of enterocytes of the terminal ileum and is actively transported into the enterocyte.

    f. In the enterocyte, cobalamin is released and binds to transcobalamin II (TCII). The TCII–cobalamin complex is transported to high-affinity receptors on tissues. The complex enters the cell, and the cobalamin is released.

B. Etiology of cobalamin deficiency

    1. Cobalamin deficiency can result from defects at any step of cobalamin metabolism.

    2. Possible causes of cobalamin deficiency:

        a. Inadequate dietary intake (e.g., strict vegetarian diet, breast-fed infants of mothers with subclinical cobalamin deficiency)

        b. Inadequate absorption, such as lack of gastric acid or pepsin, lack of IF. (Pernicious anemia is a disorder caused by the autoimmune destruction of gastric parietal cells that results in severe atrophic gastritis and a lack of IF production.)

        c. Reduced number or function of ileal receptors for IF–cobalamin complexes (e.g., surgical resection of the terminal ileum, Crohn disease, sprue)

        d. Pancreatic insufficiency

        e. Zollinger-Ellison syndrome (i.e., inactivation of pancreatic protease by gastric acid hypersecretion)

        f. Bacterial or parasitic competition for cobalamin (e.g., blind loops of intestine, fish tapeworms, diverticulosis)

        g. Nonfunctional TCII

        h. Inactivation of cobalamin (e.g., nitrous oxide)

C. Clinical presentation of cobalamin deficiency (see III.B.2.)

D. Laboratory evaluation of cobalamin deficiency

    1. Serum cobalamin (vitamin B_{12}) level

        a. This assay is a fairly reliable measure of total body cobalamin status.

        b. Some situations may lead to levels that are falsely low (e.g., folate deficiency, pregnancy, oral contraceptives), elevated (e.g., liver disease, chronic myelogenous leukemia), or normal (e.g., nonspecific interactions with some assay kit components).

    2. Serum homocysteine and methylmalonic acid levels (Fig. 5–4)

        a. The total serum homocysteine level is elevated in patients with either cobalamin or folic acid deficiency.

        b. Methylmalonic acid (a measurable precursor of L-methylmalonyl-CoA) is elevated only in patients with cobalamin deficiency.

        c. These levels will increase before serum cobalamin levels decrease.

    3. Schilling test

        a. This test is used to determine the site of a metabolic defect that has led to cobalamin deficiency. The patient is given radiolabeled cobalamin orally and an injection of unlabeled cobalamin.

        b. Stage I. The amount of radiolabeled cobalamin excreted in a 24-hour urine collection should be greater than 8% of the orally administered dose if absorption is normal.

        c. Stage II. If stage I is less than 8%, the patient is given oral IF plus radiolabeled cobalamin. If stage I is abnormal because of low endogenous IF production (e.g., pernicious anemia), more than 8% of the radiolabeled cobalamin will be excreted in a 24-hour urine collection.

        d. Stage III. If stage II is still less than 8%, the patient is given a 7- to 10-day course of antibiotics. If the abnormal stage II test was due to intestinal bacterial overgrowth, more than 8% of an orally administered radiolabeled cobalamin dose will be excreted in a 24-hour urine collection.

FIGURE 5–4. The role of cobalamin (B_{12}) and folate in homocysteine and methylmalonic acid metabolism. These primary biochemical reactions allow differentiation between cobalamin and folate deficiencies. Methyl-tetrahydrofolate (Me-FH$_4$) donates a methyl group to homocysteine to form tetrahydrofolate (FH$_4$) and the amino acid methionine. This reaction is mediated by methyltransferase, which requires cobalamin (in the form of methylcobalamin) as a cofactor. Therefore, this biochemical reaction requires both cobalamin and folate. The biochemical conversion of L-methylmalonyl-coenzyme A (CoA) to succinyl-CoA by a mutase only requires cobalamin in the form of adenosylcobalamin as a cofactor but does not require folate.

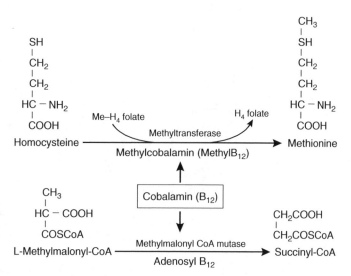

    e. If the Schilling test findings are abnormal because of pancreatic insufficiency, the coadministration of cobalamin with pancreatic extract (Viokase) will correct the excretion of orally ingested radiolabeled cobalamin.

  4. IF and parietal cell antibody studies are occasionally useful for making a diagnosis of pernicious anemia.

E. Treatment of B_{12} deficiency

  1. When possible, the underlying cause of the B_{12} deficiency should be treated.

  2. The goal of therapy is to replenish the patient's total body stores of B_{12} by administering B_{12} via an effective route.

    a. B_{12} is typically given parenterally in the form of cyanocobalamin. Various dosing schedules are used, such as 1 mg intramuscularly (IM) daily for 3–7 days, then 1 mg IM weekly for 4–8 weeks, then 1 mg IM monthly for life.

    b. Oral replacement of B_{12} can be used for some conditions, such as when the B_{12} deficiency is due to pancreatic insufficiency, in which case oral administration of pancreatic extract may be sufficient.

  3. Treating a B_{12}-deficient patient with folic acid may precipitate the neuropsychiatric manifestations associated with B_{12} deficiency.

  4. The results of treatment can be monitored over time.

    a. Reversion of megaloblastic hematopoiesis to normal hematopoiesis is evident in the bone marrow within 12–48 hours after initiation of therapy.

    b. Reticulocyte counts increase by 2–3 days and peak by 5–8 days after the initiation of therapy.

    c. Methylmalonic acid and homocysteine levels return to normal by the end of the first week of therapy.

    d. The RBC count, hemoglobin, and hematocrit normalize by 2 months.

    e. Hypersegmented PMNs remain in the blood for 10–14 days.

    f. It may take 6 months to see the maximal degree of improvement in the neurologic manifestations, and some may be irreversible.

V.   FOLIC ACID DEFICIENCY

A. Folic acid metabolism
   1. Overview
      a. Folic acid deficiency occurs most often in malnourished individuals.
      b. Total body folic acid stores are estimated to be 5–10 mg, with the liver containing most of the body's folic acid. Normal body folic acid stores are adequate for only 2–4 months.
      c. Rich sources of dietary folic acid include fresh green leafy vegetables, yeast, legumes, fruits, and animal proteins and parenchymal organs. Folic acid is thermolabile, so cooking decreases the amount of usable folic acid in a given food.
      d. Daily folic acid requirements are as follows:
         (1) Adult: 100 μg
         (2) Child: 50 μg (5–10 times that of an adult on a weight-for-weight basis)
         (3) Pregnant or lactating woman: 300–400 μg
      e. The active coenzyme forms of folic acid are derivatives of tetrahydrofolate, which acts as a methyl donor for purine and pyrimidine synthesis and for the conversion of deoxyuridine monophosphate to deoxythymidine monophosphate for DNA synthesis.
   2. Steps in folic acid metabolism
      a. Folic acid (pteroylglutamic acid) is absorbed in the small intestine.
      b. From the small intestine it makes its way to the serum, where most of the folic acid is free or loosely and nonspecifically bound to serum proteins. There is no major role for a specific transport protein for folic acid.
      c. In most tissues other than the liver, folic acid enters and remains within the cell throughout its life span. Folic acid that enters hepatic cells can later be released into the biliary circulation.
      d. Enterohepatic recirculation is important for folic acid metabolism and for redistribution of folic acid from liver stores to other tissues. Therefore, biliary drainage results in a dramatic decrease in serum folate levels.
B. Etiology of folic acid deficiency
   1. Folic acid deficiency can result from a number of abnormalities in folic acid metabolism.
   2. Possible causes:
      a. Nutritional factors (e.g., inadequate intake; increased requirements as in infancy, pregnancy, and lactation; hemolysis; psoriasis)
      b. Intestinal malabsorption (e.g., sprue, drugs, Crohn disease, HIV-related enteropathy)
      c. Drugs (e.g., ethanol, sulfa drugs, barbiturates)
      d. Defective cellular uptake of folic acid (rare)
C. Clinical presentation of folic acid deficiency (see III.B.)
D. Laboratory evaluation of folic acid deficiency
   1. Folic acid level
      a. A low serum folic acid level is diagnostic of folic acid deficiency. However, because the serum folic acid level is highly sensitive to intake (i.e., a single meal), a normal level may be reported even in the presence of total body deficiency.
      b. Measurement of RBC folic acid is a more reliable indicator of deficiency than measurement of free serum levels because it is not as readily influenced by oral intake. However, because the RBC folic acid level is 30 times

that of serum folic acid, mild hemolysis can increase the serum folic acid level and may mask a folic acid deficiency state.

2. **Serum homocysteine and methylmalonic acid levels** (Fig. 5–4)

   a. The total serum homocysteine level is elevated in patients with folic acid deficiency.

   b. Methylmalonic acid levels are normal in patients with folic acid deficiency.

E. **Treatment of folic acid deficiency**

   1. When possible, the underlying cause of the folic acid deficiency should be treated.

   2. Oral folic acid at 1–5 mg daily is usually adequate to treat deficiency, even when intestinal malabsorption of food folate is present. Therapy should be continued until complete hematologic recovery is documented.

   3. Prophylactic folic acid should be given to:

      a. All women contemplating pregnancy to prevent neural tube defects

      b. Pregnant or lactating women, who have increased daily requirements

      c. Patients with chronic hemolysis and increased erythropoiesis (see chapters 6 and 7).

   4. Folic acid supplementation decreases homocysteine levels. Therefore, elevated homocysteine levels, which have been associated with an increased risk of cardiovascular disease, should be treated with folic acid.

VI. SUMMARY

The nutritional anemias demonstrate that a number of substances obtained from foodstuffs are necessary for normal production of RBCs. Iron, cobalamin, and folic acid are the most commonly encountered nutritional substances whose deficiency is associated with anemia. Recognizing the clinical presentation and metabolism of each of these nutrients is important for recognizing and diagnosing the etiology of anemias. Therapy is generally directed at replacing the nutrient in a manner that will allow normal erythropoiesis.

CHAPTER 6

Congenital Hemolytic Anemias

• KEVIN MCDONAGH

I. INTRODUCTION

Congenital hemolytic anemias result from mutations that quantitatively or qualitatively influence the function of red blood cell proteins. These mutations can be broadly grouped into three categories: membrane defects, enzymatic defects, and hemoglobin defects. While many mutations have been described in each category, only a small number are commonly encountered in clinical practice.

II. GENERAL DIAGNOSTIC APPROACH TO CONGENITAL HEMOLYTIC ANEMIAS

Clinical findings and specialized laboratory studies are often required to precisely define the underlying disease process. This general approach is true especially in the case of congenital hemolytic anemias.

A. In all patients with hemolytic anemia, a careful **history** and **physical examination** are important.

1. The history should explore the chronicity of the problem, ethnic and racial background, family history, underlying or associated medical conditions, and new medications.

2. Jaundice is a common finding. Splenomegaly may also be associated with a wide variety of hemolytic disorders.

B. Various **laboratory abnormalities** are associated with hemolysis.

1. An elevated reticulocyte index is typical (see Fig. 4–1), consistent with a compensatory bone marrow response to anemia. Bone marrow examination is not necessary for most patients.

2. Increased lactate dehydrogenase, unconjugated bilirubin, and depressed or absent haptoglobin are also observed with hemolysis (see Table 4–2).

3. The red blood cell (RBC) morphology is frequently abnormal and provides an important clue to the underlying disease process (see Table 4–3).

4. The peripheral blood smear is rarely pathognomonic.

III. MEMBRANE DISORDERS

The features of membrane disorders are listed in Table 6–1.

A. **Hereditary spherocytosis**

TABLE 6–1 • Features of Membrane Disorders

Autosomal dominant inheritance
Marked heterogeneity in underlying mutations
Marked clinical heterogeneity
Generally mild, well-compensated hemolysis
Splenectomy is curative
Intrinsic defect
Extravascular hemolysis

---

1. **Overview.** Hereditary spherocytosis (HS) is a congenital hemolytic anemia of mild to moderate severity arising from abnormalities in RBC structural proteins that mediate **vertical interactions** with the lipid bilayer. Partial deficiencies in **spectrin, ankyrin,** or **band 3** cause HS. The inheritance pattern of HS is **autosomal dominant.** Autosomal recessive forms of the disease are rare and are usually associated with severe hemolysis. Most patients escape diagnosis until adulthood.

2. **Clinical presentation of hereditary spherocytosis.** The clinical presentation is variable from family to family, reflecting the heterogeneity of the molecular defects that underlie the disease. Members of a given kindred will exhibit a similar disease pattern. Clinical signs include the following:
   a. Jaundice
   b. Formation of pigment gallstones (from the high turnover of heme)
   c. Mild to moderate splenomegaly
   d. Leg ulcers (in patients with severe anemia)

3. **Laboratory evaluation of hereditary spherocytosis.** Typical HS patients have mild to moderate hemolytic anemia characterized by various laboratory findings.
   a. **Spherocytes** will be seen on the peripheral blood smear.
      (1) The structural protein deficiency results in the spontaneous release of lipids from the membrane and the formation of spherocytes.
      (2) Spherocytes are more rigid than normal RBCs, poorly deformable, and more susceptible to osmotic lysis. The rigidity of spherocytes leads to trapping in the spleen, where the RBCs lose additional membrane and become microspherocytes.
      (3) Ultimately, after many trips through the splenic circulation, microspherocytes are trapped in the spleen and destroyed.
   b. The anemia is characteristically well compensated by an increase in the production of new RBCs. As a result, the peripheral smear will also feature an increase in **polychromasia.**
   c. The **osmotic fragility test** is a formal laboratory test used in the diagnosis of HS. The test measures the *in vitro* lysis of RBCs suspended in solutions of decreasing osmolarity (Fig. 6–1).
      (1) Normal RBCs swell in hypotonic solutions and burst when a critical cellular volume is reached. Spherocytes are characterized by membrane loss and a decrease in the ratio of cell surface to volume; consequently, spherocytes lyse in solutions of higher osmolarity than normal RBCs. Spherocytes are more sensitive to a decrease in solution osmolarity.
      (2) Spherocytes formed by any mechanism (e.g., HS, autoimmune hemolytic anemia) will yield a positive result. Therefore, the osmotic fragility

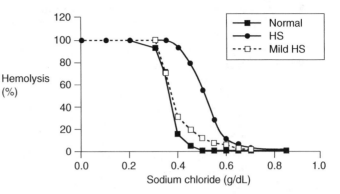

FIGURE 6–1. The osmotic fragility test. *HS,* hereditary spherocytosis. (Reprinted with permission from Bunn HF, Rosse W. H*emolytic Anemias and Acute Blood Loss.* Figure 108–1. Harrison's online, 2002.)

test is not diagnostic of HS, only confirmatory. At least 1%–2% spherocytes must be present for the findings to be abnormal.

4. **Treatment of hereditary spherocytosis. Splenectomy** is curative but is typically recommended only in patients with severe anemia. After splenectomy, spherocytes are present on the peripheral blood smear, but RBC survival is relatively normal.

B. **Hereditary elliptocytosis**

1. **Overview.** Hereditary elliptocytosis (HE) is characterized by mild to moderate hemolytic anemia associated with an autosomal dominant inheritance pattern. HE results from defects in RBC structural proteins that mediate **horizontal interactions** in the RBC cytoskeleton. In most patients, the molecular defect resides in the α- or β-spectrin gene and interferes with the normal polymerization of spectrin molecules. Homozygosity for mutations that cause HE is associated with a severe hemolytic disorder called **hereditary pyropoikilocytosis.**

2. **Clinical presentation of hereditary elliptocytosis.** The clinical features and natural history of HE are similar to those of HS (see III.A.2.), including marked variability in the severity of the hemolysis depending on the specific mutation.

3. **Laboratory evaluation of hereditary elliptocytosis.** Elliptocytes are seen on the peripheral blood smear. The elliptical shape results from deformation of the RBC as it traverses the microcirculation, with a failure to revert to the normal biconcave disk morphology.

4. **Treatment of hereditary elliptocytosis.** RBC destruction occurs in the spleen, so **splenectomy** is curative.

IV. METABOLIC ENZYME DISORDERS

A. **Overview.** Specific enzyme deficiencies have been identified in the glycolytic pathway and the hexose monophosphate shunt. Many of these abnormalities have a disproportionate impact on RBC metabolism. Only two enzyme defects, glucose-6-phosphate dehydrogenase (G6PD) deficiency and pyruvate kinase (PK) deficiency, occur with any significant frequency.

B. **Glucose-6-phosphate dehydrogenase deficiency** (Table 6–2)

1. **Epidemiology of glucose-6-phosphate dehydrogenase deficiency.** G6PD deficiency is the most common human enzymopathy, affecting nearly 10% of the world's population (more than 400 million people).

TABLE 6–2 • Features of Glucose-6-Phosphate Dehydrogenase Deficiency

X-linked inheritance pattern
Common in individuals of African descent
Self-limited hemolysis precipitated by stress, infection, or drugs
Intrinsic and extrinsic defect
Intravascular and extravascular hemolysis

a. The geographic distribution of G6PD deficiency coincides with the distribution of tropical malaria. The **malaria hypothesis** proposes that the high prevalence of certain hereditary disorders (e.g., G6PD deficiency, α- and β-thalassemia trait, sickle cell trait) in malaria-endemic regions is due to a heterozygote survival advantage driven by the selective pressure of malaria.

b. Males of African ancestry are the most common group affected by this disorder.

c. **Heterozygous females** are hematologically normal. However, heterozygous females with **skewed X chromosome inactivation (lyonization)** may have disproportionately low levels of G6PD and may be prone to mild hemolytic attacks.

d. **Homozygous females,** while rare, have disease features similar to those of affected males.

e. G6PD deficiency may be observed in other ethnic groups originating from tropical climates.

   (1) A G6PD variant (G6PD^{Med}) observed in individuals from the Mediterranean (notably Sardinians and Sephardic Jews) is associated with marked G6PD instability and chronic hemolysis.

   (2) A milder, generally asymptomatic G6PD deficiency is seen in individuals from southern China.

2. **Pathophysiology of G6PD deficiency.** Deficiency in G6PD activity becomes clinically apparent as acute hemolysis when the RBC is exposed to oxidant stress. In G6PD hemolytic anemias, the hemolysis is commonly **extravascular** (i.e., in the spleen). However, with extremely severe oxidant stress, **intravascular** hemolysis may occur, with increases in free plasma hemoglobin (Hb) and hemoglobinuria.

   a. Classically, oxidant stress is induced by exposure to a variety of chemicals or medications (Table 6–3). Acute viral or bacterial infection, acidosis (e.g., diabetic ketoacidosis), and liver disease may also precipitate acute hemolysis.

   b. Glutathione stores are rapidly depleted, resulting in oxidative damage to RBC components, including Hb, membrane structural proteins, and membrane lipids.

   c. Precipitates of oxidized, denatured Hb (**Heinz bodies**) attach to the membrane and contribute to membrane damage. Heinz bodies are not apparent on Wright-stained blood smears but can be visualized on staining with crystal violet.

   d. RBCs containing Heinz bodies are recognized as abnormal by the spleen, where reticuloendothelial cells pit Heinz bodies from the membrane, forming microspherocytes and RBC fragments.

      (1) The classic RBC morphology in **Heinz body hemolytic anemia** is char-

TABLE 6–3 • Drugs That Provoke Hemolytic Episodes in Individuals Deficient in Glucose-6-Phosphate Dehydrogenase
Acetanilid
Methylene blue
Nalidixic acid
Naphthalene (mothballs)
Niridazole
Nitrofurantoin
Pamaquine
Pentaquine
Phenylhydrazine
Primaquine
Sulfacetamide
Sulfamethoxazole
Sulfanilamide
Sulfapyridine
Thiazolsulfone
Toluidine blue
Trinitrotoluene

acterized by RBCs containing a membrane bleb or indentation (**bite cell**), formed after the removal of precipitated Hb from the membrane.

(2) Microspherocytes are present but usually few.

   e. The damaged RBC is prone to being trapped and destroyed in the spleen and has a markedly shortened lifespan.

3. **Variants of G6PD deficiency.** More than 400 variants of G6PD have been described, although most are uncommon. In most cases, the mutation results in an amino acid substitution that alters enzyme function or stability. The variants can be differentiated from the normal enzyme by protein gel electrophoresis. The most common variant is **G6PD A−**.

   a. G6PD A− is inherited as an **X-linked recessive trait. The G6PD A− allele is carried by 11% of American men of African ancestry.**

   b. The G6PD A− protein is produced in normal amounts in RBCs and demonstrates normal enzyme kinetics.

   c. The **G6PD A− enzyme is unstable** and loses activity as the RBC ages. **The activity of G6PD is inversely correlated with RBC age.**

   (1) Young RBCs just released from the bone marrow contain almost normal G6PD activity, while senescent RBCs (120 days old) may have little residual functional enzyme.

      (a) Because G6PD activity is essentially normal in younger RBCs, the hemolysis that occurs in G6PD A− deficiency is **self-limited** and leads to elimination of only the oldest RBCs.

      (b) G6PD activity in the RBCs that survive an acute hemolytic attack will be normal, so **measurement of G6PD activity immediately after a hemolytic attack may yield a false-negative result.**

      (c) Confirmation of the clinical diagnosis is accomplished by measurement of G6PD activity after the patient has recovered.

(2) All RBCs are uniquely susceptible to enzymopathies because they are unable to synthesize additional protein after being released into the circulation.

(3) RBC lysates prepared from the venous blood of affected males contain approximately 15%–50% of the G6PD activity in venous blood from unaffected individuals. In normal conditions, this activity is sufficient to preserve adequate intracellular glutathione reserves, and RBC survival is essentially normal.

C. **Pyruvate kinase deficiency**

1. PK deficiency is the only disorder of the glycolytic pathway with more than a handful of case reports. It accounts for more than 90%–95% of all described glycolytic defects.

2. PK deficiency is inherited as an **autosomal recessive** disorder.

3. It is characterized by chronic hemolysis with poikilocytosis and xerocytosis (cellular dehydration) on the peripheral blood smear. Spherocytes are typically absent. It and other enzymopathies of the red cell glycolytic pathway are considered as congenital nonspherocytic hemolytic anemias.

4. The location of the block in the glycolytic pathway results in **increased 2,3-diphosphoglycerate levels** (two to three times normal) and a right shift in the oxyhemoglobin dissociation curve (decreased affinity). The right shift facilitates oxygen delivery at the tissue level. Consequently, the anemia is generally well tolerated except in the most severe cases.

5. The diagnosis of PK deficiency—or any glycolytic enzymopathy—is made by direct measurement of enzyme activity in RBCs.

6. **Splenectomy** is useful in patients with severe disease.

V. CONGENITAL HEMOLYTIC DISORDERS OF HEMOGLOBIN

A. **Overview.** Abnormalities in Hb may be associated with hemolysis. These hemolytic disorders can be further subdivided into **quantitative defects** of Hb synthesis (e.g. the **thalassemias**) or **qualitative (structural) defects** of Hb (e.g., sickle cell anemia).

B. **Thalassemias**

1. **Overview.** The thalassemias constitute a genetically heterogeneous disease category characterized by a **globin chain imbalance**. Normally, the production of α- and β-globin chains within an RBC is equivalent and tightly regulated. Mutations that partially or completely inactivate production of a globin chain create an imbalance in the ratio between the α- and β-globin chains.

2. **Thalassemia trait.** In the case of α-thalassemia trait and β-thalassemia trait, the globin chain imbalance is sufficient to reduce the net production of Hb within RBCs, but RBC production and survival are generally normal. Therefore, α- and β-thalassemia traits are characterized by microcytosis with normal or mildly decreased RBC production and normal RBC survival.

3. **Thalassemia major.** Severe forms of thalassemia are characterized by a profound imbalance in globin chain synthesis and defects in either RBC production (β-thalassemia) or RBC survival (α-thalassemia).

a. β-**Thalassemia major** (also known as **Cooley's anemia**) results from mutations that impair the production of globin chains from both β-globin genes. As a consequence, RBCs contain a marked excess of free α-globin chains.

(1) In the absence of their preferred β-globin partner, α-globin chains form insoluble tetramers. The α-globin tetramers precipitate while RBCs mature in the bone marrow and lead to RBC membrane damage and

destruction of RBC precursors within the marrow. Thus, the profound, transfusion-dependent anemia observed in β-thalassemia major results from **ineffective erythropoiesis**.

(2) Production of low levels of β-globin from a thalassemia allele (β^+-thalassemia) or the fetal γ-globin gene may partially correct the globin chain imbalance and allow the escape of some RBCs into the circulation.

(3) In untransfused patients with β-thalassemia major, the peripheral blood smear shows markedly microcytic and hypochromic cells with severe distortion in RBC shape. These cells are prematurely destroyed in the spleen.

(4) Curative therapy for β-thalassemia major requires permanent replacement of the defective RBC precursors (allogeneic stem cell transplantation). Experimental approaches to treatment include replacement of the defective gene (gene therapy) or reactivation of Hb F (γ-globin gene) with drugs (e.g., hydroxyurea, 5-azacytidine, butyrate).

b. Severe α-thalassemia (**α-thalassemia major**) occurs with impairment of α-globin synthesis from three or four of the four α-globin genes.

(1) **Hb H disease** is a moderate to severe hemolytic anemia associated with impairment in α-globin production at three of the four α-globin genes.

(a) The deficiency in α-globin synthesis results in an excess of free β-globin chains.

(b) The β-globin chains tetramerize to form Hb H (β_4).

(c) In contrast to insoluble α-globin tetramers, Hb H is somewhat stable but becomes insoluble as the RBC ages in the circulation.

(d) With time, Hb H precipitates to form **Heinz bodies,** which bind to and damage the RBC membrane.

(e) RBC destruction occurs in the spleen. Therefore, splenectomy is an effective treatment for patients with severe Hb H disease.

(2) **Hb Bart's.** Deficiency of α-globin production at all four α-globin loci results in severe anemia that develops during the later stages of intrauterine development.

(a) This disorder is associated with fetal edema and wasting (**hydrops fetalis**), intrauterine fetal death, and potentially fatal complications for the mother if undetected or unanticipated.

(b) The disease takes its name from the γ-globin tetramers (**Hb Bart**) that form in the absence of α-globin chains.

C. Sickle cell disease

1. **Overview.** Structural or qualitative abnormalities of Hb may also be associated with hemolysis. In these disorders, amino acid substitutions within the α- or β-globin chain may reduce the solubility or stability of the Hb tetramer. The classic example of an Hb disorder associated with hemolysis is sickle cell disease.

2. **Pathophysiology of sickle cell disease**

a. The genetic defect in sickle cell disease is a point mutation in **codon 6** of the **β-globin gene.** The mutation results in the substitution of a hydrophobic **valine** residue for a hydrophilic **glutamic acid** residue.

(1) The new Hb has an altered electrophoretic mobility and is called **Hb S.**

(2) The **deoxygenated form of Hb S** is capable of **reversibly** polymerizing with other Hb S molecules. The rate of polymerization is logarithmically related to the **intracellular concentration of Hb S.**

(3) In patients with sickle cell trait (genotype AS), the concentration of Hb

S (usually approximately 40% of total Hb) falls below the threshold necessary to initiate pathologic polymerization *in vivo*. These patients are hematologically normal, with a normal Hb, hematocrit, and mean corpuscular volume (Table 6–4).

b. Sickle cell disease is associated with one of three distinct genotypes: **SS, SC, or sickle-β-thalassemia** (Table 6–4). **SS disease** is the most common and most severe of the sickle cell disorders.

(1) Polymerization of Hb S occurs in **microvascular beds,** where **hypoxia** and **acidosis** induce Hb to release oxygen, increasing the intracellular concentration of the deoxygenated form of Hb S. The polymerization of Hb S induces deformation of the RBC membrane and impairs transit of the RBC through the microvasculature. The polymerization of Hb S is **reversible** after return of the RBC to the arterial circulation.

(2) After multiple cycles of Hb S polymerization and RBC deformation, the RBC accumulates additional biochemical defects, including impairment in Na^+/K^+ and water homeostasis leading to **cellular dehydration.**

(3) Cellular dehydration further increases intracellular Hb S concentration, thus reducing the threshold for Hb S polymerization.

(4) Ultimately, the RBC becomes irreversibly damaged and trapped in microvascular beds, where it is lysed (intravascular hemolysis).

c. Why do heterozygous patients with the SC genotype have sickle cell disease, while individuals with sickle cell trait (AS genotype) do not sickle? The explanation is found in the effect of Hb C on the hydration status of the RBC. Hb C inhibits ion exchange across the RBC membrane, resulting in cellular dehydration and an associated increase in intracellular Hb concentration, hence Hb S concentration.

TABLE 6–4 • Clinical Features of Sickle Hemoglobinopathies

Condition	Clinical Features	Hb (g/dL)	MCV (fL)	Electrophoresis
Sickle cell trait	None; rare painless hematuria	Normal	Normal	Hb S/A: 40/60
Sickle cell anemia	Vasoocclusive crises with infarction of spleen, brain, marrow, kidney, lung; aseptic necrosis of bone; gallstones; priapism; ankle ulcers	7–10	80–100	Hb S/A: 100/0 Hb F: 2%–25%
Sickle-β°-thalassemia	Vasoocclusive crises; aseptic necrosis of bone	7–10	60–80	Hb S/A: 100/0
Sickle-β^+-thalassemia	Rare crises and aseptic necrosis	10–14	70–80	Hb S/A: 60/40
Hemoglobin SC	Rare crises and aseptic necrosis; retinopathy; painless hematuria	10–14	80–100	Hb S/A: 50/0 Hb C: 50%

Hb, hemoglobin.
Reprinted with permission from Benz E. *Hemoglobinopathies* Table 106–2, Harrison's Online 2002.

3. Clinical presentation of sickle cell disease
   a. Sickle cell disease is characterized by periodic episodes of acute vascular occlusion (**painful crisis**) that have their onset in the first or second year of life. Painful crisis may be precipitated by events that impair tissue oxygenation, perfusion, or acid–base status. Infection, especially pneumonia, and systemic dehydration are common precipitating events.
   b. Vascular occlusion may lead to severe impairment of organ perfusion with resulting organ dysfunction or death, including **bone infarcts, avascular necrosis, acute chest syndrome, stroke,** and **cutaneous ulcers**.
   c. In patients with the **SS genotype**, recurrent **splenic infarction** results in complete splenic involution at a young age. Evidence of impaired or absent splenic function is documented on the peripheral blood smear by the appearance of **Howell-Jolly bodies**.
   d. Patients with **SS disease** are especially susceptible to infection with **encapsulated bacteria,** and daily **antibiotic prophylaxis** is a standard component of treatment of children.
   e. Patients with **SC** and **sickle-β-thalassemia** genotypes have a milder form of sickle cell disease than SS patients. In the case of sickle-β-thalassemia, this is because the net reduction in intracellular Hb concentration that accompanies thalassemia trait also reduces Hb S concentrations.
      (1) Painful crisis is generally less frequent, though it may be severe in some individuals.
      (2) Autosplenectomy does not occur in these two genotypes.
   f. Patients with **SC and sickle-β-thalassemia** are prone to **splenic sequestration crisis,** seen only in children less than 5 years of age with SS disease.
   g. Patients with **SC disease** have a significant increase in risk for retinal vascular damage (**retinopathy**), which may lead to blindness.
4. Treatment of sickle cell disease
   a. Treatment for patients with sickle cell disease is largely supportive. **Hydration** and pain medication are used to treat acute painful crisis.
   b. Especially serious forms of vascular occlusion (e.g., stroke, acute chest syndrome, sequestration crisis, priapism) are often treated with **exchange transfusion**. Chronic RBC transfusion is also recommended in children at high risk for stroke as defined by transcranial Doppler ultrasound.
   c. In young individuals with severe clinical disease and a matched sibling donor, **allogeneic stem cell transplantation** can be curative.
   d. Because increased levels of **Hb F** inhibit Hb S polymerization, medications that increase γ-globin synthesis may be useful in decreasing the frequency of acute painful crisis. **Hydroxyurea,** an inhibitor of ribonucleotide reductase, has been shown to increase Hb F levels and is approved for the treatment of patients with frequent painful crisis.

VI. SUMMARY

Congenital hemolytic anemias result from heritable defects in components of the red blood cell membrane, metabolic pathways, or hemoglobin. Important clues to the diagnosis are obtained from the family history and the peripheral blood smear.

CHAPTER 7

Acquired Hemolytic Anemias

- SCOTT D. GITLIN

I. INTRODUCTION

Hemolytic anemias result from a shortened red blood cell (RBC) survival rate as a result of an increased rate of RBC destruction. Hemolytic disorders are generally limited to conditions in which the rate of RBC destruction is increased while the ability of the bone marrow to respond to the anemia remains intact. Bone marrow can increase its production rate 6–8 times normal; therefore, hemolytic disorders can be present in the absence of anemia. When bone marrow erythropoiesis cannot keep up with the shortened length of RBC survival, hemolytic **anemia** results.

II. PRINCIPLES OF HEMOLYTIC ANEMIAS

A. **Classification.** A number of methods are used to classify hemolytic disorders, all of which are useful in defining the cause of hemolysis.
   1. **Congenital or acquired.** One approach characterizes hemolytic disorders as either congenital (i.e., inherited) or acquired.
      a. Congenital hemolytic anemias are discussed in Chapter 6.
      b. **Acquired hemolytic disorders** can be further classified according to the general pathophysiologic cause (Table 7–1).
   2. **Intravascular or extravascular site of RBC destruction.** Hemolytic anemias can also be classified according to the site of hemolysis (i.e., where the RBCs are removed from the circulation). This method is clinically useful because clinical and laboratory findings may determine the site of hemolysis.
      a. **Intravascular hemolysis** occurs when the RBCs are destroyed within the blood circulation.
         (1) **Clinical presentation.** Disorders of intravascular hemolysis often present with fever, chills, tachycardia, and backache.
         (2) **Laboratory evaluation.** These patients typically demonstrate hemoglobinemia (free hemoglobin in the blood), hemoglobinuria (free hemoglobin in the urine), and hemosiderinuria (hemosiderin in the urine). Serum haptoglobin levels decrease markedly. In severe cases of hemolysis, elevations of free hemoglobin may be detected in the blood serum and urine; renal failure can develop from hemoglobinuria. Hemosiderin can be measured in the urine approximately 7 days after a hemolytic event and is a reliable indicator of chronic intravascular hemolysis.

TABLE 7–1 • Causes of Acquired Hemolytic Anemias

Immunohemolytic
  Transfusion of incompatible blood
  Hemolytic disease of the newborn
  Warm-antibody autoimmune hemolytic anemia
  Cold-antibody autoimmune hemolytic anemia
Traumatic and microangiopathic
  Prosthetic valves and other cardiovascular abnormalities
  Hemolytic uremic syndrome
  Thrombotic thrombocytopenic purpura
  Disseminated intravascular coagulation
  Immunologic phenomena (e.g., graft rejection, immune complex formation)
  Cancer
Infectious agents
  Protozoa (e.g., malaria, toxoplasmosis, leishmaniasis, trypanosomiasis, babesiosis)
  Bacteria (e.g., bartonellosis, clostridia, cholera, typhoid fever)
Chemicals, drugs, and venoms
Physical agents
  Burns
Hypophosphatemia
Paroxysmal nocturnal hemoglobinuria
Spur cell anemia (liver disease)
Vitamin E deficiency in newborns

All of these acquired disorders are caused by extrinsic factors that affect red blood cell survival, except for paroxysmal nocturnal hemoglobinuria, which is the result of an intrinsic defect.

   b. **Extravascular hemolysis** occurs when RBCs are removed from the blood circulation by tissue macrophages, primarily in the spleen. This is the most common form of hemolytic anemia.
      (1) **Clinical presentation.** These patients often develop jaundice and splenomegaly because of destruction of RBCs, release of unconjugated bilirubin into the blood circulation, and sequestration of RBCs in the spleen.
      (2) **Laboratory evaluation.** Haptoglobin levels are typically normal or slightly decreased. Unconjugated hyperbilirubinemia is typically present.
 B. **Laboratory tests.** Laboratory findings reflect the severity of hemolysis and the response of the bone marrow to the anemia.
   1. **Hemoglobin and hematocrit.** These studies determine the severity of the hemolytic process and the ability of the bone marrow to compensate.
   2. **RBC mean corpuscular volume.** The mean corpuscular volume (MCV) is often normal to elevated because of an increased number of reticulocytes, which are physically larger than mature RBCs.
   3. **Reticulocyte count.** Elevation of the number of reticulocytes indicates increased bone marrow erythropoiesis, which results from attempts by the bone marrow to correct the deficiency of RBCs in the circulation.
   4. **Peripheral blood smear.** Review of the peripheral blood smear typically reveals polychromatophilia (blue-tinged RBCs in the blood circulation) resulting from an increased number of reticulocytes and may also reveal nucleated RBCs. The presence of microspherocytes or fragmented RBCs may help narrow the differential diagnosis as to the cause of the hemolytic anemia.

5. **Bone marrow aspiration.** The bone marrow typically reveals erythroid hyperplasia, often with megaloblastoid features (i.e., cells that have immature-appearing nuclei with less dense chromatin, mature-appearing cytoplasm, and a cell volume that is above normal).

6. **Serum unconjugated bilirubin and lactate dehydrogenase.** The serum unconjugated bilirubin and lactate dehydrogenase (LDH) may be elevated because of release of these substances from the contents of destroyed RBCs.

7. **Plasma haptoglobin.** Haptoglobin is a hemoglobin-binding protein that is removed from the circulation after it binds to free hemoglobin. Therefore, it is decreased with intravascular hemolysis.

8. **Plasma hemoglobin.** The free hemoglobin in plasma is elevated in some cases of intravascular hemolysis and is associated with hemoglobinuria.

9. **Hemosiderinuria.** Hemosiderin appears in the urine when renal tubule epithelial cells containing absorbed iron defoliate into the urine (i.e., after approximately 7 days of intravascular hemolysis).

10. **Direct antiglobulin test, or direct Coombs test** (Fig. 7–1). The direct antiglobulin test (DAT) detects immunoglobulin G (IgG) or complement (i.e., C3) bound to the RBC membrane, the hallmark of autoimmune hemolytic anemia. This test detects only the presence of IgG or C3 complement, not any other types of antibody or complement on the RBC. Although the titer of the autoantibody can be determined, it does not predict the severity of disease.

11. **Indirect antiglobulin test, indirect Coombs test** (Fig. 7–2). The indirect antiglobulin (Coombs) test detects RBC autoantibodies in the serum of patients with immune-mediated hemolytic anemia. Additional studies are needed to differentiate between autoantibodies and alloantibodies. In addition to its use in the evaluation of patients with immune-mediated hemolytic anemia, this test is used to detect blood incompatibility for blood transfusions.

12. **Cold agglutinin test.** This test detects cold agglutinating antibodies (i.e., immunoglobulin M, or IgM) in serum. Varying dilutions of the patient's serum are incubated with normal RBCs at 4°C and the extent of RBC agglutination is scored. An agglutinating antibody in the reaction leads to agglutination of the RBCs.

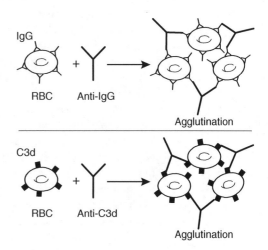

FIGURE 7–1. Direct antiglobulin test, or direct Coombs test. The direct antiglobulin test is performed by washing the patient's RBCs free of plasma and adding the antiglobulin reagent (polyspecific rabbit anti-IgG or anti-C3 antibody). The sample is mixed, centrifuged, and read for the presence or absence of agglutination. Each reagent interacts with IgG or C3d, respectively, on the surface of the cell. (Adapted with permission from Schwartz RS, Berkman EM, Silberstein LE. Autoimmune hemolytic anemias. In: Hoffman R et al., eds. *Hematology: Basic Principles and Practice.* 3rd ed. New York: Churchill Livingstone, 2000:617.)

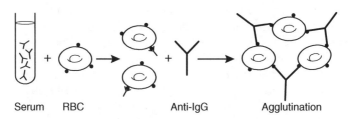

FIGURE 7–2. Indirect antiglobulin test, or indirect Coombs test. The indirect antiglobulin test is performed by incubating the patient's serum with normal RBCs, washing the cells to remove the serum, adding the antiglobulin reagent, and reading for agglutination. (Adapted with permission from Schwartz RS, Berkman EM, Silberstein LE. Autoimmune hemolytic anemias. In: Hoffman R et al., eds. *Hematology: Basic Principles and Practice*. 3rd ed. New York: Churchill Livingstone; 2000:618.)

III.   IMMUNE-MEDIATED HEMOLYTIC DISORDERS

A. **Classification.** Autoimmune hemolytic anemias (AIHAs) are a group of disorders that are the result of antibody or complement binding to specific antigens on the RBC membrane, which leads to a shortened RBC life span. These disorders can be primary (i.e., idiopathic) or secondary (e.g., underlying disease, drugs). Antierythrocyte antibodies can be divided into three general categories:

1. **IgG warm autoantibodies** bind to RBCs at 37°C but fail to agglutinate the RBCs.
2. **Cold agglutinins** almost always are of the IgM subtype and clump RBCs at cold temperatures.
3. **Donath-Landsteiner (IgG) antibodies** bind to RBC membranes in the cold and activate the hemolytic complement cascade when the RBCs are warmed to 37°C. These antibodies can be directed against self-antigens (autoantigens), non–self antigens (allogeneic antigens), or neoantigens (antigenic complexes not normally found on the surface of RBCs).

B. **Autoimmune hemolytic anemia: warm-antibody type**

1. **Overview.** Warm-antibody type AIHAs account for approximately 70% of AIHAs. This group of diseases results from the binding of IgG to the RBC membrane. These IgG-bound RBCs either are trapped by macrophages as they pass through the spleen or may first have part of their membrane removed, which results in the RBC taking the form of a spherocyte. A spherocyte is the structure that has the smallest amount of RBC membrane to hold the contents of the cell. Spherocytes are cleared by both extravascular (most common) and intravascular mechanisms.

2. **Etiology of warm-antibody type autoimmune hemolytic anemia**

   a. There are a number of potential causes of warm-antibody type AIHA that can be either idiopathic (i.e., primary) or secondary.

   b. Secondary causes:

      (1) Lymphoproliferative diseases (e.g., chronic lymphocytic leukemia, non-Hodgkin lymphoma)

      (2) Connective tissue diseases (e.g., systemic lupus erythematosus)

      (3) Immune deficiency disorders (e.g., AIDS, common variable immuno-deficiency)

      (4) Drugs (e.g., penicillin, quinidine, methyldopa, cephalosporins)

3. **Clinical presentation of warm-antibody type autoimmune hemolytic anemia**

   a. These patients can present with a variety of symptoms, including jaundice and symptoms associated with anemia (e.g., fatigue, shortness of breath, light-headedness). Some patients remain asymptomatic if the hemolysis is mild and well compensated for by an increase in RBC hematopoiesis.

b. Physical examination may reveal mild jaundice, pallor, increased respiratory rate, and splenomegaly. There may also be signs related to an underlying autoimmune disorder, such as fever, lymphadenopathy, skin rash, hypertension, renal failure, petechiae, or ecchymoses.

c. Laboratory tests:

(1) **Hemoglobin and hematocrit** can vary from normal to low.

(2) **MCV** is elevated because of an increase in the number of reticulocytes and a possible relative folic acid deficiency (if hemolysis is chronic and no folic acid replacement is provided).

(3) **Peripheral blood smear** reveals polychromasia of RBCs because of an increased number of reticulocytes; macrocytosis, nucleated RBCs, and microspherocytes may be present.

(4) **Bone marrow biopsy** shows hyperplasia.

(5) **Serum bilirubin and urobilinogen (urine)** are typically elevated.

(6) **DAT** is usually positive.

4. **Treatment of warm-antibody type autoimmune hemolytic anemia.** Treatment varies with the severity of anemia and the underlying cause. For this reason, evaluation of the patient for possible underlying disorders is important in directing the choice of therapy.

a. If the hemolytic anemia is well compensated for by bone marrow erythropoiesis, no specific therapy may be needed.

b. All patients should receive **folic acid** because of the increased demand that results from erythroid hyperplasia (i.e., increased cell division).

c. Whenever possible, an underlying secondary disease that may be causing the hemolytic process should be treated. Successful treatment of the secondary cause often leads to resolution of the hemolytic process.

d. When treatment of the underlying cause is unsuccessful, a variety of therapeutic approaches may be used. These approaches may also be used for idiopathic warm-antibody type AIHA when treatment of hemolysis is needed.

(1) **RBC transfusions** are administered only in severe, potentially life-threatening situations. There is concern that administration of allogeneic RBCs may heighten the hemolytic process. If a blood transfusion is needed, the patient should be monitored closely for adverse events.

(2) **Corticosteroids** (e.g., prednisone) are the mainstay of treatment. They are thought to interfere with the reactivity of the antibody and with the synthesis and function of the Fc receptors on macrophages that bind and destroy antibody-coated RBCs. With long-term treatment, corticosteroids can also decrease autoantibody production.

(3) **Splenectomy** is generally reserved for patients who fail to respond to corticosteroids, who are dependent on prednisone doses greater than 10–20 mg/day (or the equivalent of another corticosteroid), or who have intractable side effects from corticosteroids. Approximately 50%–60% of patients have a good to excellent initial response to splenectomy.

(4) **IV immunoglobulin (IVIG)** may increase RBC survival by saturating Fc receptors on macrophages.

(5) Other agents used in cases of warm-antibody type AIHA include **immunosuppressive therapy, danazol,** and **Vinca alkaloids.**

C. **Cold agglutinin disease**

1. **Overview.** Cold agglutinin disease is a group of disorders caused by IgM autoantibodies directed against RBCs (i.e., cold agglutinins) that preferentially bind to RBCs at cold temperatures (4°C–18°C). These autoantibodies are usually directed against the I/i antigen. After binding to an RBC, the pathogenic IgM autoantibody activates the complement cascade on the RBC membrane, which leads to binding of C3b complement to the RBC surface and eventual phagocytosis by hepatic macrophages. The severity of disease depends on the titer of the autoantibody and its ability to initiate complement activation. Most healthy people have low titers of cold agglutinins in their serum with no clinical sequelae. Cold agglutinin disease accounts for approximately 15% of AIHAs.

2. **Etiology of cold agglutinin disease.** There are two clinical forms of cold agglutinin disease:

a. The **chronic** form is the most common and occurs in older persons (fifth to eighth decade). Many of these patients have an underlying B-lymphocyte neoplasm (e.g., chronic lymphocytic leukemia, lymphoma, Waldenström macroglobulinemia).

b. The **acute** form is less common and is always self-limited. This form occurs as a rare complication of several infectious diseases, most notably *Mycoplasma pneumoniae* (anti-I) and Epstein-Barr virus (infectious mononucleosis) (anti-i). These patients tend to be much younger than those with the chronic form of the disease.

3. **Clinical presentation of cold agglutinin disease**

a. The major symptom in cold agglutinin disease is **cold-induced acrocyanosis** (i.e., blue color of the fingertips, toes, nose, and ear lobes).

b. Patients may also have symptoms related to anemia, which tends to be mild and stable, and possibly cold-associated hemoglobinuria.

c. Physical examination demonstrates findings consistent with anemia and may include jaundice and splenomegaly.

4. **Laboratory evaluation of cold agglutinin disease**

a. Laboratory studies reveal decreased hemoglobin and other findings seen in hemolytic anemias (i.e., reticulocytosis, polychromatophilia, spherocytosis, erythroid hyperplasia in the bone marrow, elevations in serum bilirubin and LDH).

b. The peripheral blood smear usually demonstrates RBC agglutination, spherocytes, and polychromatophilia.

c. The DAT is positive for C3 complement only.

d. The cold agglutinin test can confirm the diagnosis and determine the titer of the autoantibody present in the patient's serum.

5. **Treatment of cold agglutinin disease**

a. Therapy is directed at the underlying disease, when possible, and avoiding cold exposure.

b. The need to initiate a specific therapy is dictated by the severity of the anemia and symptoms. The postinfectious form of cold agglutinin disease often resolves spontaneously several weeks after infection.

c. Glucocorticoids are rarely helpful.

d. Splenectomy is usually not indicated.

e. Combination chemotherapy may be helpful in severe or refractory cases.

A. **Paroxysmal cold hemoglobinuria**

 1. **Overview.** Paroxysmal cold hemoglobinuria (PCH) is a rare disorder (about 1% of AIHAs) that occurs most frequently in children after a recent viral disorder. PCH also occurs in people with tertiary or congenital syphilis. The antibodies that cause PCH are thought to be a response to microorganism antigens, which induce antibodies that cross-react with the P blood group system. There may be a genetic predisposition for producing these antibodies. These antibodies (known as Donath-Landsteiner antibodies) are IgG and usually are polyclonal. The pathogenesis of PCH is thought to be due to this circulating IgG antibody that binds to RBCs at cold temperatures, fixes complement, and then destroys the RBCs by complement lysis upon warming.

 2. **Clinical presentation of paroxysmal cold hemoglobinuria**

    a. These patients present with paroxysms of fever, back pain, leg pain, abdominal cramps, and rigors that occur after exposure to cold temperatures.

    b. These symptoms are followed by hemoglobinuria, which may lead to renal failure.

 3. **Laboratory evaluation of paroxysmal cold hemoglobinuria**

    a. **Donath-Landsteiner test** detects Donath-Landsteiner antibody.

    b. **Hemoglobin and hematocrit** are decreased in proportion to the severity of anemia.

    c. **Reticulocyte count** is often low early in episode and elevated in recovery phase.

    d. **Peripheral blood smear** typically reveals anisocytosis, poikilocytosis, polychromatophilia, spherocytes, and nucleated RBCs.

    e. **Serum free hemoglobin** is elevated.

    f. **Haptoglobin** is decreased.

    g. **Urine studies** reveal elevated hemoglobin and methemoglobin.

    h. **DAT** is typically negative.

 4. **Treatment of paroxysmal cold hemoglobinuria**

    a. PCH is a self-limited disease that resolves spontaneously in 2–3 weeks.

    b. Treatment is directed at supportive measures and avoidance of cold temperatures.

A. **Drug-induced immune hemolytic anemia.** Four distinct mechanisms of drug-induced immune hemolytic anemia have been identified. They appear to be drug specific.

 1. **Hapten mechanism** (Fig. 7–3). Clinically, the DAT is positive for IgG, and hemolysis occurs only when the offending drug (e.g., penicillin) is present.

 2. **Immune complex mechanism** (Fig. 7–4). This process typically involves an IgM antibody; therefore, the clinical presentation is associated with intravascular hemolysis. This is the most common mechanism for drug-induced (e.g., quinidine, phenacetin) immune hemolytic anemias. The DAT is positive for complement (C3) only.

 3. **Autoantibody mechanism** (Fig. 7–5). The DAT is positive for IgG. As many as 20% of patients treated with methyldopa have a positive DAT, but fewer than 1% of these patients demonstrate hemolysis. The DAT may take several months to turn positive and may persist for several months after the offending drug (e.g., methyldopa, ibuprofen) is discontinued.

 4. **Immunogenic drug–RBC complex mechanism** (Fig. 7–6)

 5. **Non–immune protein adsorption mechanism.** Proteins (e.g., drugs) may nonspecifically attach to the RBC membrane without causing RBC destruction. The importance of this mechanism of drug–RBC interaction is the aware-

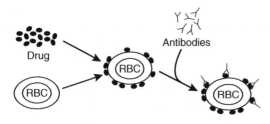

FIGURE 7–3. Hapten mechanism of drug-induced immune hemolytic anemia. The implicated drug forms an antigenic complex with a protein on the RBC membrane. An antibody directed against the complex leads to destruction of that RBC. (Adapted with permission from Schwartz RS, Berkman EM, Silberstein LE. Autoimmune hemolytic anemias. In: Hoffman R et al., eds. *Hematology: Basic Principles and Practice.* 3rd ed. New York: Churchill Livingstone; 2000:625.)

ness that this interaction can lead to a positive DAT. Examples include cephalosporins (primarily first generation), albumin, and immunoglobulins (e.g., IVIG).

IV. NONIMMUNE HEMOLYTIC ANEMIAS

A. **Overview.** The nonimmune hemolytic anemias are generally the result of extrinsic factors or effects on otherwise normal RBCs. Many physical, chemical, and infectious causes make up the differential diagnosis for the nonimmune hemolytic anemias.

B. **Fragmentation hemolysis**

1. **Overview.** Fragmentation hemolysis occurs when mechanical trauma or shear stress disrupts the physical integrity of the RBC membrane.

2. **Etiology of fragmentation hemolysis**

a. Damaged microvasculature with the resulting disorder commonly referred to as microangiopathic hemolytic anemia, such as thrombotic thrombocytopenic purpura, hemolytic uremic syndrome, preeclampsia and eclampsia, HELLP syndrome (hemolysis, elevated liver enzymes, low platelet count), malignancy, vasculitis, disseminated intravascular coagulation, renal allograft rejection, malignant hypertension

b. Arteriovenous malformations (e.g., arteriovenous shunts)

c. Cardiac abnormalities (e.g., prosthetic heart valves)

d. Drugs (e.g., cyclosporine, cancer chemotherapy agents, ticlopidine, clopidogrel, cocaine)

3. **Clinical presentation of fragmentation hemolysis.** Except in cases of extreme intravascular fragmentation, these patients typically demonstrate the same clinical findings associated with extravascular hemolysis. These findings include pallor, jaundice, and a loss of a feeling of well-being.

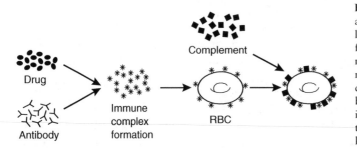

FIGURE 7–4. Immune complex mechanism of drug-induced immune hemolytic anemia. An antigenic complex is formed by the offending drug or drug metabolite and a plasma protein. Formation of this complex leads to production of an antidrug antibody that binds to the antigenic complex, forming an immune complex that adheres to RBCs, activates complement, and leads to destruction of the RBC.

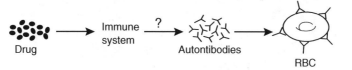

FIGURE 7–5. Autoantibody mechanism of drug-induced immune hemolytic anemia. The offending drug induces the formation of an autoantibody that reacts against a protein on the RBC membrane, typically against an Rh blood group antigen. Interaction of this antibody with the RBC membrane antigen destroys the RBC. (Adapted with permission from Schwartz RS, Berkman EM, Silberstein LE. Autoimmune hemolytic anemias. In: Hoffman R et al., eds. *Hematology: Basic Principles and Practice*. 3rd ed. New York: Churchill Livingstone; 2000:625.)

    4. Laboratory evaluation of fragmentation hemolysis
      a. Laboratory findings are similar to those for extravascular hemolysis; some intravascular hemolysis findings may be present.
        (1) Hemoglobin and hematocrit are decreased depending on severity of anemia.
        (2) MCV is normal to elevated depending on the extent of increase in reticulocytes.
        (3) Reticulocyte count is elevated to reflect increased bone marrow erythropoiesis.
        (4) Peripheral blood smear typically reveals polychromatophilia and fragmented RBCs.
        (5) Serum unconjugated bilirubin and LDH are elevated.
        (6) Plasma haptoglobin is decreased.
        (7) Plasma hemoglobin is elevated.
        (8) Hemosiderinuria may be present.
        (9) DAT is negative.
      b. Diagnosis depends on examination of the peripheral blood smear, which reveals fragmented RBCs (i.e., schistocytes, helmet cells, microspherocytes) and polychromatophilia.
    5. Treatment of fragmentation hemolysis
      a. Therapy is directed at the underlying condition.
      b. Iron and folic acid supplementation and RBC transfusions are administered as necessary.
  C. Hypersplenism
    1. Overview. Hypersplenism is a functional state of hyperactivity of the spleen, including its cellular sequestration activity. For this reason, hypersplenism can lead to a decrease in the life span of RBCs, leukocytes, and platelets. Splenomegaly is an anatomic term for enlargement of the spleen. All of the activities of the spleen are accentuated in a large spleen; therefore, hypersplenism is

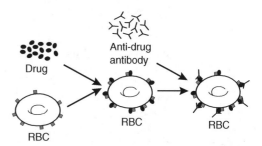

FIGURE 7–6. *In vivo* sensitization mechanism of drug-induced immune hemolytic anemia. The drug or a metabolite forms an immunogenic drug–RBC complex in association with a specific RBC antigen. This drug–RBC antigen complex conveys specificity to an antidrug antibody that interacts with the drug on the RBC membrane, destroying the RBC.

often associated with splenomegaly. Anemia in these patients is the result of increased RBC destruction and splenic sequestration.

2. **Differential diagnosis of hypersplenism.** The differential diagnosis of hypersplenism is dominated by causes of splenomegaly (Table 7–2).

3. **Treatment of hypersplenism**
   a. Therapy is directed at the underlying cause of the splenomegaly or hypersplenism.
   b. Anemia and pancytopenia are not usually severe; if they are severe, splenectomy typically leads to improvements in the blood counts.

D. **Infection**
   1. **Direct parasitization** (e.g., malaria, babesiosis, bartonellosis) can result from an organism infecting the RBC, which leads to intravascular or extravascular hemolysis, or attaching to the RBC membrane, which leads to RBC destruction.
   2. **Immune mechanisms,** such as *Mycoplasma pneumoniae*, Epstein-Barr virus (mononucleosis), are discussed earlier in the text (see III.C.2.b.).
   3. **Induction of hypersplenism** can occur as a sequela of some infections (e.g.,

---

TABLE 7–2 • Causes of Hypersplenism

Vascular congestion
  Right heart failure
  Hepatic vein thrombosis (Budd-Chiari syndrome)
  Cirrhosis
  Portal vein obstruction
  Splenic vein thrombosis
Infection
  Bacterial endocarditis
  Tuberculosis
  Parasites
  Viruses
  Fungi
Inflammatory diseases
  Systemic lupus erythematosus
  Rheumatoid arthritis
Hemolytic anemias
  Congenital (thalassemias, hereditary spherocytosis)
  Acquired (autoimmune)
Neoplasms
  Lymphomas
  Hairy cell leukemia
  Chronic lymphocytic leukemia
  Myeloproliferative disorders (e.g., chronic myelogenous leukemia,
    polycythemia vera, essential thrombocytosis, myelofibrosis)
Storage disorders
  Gaucher disease
  Mucopolysaccharidoses
Benign structural abnormalities
  Cysts
  Hamartomas
Other
  Amyloidosis
  Sarcoidosis

malaria, schistosomiasis) by immune-mediated and non–immune-mediated mechanisms.

4. **Altered RBC surface topology** (e.g., *Haemophilus influenzae*) caused by interactions between the microorganism and the RBC surface can lead to hemolysis.

5. **Release of toxins and enzymes** by a microorganism (e.g., *Clostridium*, *Escherichia coli* 0192) can cause direct damage to the RBC membrane, which leads to shortened RBC survival.

E. **Other causes of nonimmune hemolytic anemias.** A number of other causes of non-immune hemolytic anemia are uncommon compared to the causes discussed earlier, and each occurs via a different mechanism. These causes include the following:

1. Liver disease
2. Severe burns (heat denaturation)
3. Copper deficiency (Wilson disease)
4. Drug-induced oxidative damage

V. PAROXYSMAL NOCTURNAL HEMOGLOBINURIA

A. **Overview.** Paroxysmal nocturnal hemoglobinuria (PNH) is an acquired clonal disorder of the hematopoietic stem cell that results in the production of blood cells (i.e., erythrocytes, granulocytes, monocytes, platelets) with characteristic defects, including an unusual susceptibility to complement-mediated hemolysis. This defect is due to a somatic mutation of the *pig-a* gene, which affects the biosynthesis of a glycosylphosphatidylinositol (GPI) linkage that is required to attach a number of RBC membrane proteins to the RBC membrane. PNH occurs from the second decade of life onward; incidence increases with age.

B. **Etiology of paroxysmal nocturnal hemoglobinuria.** PNH is caused by an acquired abnormality (mutation) of the *pig-a* gene on the short arm of the X chromosome. PNH is associated with other diseases, including the following:

1. Aplastic anemia
2. Myelodysplastic syndromes
3. Acute myeloblastic leukemia

C. **Clinical presentation of paroxysmal nocturnal hemoglobinuria.** Patients may show these signs:

1. Hemolytic anemia
2. Pancytopenia
3. Iron deficiency (due to hemoglobinuria and hemosiderinuria)
4. Venous thrombosis

D. **Laboratory evaluation of paroxysmal nocturnal hemoglobinuria**

1. There is typically evidence of anemia due to intravascular hemolysis with normal RBC morphology on peripheral blood smear.
2. Bone marrow morphology is variable.
3. The leukocyte alkaline phosphatase (LAP) score is low.
4. Two studies that are often useful in making the diagnosis of PNH are the sucrose hemolysis test (sensitive) and the Ham (acidified serum lysis) test (specific). These tests are based on *in vitro* activation of alternate complement pathways.
5. Flow cytometry can be used to analyze cells for GPI-linked antigens.

E. **Treatment of paroxysmal nocturnal hemoglobinuria**

1. Correct the anemia (e.g., glucocorticoids, anabolic steroids, iron replacement, folic acid supplementation)
2. Treat or prevent thrombosis (e.g., anticoagulants, thrombolytics)

3. Modify bone marrow hematopoiesis by bone marrow transplantation (allogeneic) or by attempting to stimulate hematopoiesis with antithymocyte globulin.

VI.   SUMMARY

Premature destruction of RBCs can vary in severity and can occur by any of several mechanisms. RBC destruction that is adequately compensated for by increased production of RBCs usually does not require immediate intervention but still requires identification (and treatment, when possible) of the underlying cause. Hemolytic anemia occurs when the bone marrow cannot adequately compensate for the destruction of the RBCs and often requires therapeutic intervention. An understanding of the clinical and laboratory presentations and the possible etiologies of hemolytic anemias will allow for characterization, diagnosis, and selection of appropriate therapy. The primary goals of therapy are to treat significant symptoms and causative conditions, disrupt with the hemolytic process when possible, and allow the bone marrow to compensate for the RBC destruction as much as possible.

CHAPTER 8

Principles of Hemostasis

- ALVIN H. SCHMAIER

I. INTRODUCTION

The biochemical and cellular systems that have evolved in man to prevent excessive bleeding or clotting are complex. This chapter is a concise general synthesis of the contributing factors (proteins, cells, and blood vessels) that interact to keep a balance between bleeding and clotting in life. Chapters 9 to 13 discuss the approach to a bleeding or clotting patient and specific disorders where those conditions arise.

II. THE HEMOSTATIC SYSTEM

A. Overview
1. **Hemostasis.** Cessation of bleeding (hemostasis) occurs within the intravascular compartment lined with endothelium. Normal hemostasis and thrombosis involve a number of factors, including platelets, granulocytes, and monocytes, as well as the **coagulation** (clot forming), **fibrinolytic** (clot lysing), and **anticoagulant** (regulating) protein systems. Each of the three protein systems balances the activities of the others. In addition, the integrity of the vessel wall endothelium is contributory. In general, the vessel wall, which in the intravascular compartment is lined by endothelium, is constitutively an anticoagulant surface. When injured, either physically or by an inflammatory state, the endothelium can be a locus for procoagulant and antifibrinolytic activity (see II.B.3.).
2. **Components.** The physiologic hemostatic system has two limbs.
   a. The first is a large group of proteins that participate in clot formation (**coagulation**), dissolution (**fibrinolysis**), and regulation (**anticoagulation**).
   b. The second is a cell component that consists mostly of platelets but also includes granulocytes, monocytes, and endothelial cells.
3. **Regulation.** Physiologic hemostasis is a tightly regulated balance between the formation and dissolution of hemostatic plugs. The **coagulation system** is a group of proteins that participate in clot formation. The **fibrinolytic system** is a group of proteins that participate in clot dissolution. The **anticoagulation system** is a group of proteins that regulate the coagulation and fibrinolytic systems. The proteins of the anticoagulation system join those of the fibrinolytic system to prevent or counterbalance coagulation reactions. Thus, the hemostatic system is tightly modulated by a series of enzymes and scaffolding proteins.

B. Process
1. When a vessel wall is injured, subendothelial cell collagen is exposed, and platelets adhere to the site of injury. Von Willebrand factor helps platelets ad-

here to the vessel wall. This adhesion event activates platelets, initiating a signaling cascade within them. The stimulated platelets release the contents of their granules and help to generate thrombin on their surfaces. As a result, the platelets aggregate and a hemostatic plug forms (Fig. 8–1).

2. Adjacent to the site of injury, tissue factor (TF) is up-regulated in the subendothelium and forms a complex with factor VIIa. The complex activates factor IX to factor IXa, which converts zymogen factor X to enzymatically active factor Xa. In the presence of factor V, factor Xa activates prothrombin (factor II) to thrombin (factor IIa), which is the major clot-forming enzyme. Thrombin proteolyses fibrinogen to form fibrin, which is the protein basis of a clot. Thrombin is also a major activator of platelets, along with collagen, adenosine diphosphate, platelet-activating factor, and epinephrine.

3. Physiologically important coagulation and fibrinolytic reactions are likely to occur on the surface of cells in the intravascular compartment. At rest, these endothelial cells provide an anticoagulant surface. The anticoagulant nature of the endothelial cell membrane is made up by antithrombin–glycosaminoglycan interactions, tissue plasminogen activator release, nitric oxide and prostacyclin formation, and thrombomodulin expression for protein C activation. However, when stimulated, these endothelial cells become a nidus for procoagulant activity. The procoagulant activity of endothelial cells is indicated by their increased expression of TF and factor VIIa, increased synthesis of factor V and carboxypeptidase U (thrombin-activatable fibrinolysis inhibitor, or TAFI),

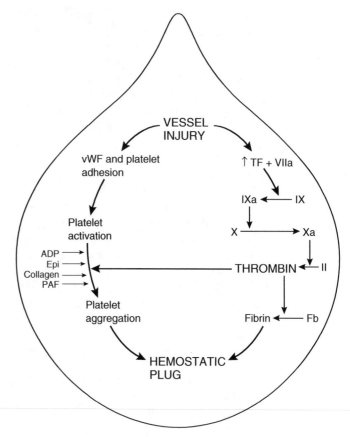

FIGURE 8–1. The hemostatic response to vessel injury. *ADP*, adenosine diphosphate; *Epi*, epinephrine; *Fb*, fibrinogen; *PAF*, platelet-activating factor; *TF*, tissue factor; *vWF*, von Willebrand factor.

and saturation of thrombomodulin with Protein C. Critical protein activation and inhibition reactions also occur on the membranes of granulocytes and monocytes.

III. COAGULATION PROTEIN SYSTEM

A. **Coagulation proteins** (Fig. 8–2)
   1. **Phospholipid-bound proenzymes (zymogens)** make up the physiologically important hemostatic system.
      a. These proteins are vitamin K–dependent. Vitamin K is required for an essential γ-carboxylation reaction that takes place on each of these proteins' glutamic acid residues on their amino terminal ends, making them α-carboxyglutamic acid. This carboxylation reaction allows these proteins to bind to lipid and cell membranes, where they are activated. Without this carboxylation reaction, these proteins do not function normally in the hemostatic system.
      b. These proenzymes include factor X (58,000 Kd), factor IX (Christmas factor, 56,000 Kd), factor VII (50,000 Kd), and factor II (prothrombin, 72,000 Kd).
   2. **Surface-bound proenzymes (zymogens)** are part of the plasma kallikrein/kinin system.
      a. Surface-bound proenzymes include factor XII (Hageman factor, 80 Kd), prekallikrein (Fletcher factor, 88,85 Kd), and factor XI (160 Kd).
      b. These protein zymogens are also known as the contact system because factor XII autoactivates when associated with a negatively charged surface (e.g., a glass tube). The initiation of activation of factor XII on a negatively charged surface induces a series of proteolytic reactions known as the **coagulation cascade** *in vitro* (Fig. 8–2). These reactions *in vitro* cause thrombin to form and fibrinogen to be proteolyzed to form a clot.
      c. The autoactivation phenomena of factor XII allow for a common laboratory test, the activated partial thromboplastin time, to be used to assess the integrity of the coagulation system. However, deficiencies of factor XII and prekallikrein are not associated with a bleeding state. Activation of this cascade through factor XII is not necessary for normal hemostasis.

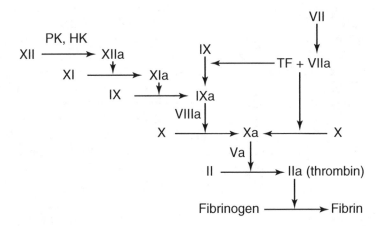

FIGURE 8–2. The coagulation cascade. *HK*, high-molecular-weight kininogen; *PK*, prekallikrein; *TF*, tissue factor.

      d. The proteins of the plasma kallikrein–kinin system participate in blood pressure regulation and fibrinolysis.

   3. Hemostatic cofactors and substrates of the enzymes of the coagulation system may act as receptors for coagulation proteins and as cofactors to accelerate the reactions that they maintain. Each cofactor or substrate also functions as a substrate of one or more enzymes that participate in their formation.

      a. **Factor VIII** (antihemophilic factor) is a 330,000-kd protein. When activated to factor VIIIa, it is a cofactor for factor IXa in the activation of factor X. Its absence is associated with hemophilia A, the most severe clinically recognized bleeding disorder.

      b. **Factor V** is a 330,000-kd protein. When activated to factor Va, it is a cofactor for factor Xa in the activation of factor II (prothrombin) to thrombin.

      c. **Fibrinogen** is a 330,000-kd protein that is the main substrate of thrombin (factor IIa) and a cofactor for platelet aggregation. When it is proteolyzed by thrombin, a fibrin monomer is formed. This monomer associates end to end and side to side to form a fibrin clot. The clot is stabilized by **factor XIII**, a tissue transglutaminase that cross-links the strands of associating fibrin.

      d. **Tissue Factor (TF)** is a 47,000-kd protein that is an essential cofactor for activated factor VIIa. It is found in most tissues and cells. Up-regulation of TF results in the formation of complexes with factor VII/VIIa that produce the initiation of hemostatic reactions.

      e. **High-molecular-weight kininogen** (Fitzgerald or Williams factor) is a 120,000-kd protein that acts as a cofactor for the activation of factor XII, prekallikrein, and factor XI on artificial surfaces and endothelial cell membranes. It is a substrate of kallikrein and activated factors XII and XI and is the parent compound for bradykinin, a biologically active peptide that regulates blood pressure and vascular biology. On endothelial cells, high-molecular-weight kininogen is a receptor for prekallikrein and factor XI. Deficiency of it is not associated with bleeding.

  B. Critical protein assemblies in hemostatic reactions. The proteins of the coagulation system that are essential for hemostasis were identified by observation of patients and by mouse knockout studies. Deficiencies in coagulation factors VIII and IX result in the most severe bleeding disorders that occur in patients who survive gestation and birth. Patients who have congenital deficiencies of coagulation factors VII, X, V, and II are few, and those who have defects have moderately severe bleeding states. However, these individuals must have some small amounts of functional coagulation factor to have survived gestation and birth. Mice who have genetic knockouts of factors VII, X, V, II, and TF die of massive hemorrhage during gestation or at birth. Directly or indirectly, all of these proteins participate in two critically important assemblies that are essential for normal hemostasis.

   1. Tenase assembly is the ability of activated factors VIII and IX to assemble on phospholipid surfaces or cell membranes to accelerate the activation of factor X to factor Xa. When all of these components are present, the rate of factor X activation by factor IXa is increased 1.4×10^8 over the rate of factor IXa activation of factor X alone (Fig. 8–3).

   2. Prothrombinase assembly is the ability of factor Xa and thrombin-activated factor Va to assemble on phospholipid membranes or cell membranes to ac-

FIGURE 8–3. The activation mechanism of factor X.

$$X \xrightarrow[\text{Phospholipids, cell membranes}]{\text{IXa, VIIIa}} Xa$$

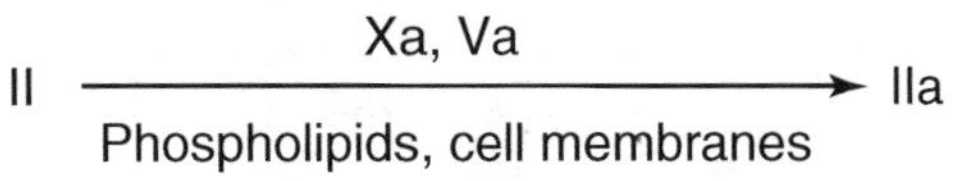

FIGURE 8–4. The activation mechanism of prothrombin (factor II).

$$II \xrightarrow[\text{Phospholipids, cell membranes}]{\text{Xa, Va}} IIa$$

celerate the activation of factor II (prothrombin) to factor IIa (thrombin). When all of these components are present, the rate of factor II activation by factor Xa is increased 1.7×10^8 over the rate of factor Xa activation of factor II alone (Fig. 8–4).

3. Because tenase and prothrombinase in the coagulation system are critical regulatory points in the physiologic hemostatic system, they are targeted by a number of anticoagulant agents that are in use or being developed.

IV. THE FIBRINOLYTIC AND ANTICOAGULATION SYSTEMS

A. The **fibrinolytic protein system** consists of the zymogen plasminogen and its naturally occurring activators. Plasminogen is activated to the main clot-lysing enzyme (plasmin) by endogenous tissue plasminogen activator, single-chain urokinase plasminogen activator, and two-chain urokinase plasminogen activator. These activators are found in the endothelium and in granulocytes and monocytes. Formed plasmin degrades fibrinogen, soluble fibrin, and cross-linked insoluble fibrin clots (Fig. 8–5).

B. Two **anticoagulant systems** regulate **coagulation proteins** and help to inhibit clot formation. These systems are the protein C and protein S system and the plasma serine protease inhibitor system. Antithrombin is the main serine protease inhibitor of coagulation reactions.

1. When activated, **protein C,** a 62-kd vitamin K–dependent protein, is an enzyme that functions as an inhibitor. Activated protein C inactivates factors Va and VIIIa to decrease the rate of thrombin formation. **Protein S,** a 69-kd vitamin K–dependent protein, is not an enzyme. It is a cofactor, or receptor, for activated protein C on cell membranes. The enzyme uses this cofactor as a receptor to localize its activity to perform its inhibitory function. Protein C is activated to an enzyme by thrombin located on an endothelial cell membrane protein known as thrombomodulin (Fig. 8–6).

2. **Antithrombin** is a 58-kd serine protease inhibitor that inhibits each of the hemostatic enzymes: IIa, Xa, VIIa, IXa, XIa, kallikrein, and XIIa. It exerts its anticoagulant effect primarily by inhibiting factors IIa and Xa. Antithrombin gives heparin its anticoagulant properties. In the presence of heparin, antithrombin is 1000-fold more effective as an inhibitor of factor IIa.

3. Other serine protease inhibitors of hemostatic and fibrinolytic enzymes include **C1 esterase inhibitor,** the most potent inhibitor of factor XIIa, kalli-

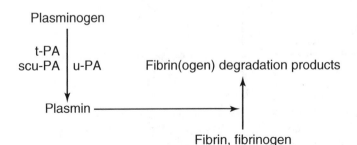

FIGURE 8–5. The fibrinolytic system. *scu-PA,* single-chain urokinase plasminogen activator; *t-PA,* tissue plasminogen activator; *u-PA,* two-chain urokinase plasminogen activator.

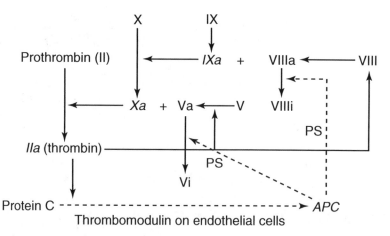

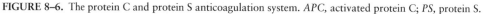

FIGURE 8–6. The protein C and protein S anticoagulation system. *APC*, activated protein C; *PS*, protein S.

krein, and factor XIa in plasma. Likewise, α_2-antiplasmin is the most potent regulator of plasmin. **Plasminogen activator inhibitor-1** is the major regulator of tissue and urokinase plasminogen activators. **Tissue Factor pathway inhibitor (TFPI)**, a Kunitz-type serine protease inhibitor, is the most potent inhibitor of factor VIIa–TF complex. Under physiologic conditions, TFPI prevents this complex from activating factor X directly. Another Kunitz-type serine protease inhibitor, the **amyloid β-protein precursor,** in platelets and brain tissue regulates factors XIa, IXa, Xa, and the VIIa–TF complex. Factor Xa is also modulated by the serine protease inhibitor **protein Z inhibitor** and its vitamin K–dependent cofactor, **protein Z.** Last, thrombin is regulated by another serine protease inhibitor, **heparin cofactor II.**

V.   CURRENT HYPOTHESIS FOR INITIATION OF THE HEMOSTATIC SYSTEM

Many proteins participate in coagulation reactions *in vitro*. However, fewer proteins are critical for hemostatic reactions *in vivo*. A new hypothesis to replace the coagulation cascade hypothesis is presented for hemostatic reactions (Fig. 8–7).

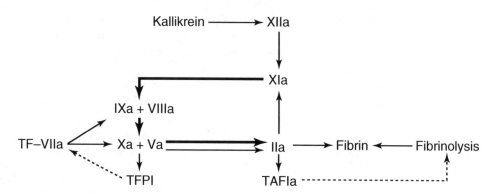

FIGURE 8–7. Revised view of the hemostatic system. *TAFIa*, activated thrombin-activatable fibrinolysis inhibitor; *TF*, tissue factor; *TFPI*, tissue factor pathway inhibitor. (Adapted with permission from Meijers JCM et al. High levels of coagulation factor XI as a risk factor for venous thrombosis. *N Engl J Med* 2000;342:696–701.)

A. Coagulation is initiated by TF, which binds to factor VIIa. This complex activates factor IX or factor X, which leads to the activation of prothrombin and the formation of fibrin.

B. TF-dependent coagulation reactions are rapidly inhibited by TFPI. However, if the stimulus for thrombin formation is strong, coagulation is maintained through the activation of factor XI by thrombin.

C. Activation of factor XI results in increased activation of factor IX and eventually increased formation of thrombin.

D. Through the tenase assembly (factors IXa and VIIIa) and the prothrombinase assembly (factors Xa and Va), the additional thrombin that is required to down-regulate fibrinolysis is generated by the activation of **thrombin activable fibrinolysis inhibitor (TAFI)**, or carboxypeptidase U.

E. Activated TAFI (TAFIa) down-regulates fibrinolysis by inactivating plasminogen.

F. The sum of increased thrombin formation and decreased clot lysis leads to a hemostatic fibrin clot.

VI. SUMMARY

The hemostatic, anticoagulant, and fibrinolytic protein pathways interact in a highly regulated fashion on the surface of activated platelets to prevent excessive bleeding and on the surface of endothelial cells to prevent thrombosis. The reactions and interactions that occur between these proteins and cells have the job of keeping blood flowing, but not to the extent that there is excessive bleeding.

SUGGESTED READING

Colman RW et al. Overview of hemostasis. In: Colman RW et al., eds. *Hemostasis and Thrombosis*, 4th ed. Philadelphia: Lippincott Williams & Wilkins, 2001: 3–16.

Meijers JCM et al. High levels of coagulation factor XI as a risk factor for venous thrombosis. *N Engl J Med* 2000;342:696–701.

Rodgers GM, Bithell TC. The diagnostic approach to the bleeding disorders. In: *Wintrobe's Clinical Hematology*. Baltimore: Williams & Wilkins, 1999:1557–1578.

Schafer AI. Approach to bleeding. In: Loscalzo J, Schafer AI, eds. *Thrombosis and Hemorrhage*. Baltimore: Williams & Wilkins, 1998:459–473.

CHAPTER 9

Approach to the Bleeding Patient

• ALVIN H. SCHMAIER

I. INTRODUCTION

This chapter aims to provide a simple diagnostic framework in which the physician can approach most patients with abnormal bleeding in a logical fashion to recognize the underlying cause. This diagnostic approach to bleeding disorders is based upon a full understanding of what the current screening assays for bleeding states measure.

II. PATHOGENESIS OF BLEEDING DISORDERS

When faced with a patient who has a bleeding disorder, the physician must use an analytic approach to determine the cause of the problem.

A. All bleeding disorders are caused by one of three defects:
1. **Plasma protein defect** (i.e., a defect in one or more plasma coagulation, fibrinolytic, or anticoagulant proteins)
2. **Platelet abnormality** (i.e., a defect in this hemostatic cell fragment)
3. **Defect in platelet–endothelial cell interactions** (i.e., a defect in the adhesive interactions between platelets and the vessel wall)

B. **Coagulation protein defects** that lead to bleeding can be classified as follows:
1. **True protein deficiency.** Insufficient protein is present for its required function.
2. **Inhibition of an active region of a protein.** The protein is present, but an inhibitor to its function arises. These inhibitors are usually immunoglobulins, but other forms are seen.
3. **Production of an abnormal protein molecule.** The protein is present, but as result of a mutation, missense, or deletion, an active portion of the protein is altered so that it cannot participate in its physiologic functions.
4. **Enhanced clearance of the protein.** An antibody arises against the protein, and the antigen–antibody complex is recognized as foreign, resulting in the complex being removed from the circulation. The resultant increased clearance of the protein gives the appearance of a deficiency.

III. CLINICAL PRESENTATION OF BLEEDING DISORDERS

The clinical presentation of bleeding disorders is presented in Table 9–1.

TABLE 9–1 • Clinical Presentation of Bleeding Disorders

	Hemophilioid State	Purpura
Bleeding source	Small artery	Capillary
Relation to trauma	Frequent	Rare
Presenting signs	Hematoma, ecchymosis	Ecchymosis, petechiae
Underlying cause	Factor deficiencies (e.g., VIII, IX, XI)	Platelet defects, vWF
Bleeding time	Normal	Abnormal

vWF, von Willebrand factor.

IV. COAGULATION CASCADE HYPOTHESIS

This 40-year-old theory of hemostasis still has merit in explaining the mechanisms for clot formation in screening tests for coagulation reactions. It is **not a complete model of physiologic hemostasis** (see Chapter 8). In the coagulation cascade hypothesis, coagulation proteins are classified as members of the intrinsic system, the extrinsic system, or the common pathway (Fig. 9–1).

A. **Intrinsic system**
1. Factor XII
2. Prekallikrein (PK)
3. High-molecular-weight kininogen (HK)
4. Factor XI
5. Factor VIII
6. Factor IX

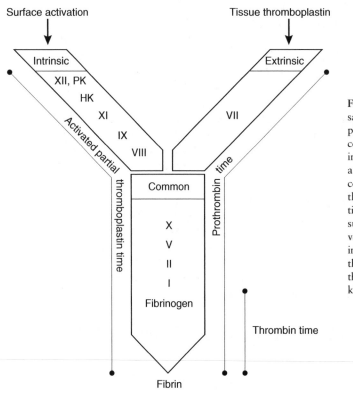

FIGURE 9–1. Plasma coagulation assays and the factors they measure. The plasma proteins involved in *in vitro* coagulation reactions can be classified into three systems: intrinsic, extrinsic, and common. The screening tests for coagulation proteins (activated partial thromboplastin time, prothrombin time, or thrombin clotting time) measure one or more of the proteins involved in *in vitro* clot formation. Knowing what finding is abnormal pinpoints the likely protein defect that will give this result. *HK*, high-molecular-weight kininogen; *PK*, prekallikrein.

B. **Extrinsic system**
  1. Factor VII
  2. Tissue factor
C. **Common pathway**
  1. Factors X and V
  2. Factor II
  3. Factor I (fibrinogen)

V. SCREENING TESTS FOR BLEEDING DISORDERS

Several screening tests are used to classify and diagnose bleeding disorders. When these assays are performed simultaneously on a sample of plasma, the results indicate almost all of the diagnostic categories for a bleeding state.

A. **Activated partial thromboplastin time (aPTT).** To perform this common coagulation assay, a mixture of a negatively charged surface, phospholipid, and plasma is incubated for a few minutes. Calcium chloride is added, and the time required for clot formation is measured. The aPTT assesses the coagulation proteins of the intrinsic system and the common pathway.

B. **Prothrombin time (PT).** To perform this common coagulation assay, tissue thromboplastin and plasma are incubated for a few minutes. Afterward, the plasma is recalcified and the time required for clot formation is measured. The PT assesses the coagulation proteins of the extrinsic system and the common pathway.

C. **Platelet count.** This assay measures the number of platelets in a microliter of blood. It is used to exclude a quantitative platelet defect as the cause of a bleeding disorder.

D. **Bleeding time.** To perform this assay, the forearm is scratched and the time until bleeding stops is measured. It assesses platelet number or function.

E. **Thrombin clotting time (TCT).** To perform this assay, purified thrombin is added to plasma to determine the time for clot formation, a direct measure of fibrinogen function.

VI. INTERPRETATION OF SCREENING TESTS OF THE PROTEINS IN THE COAGULATION SYSTEM

Using the coagulation cascade hypothesis and its grouping of proteins, the screening tests for bleeding disorders can be used to assess specific coagulation proteins (Fig. 9–1).

A. In the aPTT, factor XII is activated by exposure to an artifical negatively charged surface. The aPTT measures the proteins of the intrinsic system (factor XII, PK, HK, factor XI, factor IX, and factor VIII) and the proteins of the common pathway (factors X, V, and II and fibrinogen).

B. The **PT** measures the extrinsic system of coagulation, which consists of activated factor VII (factor VIIa) and tissue factor and the proteins of the common pathway (factors X, V, II, and fibrinogen).

C. The **TCT** measures only the ability of exogenous thrombin to proteolyze (clot) fibrinogen. It is used to characterize fibrinogen function.

VII. DIFFERENTIAL DIAGNOSIS OF PROLONGED aPTT ONLY

The following approach can be used to evaluate patients who have an isolated prolonged aPTT.

A. **Disorders associated with bleeding**

1. Factor VIII deficiency or defect is sex-linked and may be congenital or acquired. Congenital factor VIII deficiency occurs only in males. Acquired factor VIII deficiency occurs in both males and females.
2. Factor IX deficiency or defect is sex-linked.
3. Factor XI deficiency is autosomal recessive.

B. **Disorders not associated with bleeding**
1. Factor XII deficiency is autosomal recessive and is the most common type. It gives a very prolonged aPTT but is not associated with bleeding.
2. Deficiency of PK is autosomal recessive. It gives a mildly prolonged aPTT.
3. Deficiency of HK is autosomal recessive and extremely rare. It gives a very prolonged aPTT.
4. Lupus anticoagulants are antiphospholipid antibodies that interfere with coagulation reactions. These antibodies arise for many reasons and are not specific to one illness, although they are often seen in patients who have connective tissue disorders (e.g., systemic lupus erythematosus). Usually they interfere not with the protein itself but rather with the phospholipid reagents that are used in the coagulation assay. Although these antibodies prolong coagulation protein assays, they are not associated with bleeding unless hypoprothrombinemia or thrombocytopenia is present. Paradoxically, they are often associated with thrombosis because they interfere with various anticoagulation systems. When lupus anticoagulants prolong the aPTT, the diagnosis is made after other specific entities are excluded.

VIII.   DIFFERENTIAL DIAGNOSIS OF PROLONGED PT ONLY

Isolated PT prolongation usually indicates factor VII deficiency. Most of these patients have partial VII defects. Occasionally, isolated prolonged PT is seen in a patient who has dysfibrinogenemia (abnormal fibrinogen) or a deficiency in coagulation factor X, V, or II. Detection of these depends on the specific kind of reagents a clinical laboratory uses.

IX.   DIFFERENTIAL DIAGNOSIS OF PROLONGED aPTT AND PT

Usually, abnormalities in both coagulation protein screening tests are not specific protein conditions but rather reflect acquired general medical conditions (see Chapter 11). These abnormalities may be caused by many factors.
A. Medical causes include disseminated intravascular coagulation (see Chapter 11), liver disease, vitamin K deficiency, the use of anticoagulants (e.g., heparin, warfarin, low-molecular-weight heparin), and massive transfusion.
B. Dysfibrinogenemia occurs when abnormal fibrinogen molecules do not participate properly in coagulation reactions.
C. In rare cases, coagulation protein defects of the common pathway (factor X, V, or II) are seen.

X.   DIFFERENTIAL DIAGNOSIS OF PROLONGED BLEEDING TIME WITH NORMAL PLATELET COUNT

Defects in bleeding time in the presence of a normal platelet count signify abnormalities in the following:
A. **Von Willebrand factor** (von Willebrand disease) (see Chapter 10)

B. **Platelet function** (see Chapter 12)
C. **Rare connective tissue disorders,** including pseudoxanthoma elasticum, Ehlers-Danlos syndrome, and scurvy

XI. PROLONGED BLEEDING TIME AS A RESULT OF PLATELET DEFECTS

This abnormality occurs when the number of platelets is decreased or when a true intrinsic defect in platelet function occurs.

A. **Quantitative decrease in platelet count.** As the platelet count decreases to less than $100,000/\mu L$, the bleeding time becomes prolonged.
B. **True platelet function defect** (see Chapter 12)

XII. DIFFERENTIAL DIAGNOSIS OF BLEEDING WITH NO ABNORMALITY IN THE SCREENING TESTS

These entities are rare and mainly consist of abnormalities of the fibrinolytic system (e.g., defects in α_2-antiplasmin or plasminogen activator inhibitor) or abnormalities in factor XIII.

A. Factor XIII deficiency may be congenital or acquired. Patients bleed excessively as a result of surgery or trauma. Deficient middle-aged adults have a high incidence of spontaneous intracerebral hemorrhage.
B. α_2-Antiplasmin deficiency is the absence of the major serine protease inhibitor (serpin) of plasmin. These patients have a bleeding disorder that is caused by a hyperfibrinolytic state, with lysis of any clots that are formed. α_2-Antiplasmin deficiency can be acquired as a result of consumption in disseminated intravascular coagulation (e.g., acute promyelocytic anemia).
C. Plasminogen activator inhibitor-1 deficiency is a deficiency in the major serpin inhibitor of plasminogen activators. This abnormality causes increased activation of plasminogen. A profibrinolytic state occurs as a result.
D. α_1-Antitrypsin$_{PITTSBURGH}$ is an abnormal serpin that changes α_1-antitrypsin into a potent antithrombin. It causes a severe bleeding disorder because it has exceedingly tight binding and potent inhibition of the activity of thrombin. Thus, any thrombin that forms is rapidly neutralized, so no clotting can occur.

XIII. SUMMARY

Understanding what the aPTT, PT, platelet count, and bleeding time measure allows the physician recognize the underlying cause of most bleeding disorders that one may encounter in clinical practice. It is of great clinical value to fully understand the results of these assays.

SUGGESTED READING

Greaves M, Preston FE. Approach to the bleeding patient. In: Colman R et al. *Hemostasis and Thrombosis.* Philadelphia: Lippincott Williams & Wilkins, 2001: 783–793.

Rodgers GM, Bithell TC. The diagnostic approach to the bleeding disorders. In: Lee GR et al. *Wintrobe's Clinical Hematology.* Baltimore: Williams & Wilkins, 1999:1557–1578.

Schafer AI. Approach to bleeding. In: Loscalzo J, Schafer AI. *Thrombosis and Hemorrhage.* Baltimore: Williams & Wilkins, 1998:459–473.

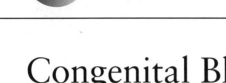

CHAPTER **10**

Congenital Bleeding Disorders

• PAULA BOCKENSTEDT

I. INTRODUCTION

The most frequently encountered congenital bleeding disorders are deficiencies in factors VIII, IX, and XI (known as hemophilia A, B, and C, respectively) and von Willebrand disease (vWD); therefore, this chapter describes these disorders in detail. Factor VIII and IX deficiencies are the most common congenital bleeding disorders because they are sex-linked defects (i.e., on the X chromosome). Unique features of the rarer deficiencies of fibrinogen and factors II, V, VII, X, and XIII are also discussed in this chapter.

II. PATHOPHYSIOLOGY OF CONGENITAL BLEEDING DISORDERS

A. Deficiencies in coagulation factors result in a decreased rate and amount of thrombin produced, resulting in a reduced rate and amount of fibrin plug formation at the site of injury.
B. The quality of the fibrin plug is poor, with decreased hydrostatic strength and greater susceptibility to fibrinolytic dissolution.

III. CLINICAL EVALUATION OF CONGENITAL BLEEDING DISORDERS

A. Deficiencies of all blood coagulation factors, with the exception of von Willebrand factor (vWF), factor XII, prekallikrein, and high-molecular-weight kininogen, result in similar bleeding manifestations that are distinct from those observed in platelet disorders (Table 10–1). Congenital deficiency in a coagulation factor is associated with the characteristic symptoms and signs of spontaneous intramuscular or intraarticular bleeding and delayed bleeding after injury.
B. The laboratory diagnosis of a specific factor deficiency is based on results obtained with screening studies, including prothrombin time (PT), activated partial thromboplastin time (aPTT), thrombin clotting time, clottable fibrinogen level, and a specific factor assay (see Fig. 9–1).

TABLE 10–1 • Patterns of Clinical Bleeding in Disorders of Hemostasis

Characteristics	Primary Hemostasis (Platelet/Vascular Problem)	Secondary Hemostasis (Coagulation Factor Problem)
Onset	Spontaneous, immediately after trauma	Delayed after trauma
Sites	Skin, mucous membranes	Deep tissues
Form	Petechiae, ecchymoses	Hematomas
Mucous membrane	Common (nasal, oral, GI, GU)	Rare
Other sites	Rare	Joint, muscle, CNS, retroperitoneal
Clinical examples	Thrombocytopenia, platelet defect, vWD, scurvy	Factor deficiency, acquired inhibitors, liver disease

CNS, central nervous system; GI, gastrointestinal; GU, genitourinary; vWD, von Willebrand disease.

IV.   DISORDERS OF THE INTRINSIC COAGULATION SYSTEM: FACTORS VIII, IX, AND XI

A. **Factor VIII deficiency (hemophilia A)**
   1. **Overview.** Factor VIII deficiency is the most common of the hemophilias, with an incidence of 1–2 cases per 10,000 male births. Factor VIII is an essential cofactor for factor IXa–mediated factor Xa production.
   2. **Genetics.** Factor VIII deficiency is inherited as a **sex-linked recessive** disorder. The sons of a hemophilic man and a normal woman do not inherit the paternal hemophilia. However, all daughters of such a union are obligate carriers (XX^h). A carrier has equal chances of having a normal (XY) or hemophilic (X^hY) son and a normal daughter or a daughter who carries the hemophilia gene on one of her X chromosomes (XX^h). All patients with hemophilia A have less than 50% factor VIII activity. Some patients have reduced activity levels and reduced factor VIII antigen levels. Some have reduced factor VIII levels but detectable immunoreactive factor VIII protein. In most patients with moderate to mild hemophilia A, the defect is a single amino acid missense mutation within a functional region of the factor VIII protein. The intrachromosomal recombination mutation resulting in inversion of intron 22 of the factor VIII gene has been shown to account for approximately 40%–50% of cases of severe factor VIII deficiency. Of newly diagnosed patients with factor VIII deficiency, 30% have no family history of hemophilia because there is an inherent de novo spontaneous mutation rate of that portion of the X chromosome.
   3. **Clinical presentation.** The hallmark of coagulation factor deficiency bleeding is the delayed and spontaneous nature of the bleeding, with predilection for soft tissue and intraarticular bleeding.
      a. Table 10–2 lists the typical bleeding symptoms encountered in a person with severe factor VIII deficiency.
      b. Bleeding symptoms of factor VIII deficiency may be expressed in females with the following traits:
         (1) Gene mosaicism (46,XX/X^hO)
         (2) Turner syndrome (X^hO)
         (3) Double heterozygote for factor VIII deficiency (X^hX^h) (daughter of a

mother who is a carrier of factor VIII deficiency and a father who has hemophilia A)

    (4) Lyonized carrier of factor VIII deficiency (XX^h)

       (a) Only one of the X chromosomes is expressed in each somatic cell. Inactivation of the second X chromosome occurs randomly in lyonization.

       (b) Most carriers of factor VIII deficiency have 50% factor VIII levels; however, some carriers have less than 50% levels as a result of lyonization and therefore exhibit symptomatic bleeding.

4. **Diagnosis.** Both history and laboratory evaluation contribute to the diagnosis of hemophilia A.

  a. **History**

    (1) Ask the patient about the types of trauma and sites of spontaneous bleeding and about interval of time between injury and bleeding.

    (2) Carefully obtain a history of the type of bleeding at the time of common surgical procedures or events (e.g., dental prophylaxis, tooth eruption, tooth extraction, ear piercing, biopsy, childbirth, circumcision).

    (3) Obtain a menstrual history, with specific attention to amount of daily bleeding and length of cycles. Occasionally symptomatic carriers of hemophilia have heavy menses.

    (4) Pay careful attention to maternal family bleeding history.

  b. **Laboratory evaluation**

    (1) Factor VIII levels less than 30% can be reliably detected using the **aPTT** as a screening test. However, routine aPTT screening alone misses some patients with hemophilia because the aPTT is not always prolonged with mildly decreased factor VIII levels (i.e., 25%–49%).

    (2) A **specific clotting factor assay** for factor VIII is called for (Table 10–3).

    (3) The PT, bleeding time, and thrombin clotting time (TCT) are normal in factor VIII deficiency.

5. **Specific problems in hemophilia A and B**

  a. **Acute hemarthrosis,** either spontaneous or traumatic, is the most frequent type of bleeding encountered in patients with severe hemophilia. Hemarthroses may occur several times a month in a patient with severe hemophilia. The release of blood proteases into the synovial space results in destruction of cartilage. Successful treatment is aimed at early recognition of joint bleeding symptoms. Self-infusion of factor concentrates before clinical signs of swelling and pain help to preserve the joint from destruction. Long-term prophylactic infusion therapy to maintain levels of approximately 1% may be sufficient to prevent intraarticular bleeds.

TABLE 10–2 · Bleeding Manifestations in Hemophilia

Bleeding after circumcision
Delayed oozing from deep lacerations
Protracted bleeding after dental extraction
Intramuscular hematomas
Intraarticular hemorrhage
Central nervous system bleeding
Hematuria

TABLE 10–3 • Predictive Value of Factor VIII Levels

Factor VIII (%)	Severity of Hemophilia	Specific Symptoms
<1	Severe	Spontaneous intraarticular and intramuscular bleeds
1–5	Moderate	Predominantly soft tissue bleeding
5–10	Mild	Risk of bleeding after surgery, trauma; reduced risk of spontaneous hemorrhage[a]

[a]Patients with factor VIII levels greater than 20% may be clinically asymptomatic until major surgery or trauma.

  b. **Chronic hemophilic arthropathy** (Fig. 10–1), a crippling disorder, imposes great socioeconomic impact on hemophilic patients. The arthropathy results from recurrent or extensive bleeding into the joint space. Cartilage destruction is severe. Synovial neovascularization also occurs. Eventually subchondral cysts form and the joint space is destroyed by collapse of underlying bony structures. Progressive loss of range of motion and function occurs. Joint replacement may be necessary.
  c. **Intramuscular hemorrhage** is the second most frequent type of bleeding in patients with severe hemophilia. Intramuscular hemorrhages are particularly damaging when they occur in closed compartments (e.g., volar aspect of the wrist or forearm, deep palmar compartments of the hand, anterior or posterior tibial compartments). Iliopsoas hemorrhage may be confused with an intraarticular hip bleed.

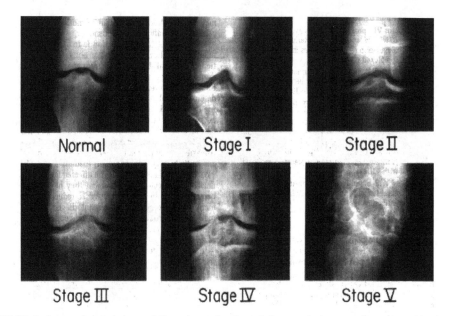

FIGURE 10–1. Stages of chronic hemophilic arthropathy. Stage I shows soft tissue swelling due to bleeding in and around the joint and no skeletal abnormalities. Stage II shows osteoporotic and epiphyseal overgrowth with an intact joint space and no bone cysts. Stage III shows subchondral cysts and minor irregularities of the joint surface with a preserved joint space. Stage IV shows cysts and joint surface irregularities that are more prominent. The joint space is narrowed as a result of cartilage damage. Stage V shows loss of joint space and marked epiphyseal overgrowth. (Reprinted with permission from White GC II, Levin J. Disorders of blood coagulation. In: Stein JH. *Internal Medicine.* Boston: Little, Brown, 1987:1012.)

    d. **Central nervous system bleeding** is the most common cause of death from bleeding in a patient with hemophilia. It may occur spontaneously with minimal head trauma (e.g., a bump on the head from a cabinet door) or after falling directly on the buttocks. Symptoms include headache and lethargy. Treatment should be administered empirically without waiting for the results of a diagnostic computed tomography scan.

    e. **Mouth, throat, and nose bleeds** are frequently caused by biting the tongue, tonsillitis, protracted coughing, or regional block anesthesia for dental work. The hematoma may cause airway compromise if it dissects under the tongue, behind the pharyngeal wall, or around the trachea.

    f. **Dental procedures** generally require factor replacement plus an antifibrinolytic agent, 1-deamino-8-D-arginine vasopressin (DDAVP) plus an antifibrinolytic agent, or an antifibrinolytic agent alone, depending on the severity of hemophilia and the extent of the dental procedure. Prior to coagulation factor replacement therapy, many patients with hemophilia died of protracted hemorrhage after a simple tooth extraction or tongue laceration.

    g. **Major surgery** requires factor replacement with all levels of factor deficiency.

    h. **Other procedures,** including routine venipuncture, intravenous catheter placement, and immunizations, can be administered without risk of major bleeding. Invasive procedures (e.g., biopsy, spinal tap, arterial blood gas sampling, deep intramuscular injection) require factor replacement therapy.

B. Factor IX deficiency (hemophilia B)

    1. **Overview.** Factor IX deficiency accounts for approximately 10% of hereditary coagulation factor deficiencies. Incidence is 1 in 30,000 live male births. Along with factor VIII deficiency, factor IX deficiency is the most severe bleeding state that allows for normal gestation and delivery.

    2. **Genetics.** Factor IX deficiency is an X-linked recessive disorder, although 30% of patients may have no other affected family members but instead carry a spontaneous new mutation in the factor IX gene. Many mutations in the factor IX gene result in reduced levels of factor IX activity and antigen or normal levels of a functionally abnormal molecule. Decreased functional factor IX levels can result from defects in splicing of the factor IX transcript, nonsense mutations, gene deletions, and abnormalities in the promoter region.

    3. **Clinical presentation.** Bleeding symptoms of factor IX deficiency are identical to those of factor VIII deficiency (Table 10–2); the diseases are indistinguishable without specific factor assays. Female carriers of factor IX deficiency may also be symptomatic [see IV.A.3.b.(4)(b)].

    4. **Laboratory evaluation.** Levels of factor IX below 50% result in a **prolonged aPTT**. A specific factor assay for factor IX is diagnostic. The predictive value of factor IX levels is identical to that of factor VIII levels (Table 10–3). The PT, thrombin clotting time, and bleeding time are normal in factor IX deficiency.

    5. **Specific problems in factor IX deficiency** are identical to problems in hemophilia A.

C. Factor XI deficiency (hemophilia C)

    1. **Overview.** Factor XI deficiency is rare, occurring in 1 of 100,000 persons.

    2. **Genetics.** Factor XI deficiency is an incompletely recessive autosomal trait. There is a high predilection of factor XI deficiency in Ashkenazi Jews of eastern European descent; however, 50% of cases of factor XI deficiency occur in other ethnic groups.

    3. **Clinical presentation.** Overall, bleeding symptoms are less than in moderate or severe factor VIII or IX deficiency.

      a. Approximately 50% of patients bleed after surgery or trauma. The remainder of factor XI–deficient patients have relatively minor symptoms and are identified only by an abnormal aPTT.

      b. Spontaneous hemarthroses are rare.

      c. Symptomatic patients typically have spontaneous nosebleeds, hematuria, and menorrhagia.

      d. Bleeding with dental extractions and urologic procedures is common.

      e. Bleeding symptoms not only show great variation among unrelated patients with the same factor XI level, they also vary over time in the same individual.

      f. Clinical symptoms tend to be similar within affected family members.

    4. Laboratory evaluation. The **aPTT is prolonged** in factor XI deficiency. The PT, thrombin clotting time, and bleeding time are normal. A specific factor XI assay is diagnostic. Functional levels of factor XI are concordant with antigenic levels, and bleeding is most likely to occur in individuals with levels below 10%.

    5. In **factor XI deficiency,** bleeding most often appears in associated mucosal surfaces, such as after dental extraction or urologic surgery.

  D. Deficiency of proteins of the intrinsic coagulation system not associated with bleeding

    1. Factor XII, prekallikrein, and **high-molecular-weight kininogen** of the plasma kallikrein–kinin system are entities that affect the aPTT, but deficiencies in each of these proteins are not associated with bleeding. The plasma kallikrein–kinin system contributes to the anticoagulant nature of the intravascular compartment and has a role in regulating blood pressure and counterbalancing the renin–angiotensin system.

    2. Factor XII autoactivates when associated with artificial negatively charged surfaces. Factor XII then initiates a cascade of events in the presence of high-molecular-weight kininogen and prekallikrein *in vitro*, resulting in thrombin and clot formation. However, *in vivo* they do not participate in hemostasis.

    3. A defect in the kallikrein–kinin system is diagnosed by a prolonged aPTT (often > 100 seconds). Specific factor assays are required to determine the exact factor deficiency.

    4. The PT, bleeding time, and thrombin clotting time are normal.

    5. No factor replacement is necessary at the time of surgery in patients with these deficiencies.

V.   DISORDERS OF THE COMMON PATHWAY: FACTORS V, X, AND II

  A. Overview. Deficiencies of these proteins are rare disorders of autosomal recessive inheritance. Incidence is less than 1 in 1 million. Deficiency results from decreased synthesis of factor or synthesis of normal amounts of a functionally impaired factor. In most cases, some functional protein is present. Most patients with a heterozygous deficiency are clinically silent.

  B. Clinical presentation. Disorders of the common pathway present with soft tissue and spontaneous bleeding, as in hemophilia in general. Only severe factor V and X deficiencies are associated with hemarthroses.

  C. Laboratory evaluation. Factors II, V, and X form the prothrombinase complex in the common pathway. The PT and aPTT are both prolonged in deficiencies of these factors. The thrombin clotting time is normal.

VI. DISORDERS OF THE EXTRINSIC COAGULATION SYSTEM: FACTOR VII DEFICIENCY

A. **Genetics.** Factor VII is inherited in an autosomal recessive pattern. Heterozygous individuals are usually asymptomatic, but homozygous individuals are clinically affected.

B. **Clinical presentation.** Factor VII levels less than 1% are generally associated with severe spontaneous hemorrhage and intraarticular bleeding, as seen in severe deficiency of factor VIII or IX. Factor VII levels as low as 10% seem to protect against severe bleeding symptoms.

C. **Laboratory evaluation.** Factor VII deficiency is the only cause of an **isolated prolonged PT**. The aPTT, bleeding time, and thrombin clotting time are normal.

VII. DISORDERS OF FIBRINOGEN

A. **Overview.** Congenital abnormalities in fibrinogen have been reported in approximately 200 patients worldwide.

B. **Genetics.** The fibrinogen genes are on chromosome 4, where three separate genes (α, β, and γ) encode for the Aα, Bβ, and γ fibrinogen chains, respectively. Sequential cleavage of fibrinopeptides A and B from fibrinogen by thrombin is important in initiating the alignment and polymerization of fibrin monomers into the hydrostatic barrier critical to clot formation. Mutations in the Aα, Bβ, and γ chains of fibrinogen can interfere with binding and proteolytic cleavage of fibrinogen to fibrin, resulting in misshapen and poorly interconnected fibrin monomers. A variety of amino acid substitutions have been described. Segmental insertions and deletions are less common causes of fibrinogen defects.

1. **Hereditary afibrinogenemia** is rare, with only 150 cases reported worldwide. Afibrinogenemia is autosomal recessive. No clottable or antigenic fibrinogen is detected. Most patients have truncating deletions in the fibrinogen α chain gene.

2. **Hereditary hypofibrinogenemia** is more common than afibrinogenemia, but some cases are actually **dysfibrinogenemia** with normal amounts of fibrinogen antigen but functionally abnormal fibrinogen. Most patients with hereditary dysfibrinogenemia are heterozygous for a genetic mutation.

C. **Clinical presentation of abnormal fibrinogen**

1. Patients with disorders in fibrinogen may have:
   a. Prolonged umbilical stump bleeding
   b. Intracranial hemorrhage (leading cause of death)
   c. Intraarticular bleeds (20%)

2. Gastrointestinal and mucosal bleeding are more frequent in hypofibrinogenemia than in hemophilia in general.

3. Most patients with fibrinogen disorders do not have crippling arthritis by adulthood, as seen in factor VIII and IX deficiencies.

4. Women with afibrinogenemia are generally unable to carry a developing fetus without aggressive fibrinogen replacement therapy.

5. Patients with congenital hypofibrinogenemia do not have spontaneous bleeds until the functional fibrinogen level is below 50 mg/dL.

6. Most patients with dysfibrinogenemia are asymptomatic and are diagnosed during routine laboratory screening.

7. The tendency to hemorrhage is associated with several factors.
   a. If the concentration of normal fibrinogen is greater than 100 mg/dL, there is a decreased tendency to hemorrhage.

      b. If the fibrinogen clotting assay and the fibrinogen antigen levels are below 100 mg/dL, there is a higher frequency of bleeding.

      c. Disorders resulting in abnormal fibrinopeptide release and fibrin cross-linking are more commonly associated with bleeding.

      d. Abnormalities in polymerization are frequently associated with thrombotic manifestations, although to date no known common thread results in the prothrombotic risk.

D. Laboratory evaluation

    1. The PT, aPTT, and thrombin clotting time are all markedly prolonged in afibrinogenemia and to a lesser extent in hypofibrinogenemia.

    2. In dysfibrinogenemia, the PT, aPTT, and thrombin clotting time are variably prolonged, with the PT and thrombin clotting time being the most sensitive screening tests. Occasionally the thrombin clotting time is shortened and may reflect a predilection to thrombosis rather than hemorrhage.

    3. A discrepancy in the ratio of the clottable fibrinogen level to the antigenic fibrinogen level is characteristic of dysfibrinogenemia.

VIII. FACTOR XIII DEFICIENCY

A. Overview. Factor XIII is a transglutaminase found in plasma and platelets that is important in forming stabilizing covalent bonds between polymerizing fibrin monomers during clot formation (Fig. 10–2). Lack of these links results in a fibrin clot, which is easily permeable to blood cells and readily degraded by tissue proteases and fibrinolytic enzymes. Inheritance is autosomal recessive. Heterozygous individuals are not generally symptomatic, but women may have a higher incidence of infertility than normal. The incidence is thought to be approximately 3–5 new cases per year in the United States.

B. Genetics. Factor XIII exists as a complex of two A subunits and two B subunits in

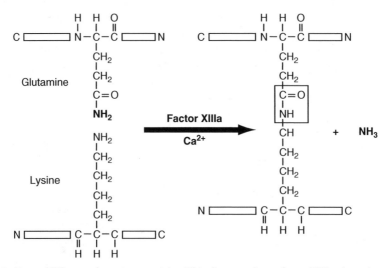

FIGURE 10–2. Factor XIII transglutaminase activity. This diagram shows factor XIIIa–dependent covalent bond formation. The cysteine on the active site of factor XIIIa forms a calcium-dependent thioester complex with a glutamine residue. A neighboring lysine residue aligned by fibrin polymerization serves as an electron acceptor, and an isopeptide γ-glutamyl ε-lysyl bond forms between the proteins. Ammonia is released as a by-product. (Reprinted with permission from Greenberg CS. Fibrin Formation and Stabilization. In: Thrombosis and Hemorrhage, Loscalzo J, Schafer AI (eds), Blackwell, Boston, 1994 Fig. 6.7, p. 117.)

plasma. The A and B subunits derive from separate genes on separate chromosomes. Most individuals with factor XIII deficiency exhibit absent or defective A and B subunits. Only one case has been described with only B subunit deficiency.

C. **Clinical presentation of factor XIII deficiency.** Factor XIII deficiency is typically associated with umbilical stump bleeding and a high incidence (25%) of spontaneous intracranial hemorrhage. Most patients present shortly after birth and die in middle age of spontaneous intracerebral hemorrhage. Poor wound healing is a characteristic manifestation of factor XIII deficiency but is seen in only 14% of patients. As in factor VIII and IX deficiencies, all forms of soft tissue and intraarticular hemorrhage are seen with trauma. Spontaneous joint hemorrhage is rare.

D. **Laboratory evaluation.** In factor XIII deficiency, the routine screening PT, aPTT, thrombin clotting time, platelet count, and bleeding time are normal. The urea clot solubility test readily demonstrates clot dissolution because of the decreased cross-links formed; however, it is not sensitive to individuals with factor XIII levels greater than 4%–10%. Only approximately 3% factor XIII activity is required for a relatively normal life free from recurrent hemorrhage.

IX. VON WILLEBRAND DISEASE

A. **Overview.** vWD is the most common congenital bleeding disorder, affecting 1% of the population worldwide. It is a heterogeneous disorder characterized by an array of variants and subtypes. vWF participates in primary hemostasis by serving as a link between the injured vascular subendothelium and platelet glycoprotein (GP) Ib-IX-V complex (GPIb-IX-V) (Fig. 10–3). The platelet adhesion function for vWF is important at conditions of high shear rate. It is also necessary as a carrier protein for factor VIII.

B. **Genetics.** To understand the classification of vWD subtypes, it is necessary to understand the basic structure of vWF.

1. Mature vWF exists as a series of oligomers ranging in size from the dimer of 550 Kd to more than 10,000 Kd. Each dimer of vWF consists of two mature vWF subunits linked by disulfide bonds at their carboxytermini.

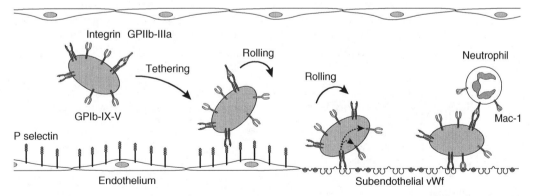

FIGURE 10–3. Role of Von Willebrand factor in primary hemostasis. In hemostasis, vWF is the major participant in the interaction of platelets with the blood vessel wall. With the help of platelet glycoprotein Ib–IX–V complex (*GPIb-IX-V*), circulating platelets may interact with the P selectin expressed on activated endothelial cells or with vWF in the subendothelial matrix. Subsequently, GPIIb-IIIa becomes activated and adhesive to vWF. GPIb-IX-V may also interact with leukocyte Mac-1 integrin in the recruitment of leukocytes to thrombotic sites. (Adapted with permission from Berndt MC et al. The vascular biology of the glycoprotein Ib-IX-V complex. *Thromb Haemost* 2001;86:179.)

2. The mature vWF subunit is divided into several homologous domains.
   a. The factor VIII binding site on vWF is contained within the first 272 amino acids of the amino terminus.
   b. The A domains contain sequences important for the binding of vWF to collagen, heparin, and receptor GPIb-IX-V on platelets.
   c. The C1 domain in the carboxy terminus contains Arg-Gly-Asp (RGD) sequences for vWF binding to platelet GPIIb-IIIa.
3. vWF is synthesized only in endothelial cells and megakaryocytes.
   a. In the endothelial cell, vWF is synthesized and released into the circulation, where it ultimately combines with factor VIII. This complex is essential for factor VIII survival and its delivery to sites of active platelet adhesion during clotting. The regulated pathway of vWF synthesis results in storage of high-molecular-weight vWF in elongated endothelial granules called Weibel-Palade bodies. These high-molecular-weight multimers are believed to be the most effective in adhesion under high-shear stress and are released in a regulated fashion.
   b. vWF is also synthesized and stored in platelet α-granules along with other adhesive GPs. During platelet activation and release, these α-granules are mobilized to the platelet surface, where vWF and other proteins are released.
C. **Clinical presentation.** The bleeding symptoms in vWD (Table 10–4) are typical of immediate platelet-type bleeding with predominant bruising, epistaxis, and mucosal bleeding. The bleeding symptoms due to injury may be delayed when factor VIII levels are less than 25%.
D. **Laboratory evaluation.** Normal vWF levels vary according to an individual's blood group.
1. Bleeding time is used to assess platelet plug formation *in vivo* by determining the time to cessation of bleeding from a small skin laceration. The bleeding time may be prolonged in vWD or other qualitative or quantitative platelet disorders as well as some disorders of connective tissue.
2. Ristocetin cofactor activity (vWF function; R:CO) is the only functional assay readily available for vWF. Ristocetin is a negatively charged antibiotic. When added to plasma, ristocetin induces a structural change in vWF, exposing the domain for binding to platelet GPIb-IX-V. The assay is based on the ability of patient plasma to induce agglutination of formalin-fixed platelets in the presence of a fixed concentration of ristocetin. The level of vWF functional activity in a blood sample is assessed by comparing its ability to induce platelet agglutination with that of various dilutions of known normal pooled human plasma.

TABLE 10–4 • Bleeding Manifestations in Von Willebrand Disease

Mucocutaneous bleeding with normal platelet count
Superficial bruising (common)
Petechiae (rare)
Gingival bleeding
Epistaxis
Menorrhagia
Gastrointestinal mucosal bleeding
Immediate bleeding after dental extraction
Postpartum hemorrhage
Spontaneous hemarthroses (rare; usually in type III von Willebrand disease)

3. Ristocetin-induced platelet aggregation is similar to the test performed for ristocetin cofactor activity, except that the patient's own platelets in plasma (i.e., platelet-rich plasma) are used and the ristocetin concentration is varied to determine sensitivity to ristocetin. Enhanced ristocetin-induced platelet aggregation may be an indicator of type IIB vWD (see IX.E.2.b.) or pseudo-vWD.

4. Plasma vWF antigen (vWF:Ag) is an immune quantitation of the amount of vWF in plasma.

5. Factor VIII activity is measured using a standard clotting factor assay based on the aPTT. Because factor VIII binds to plasma vWF, factor VIII levels generally parallel the level of vWF antigen.

6. Multimer analysis requires that patient plasma be fractionated on an agarose gel. The vWF multimers are then visualized with a radiolabeled anti-vWF antibody (Fig. 10–4).

   a. Normal vWF is seen as a complex series of bands divided into groups of low-, intermediate-, and high-molecular-weight multimers.

   b. Type I vWD is characterized by an overall decreased but normal array of vWF multimers.

   c. Type II subtypes are characterized by an abnormal multimer pattern (Fig. 10–4).

   d. Type III subtype is characterized by absence of all vWF multimers.

E. **Von Willebrand disease subtypes**

   1. **Type I vWD** accounts for 70% of cases of vWD. It is characterized by a partial deficiency in vWF. It is inherited in an autosomal dominant fashion and is characterized by concordant reductions in vWF antigen, ristocetin cofactor activity, and factor VIII activity in the range of 20%–50%. The vWF multimers are normal. Bleeding time is variably prolonged.

   2. **Type II vWD** accounts for approximately 20%–30% of cases of vWD. It is characterized by a qualitative defect in vWF and is generally also inherited in an autosomal dominant fashion. There are four subtypes of type II vWD: IIA, IIB, IIM, and IIN.

      a. **Type IIA** is the most common qualitative variant of vWD. Large and intermediate-molecular-weight vWF multimers are uniformly absent from plasma. In general, ristocetin cofactor activity is more severely reduced than vWF antigen. Most patients with type IIA vWD have a point mutation

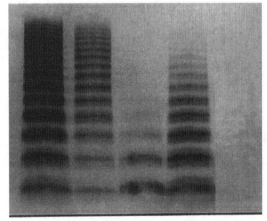

FIGURE 10–4. Von Willebrand factor multimer patterns in Von Willebrand disease. Samples of plasma from a normal individual (*NP*) and from patients with von Willebrand disease types I, IIA, IIB, and III were electrophoresed through a 1.3% agarose–sodium dodecyl sulfate gel, and the von Willebrand factor was detected by immunoblotting. (Reprinted with permission from Sadler JE. Von Willebrand disease. In: Bloom AL et al., eds. *Haemostasis and Thrombosis*. 3rd ed. Edinburgh: Churchill Livingstone, 1994:843–857.)

NP   I   IIA   IIB   III

in vWF within a 134 amino acid sequence from residue Gly742-Glu875 in the A domain. This mutation results in impaired assembly and secretion of normal vWF multimers, causing retention and loss of the large-molecular-weight multimers within the endoplasmic reticulum.

  b. **Type IIB** vWD accounts for fewer than 20% of all cases of type II vWD. The distinguishing characteristic is enhanced ristocetin-induced platelet aggregation despite low ristocetin cofactor activity. vWF antigen and factor VIII activity are low to normal. Plasma vWF multimer analysis shows loss of the highest-molecular-weight multimers only. Patients with type IIB vWD characteristically have mild to moderate thrombocytopenia. The defect has been shown to be due to point mutations in the A1 repeat, which contains the binding domain for platelet GPIb. These mutations result in gain of function for this region on the mutated vWF, resulting in increased and spontaneous binding of vWF to GPIb-IX-V complex. Plasma from patients with type IIB vWD typically shows heightened sensitivity to lower concentrations of ristocetin in the ristocetin-induced platelet aggregation assay. Type IIB must be distinguished from platelet-type vWD or pseudo-vWD. In the case of platelet-type vWD, mutations in the GPIb-IX-V receptor complex result in increased vWF platelet binding, which mimics type IIB vWD.

  c. **Type IIM** vWD is characterized by decreased ristocetin cofactor activity, not caused by loss of high-molecular-weight multimers. The type IIM variant contains large amounts of uncleaved pro-vWF in the multimer. Consequently, type IIM vWF has larger than normal plasma multimers.

  d. **Type IIN** vWD (originally called vWD Normandy) is inherited as an autosomal recessive disorder and mimics mild hemophilia A. This variant has normal vWF antigen, normal ristocetin cofactor activity, and decreased factor VIII activity. Patients with this disorder have mutations in the N terminal region of the vWF molecule within the factor VIII binding domain. Type IIN vWD is less common than classic mild hemophilia but should be considered when the family pedigree suggests autosomal recessive rather than sex-linked inheritance.

  3. **Type III** vWD is characterized by nearly complete deficiency in vWF function and antigen. Consequently, ristocetin cofactor activity and vWF antigen are undetectable and factor VIII activity is approximately 5%. In most cases, type III vWD is an autosomal recessive disorder. It is a severe bleeding disorder with spontaneous hemarthroses.

X. TREATMENT OF FACTOR DEFICIENCIES AND vWD

  A. **DDAVP** is a synthetic analogue of vasopressin. When administered intravenously or intranasally, DDAVP results in a progressive twofold to fourfold rise in vWF antigen, factor VIII coagulant activity, and ristocetin cofactor activity; this rise occurs within 30 minutes and lasts for 6–12 hours. Most patients with type I vWD or mild hemophilia A respond to this treatment.

  B. **Estrogens** are useful when trying to increase endothelial cell vWF synthesis. In the form of birth control pills, estrogens are useful in controlling the extent and duration of menstrual flow in female patients with vWD and a variety of coagulation factor deficiencies.

  C. **Fresh frozen plasma** contains all coagulation factors. However, because liters of plasma are required to replace severe deficiencies, fresh frozen plasma is not practical. Fresh frozen plasma may be used for the correction of rare deficiencies (e.g., factors II, V, X, VII, XI, XIII and fibrinogen) that may need replacement only to the 20%–25% level to improve bleeding symptoms.

D. **Cryoprecipitate** contains vWF, factor VIII, fibrinogen, and fibronectin. Cryoprecipitate is useful in treating hypofibrinogenemic states.

E. **Partially purified human plasma–derived factor concentrates** are available for the replacement of factors II, VII, IX, and X in a single concentrate formerly referred to as prothrombin complex concentrate. Prothrombin complex concentrate carries a risk of inducing disseminated intravascular coagulation. Highly purified and virally sterilized concentrates of factors IX and VIII are also available and carry little risk of inducing thrombosis at normal dosing levels. All plasma-derived concentrates have the potential to transmit viral disease. Some plasma-derived factor VIII concentrates originally immunopurified for replacement in patients with hemophilia A were found to contain significant amounts of vWF (e.g., Humate-P, Alphanate); they are the primary replacement treatment for vWD.

F. **Recombinant coagulation factor concentrates** are highly purified concentrates of commercially prepared recombinant coagulation factor proteins. Currently, recombinant concentrates are available for factors VII, VIIa, VIII, and IX.

G. **Antifibrinolytic agents** (e.g., aminocaproic acid, tranexamic acid) are drugs that bind to and inhibit the ability of plasmin to degrade fibrin clots. These drugs do not cause formation of fibrin clots but interfere with the remodeling and degradation of fibrin clots.

XI. SUMMARY

Excluding vWD, hemophilias A and B are the most common of the hereditary deficiencies and the most severe. The principles of diagnosis and treatment of hemophilia can be extrapolated to the rarer congenital coagulation factor deficiencies. All share the clinical characteristic of delayed bleeding in response to injury. Bleeding manifestations in vWD are most like those seen in platelet disorders because of the dual role played by vWF in the adhesion of platelets to the vascular subendothelium and in carrying factor VIII.

Treatment of bleeding in congenital factor deficiencies and vWD has evolved from the transfusion of fresh frozen plasma in the emergency room to patient self-administered therapies utilizing highly purified, virally sterilized plasma-derived or recombinant clotting factor concentrates. Successful gene therapy for many of these disorders, particularly hemophilia, is only a few years away.

SUGGESTED READING

Anonymous. Hemophilia management. United States Pharmacopeial Convention. *Transfusion Medicine Reviews*. 1998;12:128–40.

DiMichele D, Neufeld EJ. Hemophilia. A new approach to an old disease. *Hematol Oncol Clin North Am*, 1998;12: 1315–44.

Federici, AB. Diagnosis of von Willebrand disease. *Haemophilia*, 1998;4:654–60.

Loscalzo J, Schafer AI. *Thrombosis and Hemorrhage*. Baltimore: Williams & Wilkins:1998.

Sadler JE et al. Impact, diagnosis and treatment of von Willebrand disease. *Thromb Haemost*, 2000;84:160–74.

CHAPTER 11

Acquired Bleeding Disorders

- ALVIN H. SCHMAIER

I. INTRODUCTION

Acquired bleeding disorders are the most common ones that physicians encounter. An acquired bleeding disorder is often the result of medical treatment or a manifestation of an underlying disease state rather than specific abnormalities of the hemostatic system.

II. DIAGNOSIS

A. Acquired bleeding disorders can often be diagnosed by knowing the underlying disease. The knowledgeable physician recognizes the possible complications of an underlying disease and is vigilant in looking for a bleeding complication. For example, patients with severe gram-negative bacterial infections often get disseminated intravascular coagulation (DIC).

B. Alternatively, a bleeding disorder can prompt the physician to perform a differential diagnosis and ultimately identify an underlying disease. For example, a patient is recognized to have DIC. After a careful history and physical examination, the physician recognizes that the patient has a severe genitourinary tract infection.

C. The diagnosis of an acquired bleeding disorder can be made with the screening assays that are used to classify bleeding states. These assays are prothrombin time (PT) and activated partial thromboplastin time (aPTT). An acquired bleeding disorder usually causes prolongation of PT, aPTT, or both (Table 11–1).

III. ACQUIRED BLEEDING DISORDERS ASSOCIATED WITH PROLONGED PT AND aPTT

A. **Anticoagulation defects.** Defects in the coagulation and platelet systems for hemostasis occur in patients who are taking anticoagulant agents to treat venous thrombosis, myocardial infarction, stroke, and other conditions. For patients who take anticoagulants, management involves achieving a balance between preventing thrombosis by increasing the threshold for clot formation and preventing excessive bleeding.

1. **Medications that interfere with coagulation proteins** usually interfere with the PT and aPTT but do not prolong the bleeding time.

   a. **Heparin** is a carbohydrate polymer that forms complexes with antithrombin and other plasma protease inhibitors. These complexes inhibit the major enzymes of the hemostatic system: thrombin, factor Xa, and to a lesser

TABLE 11–1 • Laboratory Evaluation of Acquired Bleeding Disorders

Laboratory Results	Associated Disorders
Prolonged PT, aPTT	Anticoagulants
	DIC
	Liver Disease
	Vitamin K Deficiency
	Massive Transfusion
	Rare acquired inhibitors to coagulation proteins (e.g. paraproteinemias, dysfibrinogenemias, systemic amyloidosis, inhibitors to factor V, II, and X)
Prolonged aPTT with normal PT	Acquired inhibitors to factor VIII
	Acquired inhibitors to factor IX or XI
Prolonged PT with normal aPTT	Acquired inhibitor to factor VII
Abnormal bleeding time with normal PT and aPTT	Platelet defects due to drugs or toxins (e.g. renal failure)
Abnormal bleeding but normal bleeding time, PT, and aPTT	Inhibitors to factor XIII
	α_2-Antiplasmin deficiency

aPTT, activated partial thromboplastin time; DIC, disseminated intravascular coagulation; PT, prothrombin time.

extent, factors IXa, XIa, and XII and kallikrein. Because heparin inhibits activity at the level of factors Xa and IIa (thrombin), it prolongs both PT and aPTT. Usually aPTT is prolonged to a greater degree than PT.

b. **Warfarin (Coumadin)** is a vitamin K antagonist of two enzymes that are essential for carboxylation reactions of certain amino acids in coagulation factors VII, IX, X, and II and proteins C, S, and Z. Warfarin prolongs both PT and aPTT because it decreases the synthesis of factors II, VII, IX, and X and produces uncarboxylated (abnormal) forms of all the vitamin K–dependent factors. Usually, PT is more significantly prolonged than aPTT.

c. **Low-molecular-weight heparin** is a smaller, more highly purified carbohydrate polymer. It is directed primarily at factor Xa. Some preparations also inhibit the activity of thrombin. At most therapeutic doses, these preparations do not prolong the PT or aPTT. However, at higher doses, these preparations prolong both assays because they inhibit factor Xa activity.

d. **Danaparoid sodium (Orgaran)** is a mixture of dermatan sulfate, cholesterol sulfate, and heparin sulfate carbohydrates. It inhibits the activity of factor Xa. At large doses, it prolongs both PT and aPTT. At therapeutic concentrations, its effect on these assays is minor.

e. **Hirudin** and **Hirulog** bind to the active site and exosite I of thrombin (factor IIa). **Argatroban** inhibits the active site of thrombin. All agents prolong both PT and aPTT and interfere with all actions of thrombin.

2. **Medications that inhibit platelet function** prolong bleeding time but do not affect PT or aPTT.

a. **Abciximab (ReoPro), eptifibatide (Integrilin),** and **tirofiban (Aggrastat)** inhibit the activity of platelet glycoprotein IIb-IIIa ($\alpha_{IIb}\beta_3$ integrin). They prevent platelet aggregation (i.e., binding of fibrinogen to platelets). They do not interfere with plasma coagulation proteins.

b. **Aspirin** inhibits the activity of platelet cyclooxygenase I and II.

   c. **Thienopyridines (ticlopidine, clopidogrel)** inhibit the platelet adenosine
      diphosphate receptor ($P2Y_{12}$ purinergic receptor).
B. **DIC** is a clinicopathologic syndrome of activated coagulation. DIC causes bleeding or thrombosis because of a loss of balance between the clot-promoting and
   clot-lysing systems *in vivo*. The clinical spectrum ranges from a bleeding state to
   a prothrombic state. DIC is not a specific diagnosis; it always indicates underlying disease. The medical challenge is to recognize the underlying disease and in-
   stitute effective therapy. Bleeding associated with DIC is usually the result of excess fibrinolysis. Thrombosis associated with DIC is the result of excess thrombin
   formation. Biochemically, DIC is characterized by the simultaneous presence of
   thrombin and plasmin. Understanding the role of thrombin and plasmin in DIC
   explains many of the clinical and laboratory manifestations of the syndrome.
   1. **The role of thrombin.** Thrombin is a protein that acts by proteolysing other
      proteins. Thrombin interacts with other proteins, including its cell receptors,
      as an enzyme on a substrate.
      a. Thrombin cleaves fibrinogen and liberates fibrinopeptides A and B.
      b. Thrombin activates factors V, VII, XI, and XIII; protein C; and thrombin-
         activatable fibrinolysis inhibitor (TAFI) (carboxypeptidase U).
      c. Thrombin induces the aggregation and secretion of platelets. It contributes
         to their procoagulant activity.
      d. Thrombin induces chemotaxis of granulocytes and adhesion of endothe-
         lial cells and increases the permeability of endothelial cells.
      e. Thrombin stimulates platelet-activating factor, tissue plasminogen activa-
         tor, plasminogen activator inhibitor-1, the formation of nitric oxide, the
         formation of prostacyclin, the release of von Willebrand factor, and the lib-
         eration of P selectin from endothelial cells.
      f. Thrombin reduces the clearance of activated products of coagulation by
         the reticuloendothelial system.
   2. **The role of plasmin**
      a. Plasmin proteolyses factors V, VIII, and IX and HK.
      b. Plasmin cleaves platelet glycoprotein Ib-IX-V complex and liberates its ex-
         tracellular domain (glycocalicin). At low doses, plasmin activates platelets,
         but at high doses, it inhibits their activity.
      c. Plasmin forms degradation products with fibrinogen and fibrin.
      d. Plasmin liberates the D-dimer domain from insoluble cross-linked fibrin,
         which results from the formation of thrombin.
   3. **Etiology**
      a. **Acute DIC** is usually a hemorrhagic condition mostly resulting from hy-
         perfibrinolysis. It has several causes:
         (1) Infectious causes include gram-positive and gram-negative septicemia,
             typhoid fever, Rocky Mountain spotted fever, viremia, and parasites.
         (2) Obstetric causes include abruptio placentae, amniotic fluid embolism,
             hypertonic saline abortion, and eclampsia.
         (3) Malignant causes include acute promyelocytic leukemia and metasta-
             tic mucoid adenocarcinoma.
         (4) Injury-related causes include snakebite, necrotizing enterocolitis, fresh-
             water drowning, heat stroke, brain or crush injury, renal homograft re-
             jection, dissecting aortic aneurysm, and hemolytic transfusion reaction.
         (5) Other causes include homozygous protein C and S deficiency, factor V
             Leiden, severe liver disease, and heparin-induced thrombocytopenia
             and thrombosis syndrome.

       b. Subacute (or chronic) DIC is usually a prothrombic condition resulting from increased thrombin formation. It also has several causes:

         (1) A malignant cause is mucinous adenocarcinomas that may manifest as Trousseau syndrome (i.e., migratory thrombophlebitis, marantic endocarditis [fibrin on heart valves], and arterial embolization).

         (2) An obstetric cause is a retained dead fetus.

         (3) Vascular causes include connective tissue disorders, giant cavernous hemangioma, chronic renal disease, venous thrombosis, and pulmonary embolus.

  4. Laboratory evaluation

       a. Screening assays include PT, aPTT, platelet count, and fibrinogen level.

         (1) If the findings of two of these tests are abnormal, DIC is a possible diagnosis.

         (2) If the findings of three of these tests are abnormal, DIC is a probable diagnosis.

         (3) If the findings of all of these tests are abnormal, the diagnosis is considered to be DIC until another diagnosis is established.

       b. The **confirmatory tests** for DIC are the D-dimer, fibrin degradation products, and fibrin monomer assays.

         (1) The **D-dimer assay** measures plasmin-cleaved insoluble cross-linked fibrin. Insoluble cross-linked fibrin is formed when thrombin cleaves fibrinogen and leaves a soluble fibrin monomer. In the presence of thrombin-activated factor XIII, the fibrin monomer cross-links to form an insoluble, cross-linked fibrin monomer. Plasmin cleaves the insoluble cross-linked monomer to liberate the D-dimer. Therefore, the D-dimer assay indirectly detects thrombin and plasmin, which are biochemical markers of DIC.

         (2) The **fibrin degradation products assay** measures plasmin-cleaved soluble or insoluble fibrinogen or fibrin.

         (3) The **fibrin monomer assay** measures thrombin-cleaved fibrinogen only. It is the least reliable test for DIC and often produces false negative results.

  5. Treatment

       a. The underlying condition is treated first.

       b. Replacement therapy may include platelets or fresh frozen plasma for factor replacement.

       c. Heparin therapy may be useful for patients who have acral cyanosis and digital ischemia, purpura fulminans, a retained dead fetus, migratory thrombophlebitis, or acute leukemia.

C. Liver disease. The liver synthesizes all coagulation proteins and clears the activated products of coagulation.

  1. Plasma prekallikrein is the first protein that is decreased in liver disease.

  2. Factors VII and V are also decreased.

  3. Fibrinogen is one of the last hemostatic proteins to be altered in liver disease.

  4. The structural manifestations of liver disease also promote bleeding. These include portal hypertension, varices, gastritis, and hemorrhoids.

D. Vitamin K deficiency. Vitamin K plays an essential role as a cofactor for two enzymes that participate in an essential carboxylation reaction. This reaction occurs on certain amino acids on the carboxy terminal portion of factors II, VII, IX, and X and proteins C, S, and Z. This reaction is important because it allows these proteins to bind to cell membranes and participate in hemostatic reactions. Vitamin K is lipid soluble, and large amounts cannot be stored.

1. Vitamin K deficiency occurs in nutritionally depleted patients who abuse alcohol and in patients who receive long-term intravenous nutrition.
2. Warfarin also interferes with the use of vitamin K by inhibiting the two enzymes in the carboxylation sequence.
3. Antibiotics can interfere with intestinal bacteria synthesis and the absorption of vitamin K.

E. **Massive transfusion** is infusion of more than 1.5 times the patient's blood volume in 24 hours.
1. Acquired coagulopathy can occur as a result of dilution of plasma and platelets, increased concentration of the anticoagulant sodium citrate dextrose, and depletion of calcium.
2. Acquired coagulopathy is prevented by administering 1 unit of fresh frozen plasma for every 4–6 units of packed red blood cells. In addition, one ampule of calcium for every 4–6 units of transfused red blood cells or fresh frozen plasma is administered to overcome the anticoagulant effect of sodium citrate.

F. **Uncommon acquired coagulation protein defects**
1. Dysfibrinogenemias (abnormal fibrinogens) are relatively common. They are usually found in patients who have acquired liver disease as a result of alcoholism or immunologic, toxic, or viral causes. Because proteolysis of fibrinogen is the final step in the formation of clots, both PT and aPTT are prolonged in patients who have dysfibrinogenemia. This condition is usually diagnosed in patients who have a prolonged thrombin time.
2. Inhibitors to factors X, V, and II and fibrinogen influence hemostasis.
3. Hypergammaglobulinemic states include multiple myeloma (immunoglobulin G) and Waldenström macroglobulinemia (immunoglobulin M).
4. Systemic amyloidosis is usually associated with a decrease in plasma factor X or IX.
5. Heparinoids, or heparin-like anticoagulants, may be produced in patients who have an underlying malignancy.
6. Factitious bleeding disorders most often occur in an individual who is a health care professional and fakes medical illness by self-administering an anticoagulant, usually heparin or warfarin.

IV. ACQUIRED BLEEDING DISORDERS ASSOCIATED WITH PROLONGED PT OR aPTT

A. **Disorders associated with inhibitors to factor VIII** are seen in heavily transfused patients who have hemophilia A (factor VIII deficiency). Inhibitors to factor VIII also occur spontaneously in the elderly, in patients who have connective tissue disorders (e.g., systemic lupus erythematosus), in patients who have B-cell malignancies (e.g., lymphoma, myeloma), and in postpartum patients.

B. **Disorders associated with inhibitors to other coagulation proteins** occur in 5% of patients who have factor IX deficiency. Inhibitors to factor XI usually occur in heavily transfused patients who have factor XI deficiency. Inhibitors to the activity of factor VII has been reported in patients who have an underlying malignancy.

V. ACQUIRED BLEEDING DISORDERS NOT ASSOCIATED WITH PROLONGED PT AND aPTT

A. **Platelet defects** can be caused by medications (e.g., procainamide) that produce antibodies to platelet glycoproteins, such as glycoprotein Ib-IX-V complex. Platelet defects can also be caused by uremia (as a result of severe kidney failure) and the use of aspirin, nonsteroidal anti-inflammatory drugs, glycoprotein IIb/IIIa antagonists, and adenosine diphosphate receptor antagonists.

B. Acquired factor XIII deficiency is usually associated with the administration of isoniazid.

C. Acquired α_2-antiplasmin deficiency occurs in patients who have acute promyelocytic leukemia.

VI.   SUMMARY

Acquired bleeding disorders are the most common forms of bleeding that physicians encounter in their practice. When one sees a prolonged PT and aPTT, one should first think of common medical causes as outlined in detail in this chapter rather than rare hemostatic defects. This approach will serve the physician well to make the diagnosis expeditiously.

SUGGESTED READING

Colman RW, Robboy SJ, Minna JD. Disseminated intravascular coagulation (DIC): an approach. *Am J Med* 1972;52:679.

Green D. Factor VIII and other coagulation factor inhibitors. In: Loscalzo J, Schafer AI, eds. *Thrombosis and Hemorrhage*. Baltimore: Williams & Wilkins, 1998:803–815.

Grosset ABM, Rodgers GM. Acquired coagulation disorders. In: Lee Gret al., eds. *Wintrobe's Clinical Hematology*, 10th ed. Baltimore: Williams & Wilkins; 1999:1733–1780.

Schmaier AH. Disseminated intravascular coagulation. *eMedicine Journal*. http://www.emedicine.com. Accessed November 27, 2001.

Schmaier AH. Acquired disorders of blood coagulation. In: Humes HD, ed. *Kelley's Textbook of Internal Medicine*, 4th ed. Philadelphia: Lippincott Williams & Wilkins, 2000:1718–1723.

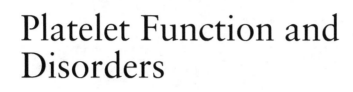

Platelet Function and Disorders

• PAULA BOCKENSTEDT AND ALVIN H. SCHMAIER

I. INTRODUCTION

Platelet disorders are best categorized by disorders of number of platelets or disorders of platelet function.

II. PLATELET BIOCHEMISTRY

A. **Platelet production and structure**
 1. Platelets are produced from megakaryocytes in the bone marrow by a process of pseudopod formation followed by septation. They have a life span of 8–10 days.
 2. Platelets are 2–3 microns in size. They do not have a nucleus but do contain mitochondria and messenger RNA.
 3. Although platelets have only two types of granules under the electron microscope, they have three kinds of functional granules: dense, alpha, and lysosomal granules (Fig. 12–1)
    a. **Dense granules** contain adenosine triphosphate (ATP), adenosine diphosphate (ADP), serotonin, and calcium.
    b. **α-Granules** contain two kinds of constituents: platelet-specific proteins and growth factors (e.g., platelet factor 4 [PF_4], β-thromboglobulin, platelet basic proteins, platelet-derived growth factor). α-Granules also contain a number of large-molecular-weight proteins that are adsorbed and packaged into the α-granule, synthesized in the α-granule, or both. These large-molecular-weight proteins include coagulation proteins (e.g., fibrinogen, factor V, von Willebrand factor [vWF], high-molecular-weight kininogen, thrombospondin) and plasma protease inhibitors (e.g., α_1-antitrypsin, C1 inhibitor, plasminogen activator inhibitor-1, α_2-antiplasmin, α_2-macroglobulin, amyloid β-protein precursor).
    c. **Lysosomal granules** contain acid hydrolases, glucuronidases, galactosidases, cathepsins, elastases, collagenases, and mannosidases.
 4. Platelets have a membrane compartment, the **open canalicular system (OCS)**. The OCS is an extensive system of internal membrane tunnels through which the contents of the platelet granules are extruded during platelet aggregation and secretion. Some platelet surface membrane proteins can move inward along the membranes of the OCS from the surface.

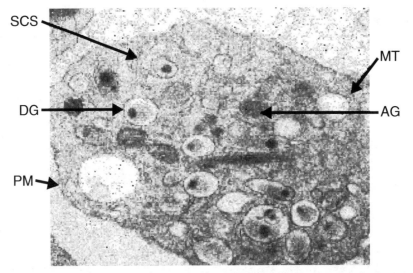

FIGURE 12–1. Electron micrograph of the ultrastructure of a platelet. In an unactivated platelet, a ring of micro-tubules (*MT*) circle the platelet. The plasma membrane (*PM*) invaginates at several points to form the surface-connected canalicular system (*SCS*). This system communicates with the dense tubular system, which is a residual of the endoplasmic reticulum. The secretory α-granules (*AG*) are recognizable because of their dense nucleoid. Dense granules (*DG*) have a central density. Mitochondria are also present in the cytoplasm. (Courtesy of Dr. Daniel Remick, Department of Pathology, University of Michigan.)

5. In patients with normal spleen size, 80% of platelets are circulating and 20% are in the spleen. In pathologic states (e.g., hypersplenism), the spleen may contain up to 90% of platelets.

B. **Role of platelets in hemostasis** (Fig. 12–2)

1. **Adhesion.** The initial event in hemostasis is the adhesion of platelets to vascular subendothelium at sites of injury; vWF provides the link between the platelet and the subendothelium. Adhesion and subsequent spreading of platelets is mediated by binding of vWF to the platelet glycoprotein (GP) Ib-IX-V complex (GPIb-IX-V). The vWF factor then binds to exposed subendothelial constituents. Collagen receptors on platelets provide additional links by binding directly to exposed collagen fibrils in the subendothelial matrix.

2. **Activation.** Once platelets adhere to the injured vessel wall, surface receptors mediate intracellular events, leading to internal phosphorylation of proteins and calcium mobilization. The platelet undergoes a shape change with protrusion of membrane-bound cytoplasmic extensions. As platelet protrusions form, the cytoskeleton is reorganized; the intracellular granules containing ADP, serotonin, and other mediators are compressed into the center of the activated platelet. These granules are released through the surface-connected canalicular system (SCS), thereby enhancing platelet plug formation by recruitment of additional platelets.

3. **Aggregation.** Platelet aggregation begins after activation-induced cytoskeletal reorganization is complete. Availability of ADP results in expression of the heterodimeric complex of platelet GPIIb-IIIa (integrin $\alpha_{IIb} \beta_3$). Subsequent binding of fibrinogen to integrin $\alpha_{IIb} \beta_3$) allows for platelet–platelet interconnection (i.e., formation of platelet aggregates).

4. **Coagulant activities of platelets.** The plasma membrane of activated platelets provides a phospholipid surface for assembly of the tenase (complex of VIIIa,

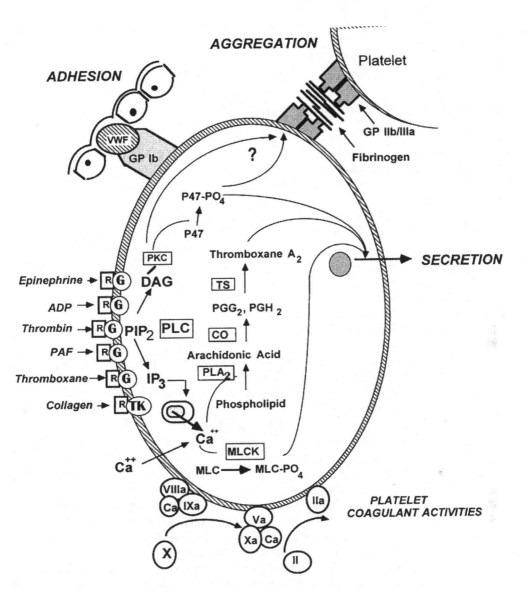

FIGURE 12–2. Mechanisms of platelet function. Adhesion to subendothelium is mediated by the glycoprotein Ib-IX-V complex (*GPIb*), which binds von Willebrand factor (*vWF*). Aggregation is mediated by the heterodimeric complex of GPIIb-IIIa (integrin $\alpha_{IIb}\beta_3$) binding fibrinogen. Various agonists, such as epinephrine, adenosine diphosphate (*ADP*), thrombin, platelet-activating factor (*PAF*), thromboxane, and collagen, bind and activate a specific receptor or receptors. Activation of these receptors activates phospholipase C (*PLC*), probably through G proteins. PLC catalyzes the cleavage of phosphatidyl 4,5-bisphosphate (*PIP$_2$*) to inositol 1,4,5-triphosphate (*IP$_3$*), which mobilizes calcium (*Ca^{++}*) from the dense tubular system to activate myosin light-chain kinase (*MLCK*). MLCK phosphorylates myosin light chain (*MLC*). Ca^{++} also activates phospholipase A$_2$ (*PLA$_2$*) to release arachidonic acid from phospholipids, which in turn is converted by cyclooxygenase (*COX*) to prostaglandin G$_2$ (PGG$_2$) and prostaglandin H$_2$ (PGH$_2$). Prostaglandin H$_2$ is then converted by thromboxane synthetase (*TS*) to thromboxane A$_2$. The other product of the cleavage of PIP$_2$ is diacylglycerol (*DAG*), which stimulates protein kinase C (*PKC*) to phosphorylate the intracellular protein P47 to P47-PO$_4$. Together, thromboxane A$_2$ and phosphorylated myosin light chain kinase (MLC-PO$_4$) stimulate secretion of products of the dense, alpha, and lysosomal granules (i.e., platelet activation). Platelet coagulant activity is generated by the assembly of factors IXa and VIIIa on the platelet membrane to allow for factor X activation (tenase) and the assembly of factors Xa and Va to allow for prothrombin (factor II) activation (prothrombinase). (Reprinted with permission from Colman RW et al. Overview of coagulation, fibrinolysis, and their regulation. In: Colman RW et al. *Hemostasis and Thrombosis.* Philadelphia: Lippincott Williams & Wilkins, 2001:6.)

IXa, and X) and prothrombinase (complex of Va, Xa, and prothrombin) complexes on the activated platelet surface. Binding of these complexes to the activated membrane surface of the platelet accelerates the biochemical reactions several thousand-fold and localizes the production of thrombin to the site of injury.

III.   TESTS OF PLATELET FUNCTION

A. The **peripheral blood smear** indicates the presence, size, and granularity of the platelets.

B. The **platelet count** is normally 150,000–400,000/μL.

C. **Bleeding time** is a diagnostic test for platelet dysfunction. A normal bleeding time is less than 9 minutes. The bleeding time will be prolonged as the platelet count decreases below 100,000/μL. It will also be prolonged in the presence of a normal platelet count when there is a qualitative platelet dysfunction.

D. **Platelet aggregation and secretion assays** are qualitative tests of platelet function.
   1. Platelet-rich plasma is stirred in cuvettes at 37°C with an agonist such as thrombin, ADP, epinephrine, collagen, or ristocetin.
      a. Correlations have been drawn between the responses to each of these agonists and specific abnormalities of platelet function.
      b. Platelet aggregation studies using these agonists identify defects in GPIIb-IIIa and GPIb-IX-V.
   2. The change in optical density of the platelet-rich plasma in response to an agonist is graphed over time (Fig. 12–3).
      a. The initial depression in the baseline tracing associated with decreased light transmission after addition of agonist is due to platelet shape change after stimulation. Platelet shape change indicates that an agonist binds to its platelet receptor.
      b. After shape change, there is a rapid rise in light transmission. When ADP or epinephrine is used as the agonist, this initial change in light transmission is called the primary wave of aggregation.
         (1) When ADP or epinephrine is used, there is a slight pause before platelets are fully aggregated during the second wave of aggregation.
         (2) When submaximal doses of an agonist are used, there may be only the primary wave followed by disaggregation.
   3. Aggregation studies also detect any stimulus–response coupling defect to weak agonists like ADP and epinephrine, which have aggregation-dependent secretion. With strong agonists, such as collagen and thrombin, that induce platelet secretion independent of aggregation, only one wave of aggregation is seen.
   4. Platelet secretion studies measure the amount of granule constituents (e.g., ATP, serotonin) released during aggregation with agonists such as thrombin, collagen, epinephrine and ADP.

IV.   CLINICAL FEATURES OF PLATELET DISORDERS

A. **Hemorrhage** occurs with falling platelet counts (i.e., <100,000/μL) (Table 12–1).

B. **Sites of bleeding:**
   1. **Cutaneous** (petechiae, purpura, ecchymosis, venipuncture sites)
   2. **Mucosal** (epistaxis, menometrorrhagia [heavy, irregular periods], hemorrhagic bullae in mouth [blood blisters], gastrointestinal bleeding)
   3. **Central nervous system**

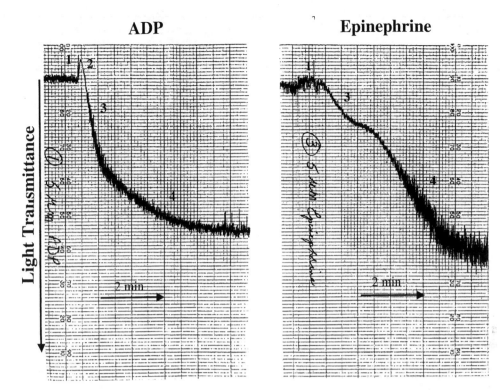

FIGURE 12–3. Changes in light transmission during normal platelet aggregation induced by adenosine diphosphate (ADP) and epinephrine. The spike to the right of 1 indicates instillation of the platelet agonist ADP or epinephrine. The decrease in light transmittance (2) to the left of the ADP-induced platelet aggregation curve indicates platelet shape change as a result of the ADP agonist binding to platelets. No shape change reaction occurs when epinephrine is the platelet agonist. The curves to the left of 3 indicate primary wave aggregation. The curves to the left of 4 indicate secondary wave aggregation, which arises as a result of release of platelet granule contents that potentiate the initial aggregatory response. When potent agonists such as collagen or thrombin are used, there is only one curve and no distinction between primary or secondary wave aggregation (data not shown).

V. QUANTITATIVE PLATELET DISORDERS

A. Thrombocytopenia

    1. **Thrombocytopenia caused by decreased production of platelets.** Failure of bone marrow megakaryocytes to replenish peripheral blood platelets adequately is due to a variety of primary hematopoietic disorders or diseases that secondarily impair hematopoiesis (Table 12–2).

      a. **Primary bone marrow disorders.** Primary bone marrow disorders that result in thrombocytopenia (Table 12–2) typically involve all cell lines and result in peripheral blood pancytopenia. Bone marrow megakaryocytes are decreased in number and abnormal in appearance.

TABLE 12–1 • Clinical Presentation Associated with Falling Platelet Counts

Platelet Count per Microliter	Clinical Manifestations
70,000–20,000	Increased bleeding with surgical procedures and trauma
< 20,000	Increased risk of spontaneous hemorrhage
< 10,000	Increased risk of spontaneous intracerebral hemorrhage

---

TABLE 12–2 • Thrombocytopenia Caused by Decreased Production

Primary bone marrow disorders
 Acquired aplastic anemia
 Fanconi anemia
 Leukemia
 Myelodysplasia
 Congenital intrauterine rubella infection
Bone marrow invasion
 Metastatic cancer
 Myelofibrosis
 Infectious diseases (e.g., tuberculosis)
Bone marrow injury
 Drugs (e.g., chemotherapeutic agents, chloramphenicol, thiazides, ethanol)
 Chemicals (e.g., benzene)
 Radiation
 Infection
Nutritional disorders
 Vitamin B_{12} deficiency
 Folate deficiency
 Copper deficiency
Hereditary thrombocytopenic syndromes
 Hypomegakaryocytic thrombocytopenia (e.g., thrombocytopenia–absent radius syndrome)
 Ineffective platelet production (e.g., May-Hegglin anomaly, Wiskott-Aldrich syndrome)

---

   b. **Bone marrow invasion.** Metastatic cancer, myelofibrosis, and infectious organisms destroy the local microenvironment important in sustaining normal bone marrow productivity. Typically, patients with these pathologic processes exhibit abnormalities in all three cell lines in the peripheral blood.
   c. **Bone marrow injury.** Rapidly dividing bone marrow progenitor cells are sensitive to the toxic and suppressive effects of drugs, chemicals, radiation, and infection (Table 12–2). Thrombocytopenia due to alcohol ingestion is common and reversible. Recovery of the platelet count begins 2–3 days after cessation of alcohol.
   d. **Nutritional disorders.** Megaloblastic anemia caused by vitamin B_{12} or folate deficiency results in defective DNA synthesis and megakaryocytes of low ploidy. These megakaryocytes produce reduced numbers of platelets, resulting in thrombocytopenia.
   e. **Hereditary thrombocytopenic syndromes.** These rare disorders are characterized by decreased numbers of bone marrow megakaryocytes or normal numbers of megakaryocytes that are ineffective in producing platelets.
     (1) **Hypomegakaryocytic thrombocytopenia** (Table 12–2) presents in early childhood and is associated with additional congenital abnormalities. Skeletal defects affecting nonterminal bones of the upper and lower extremities are common.
     (2) The second category is **ineffective platelet production** (Table 12–2). These disorders vary in clinical severity and may be associated with other congenital disorders, such as the immune deficiency seen in Wiskott-Aldrich syndrome.

2. **Thrombocytopenia caused by increased destruction: immune-mediated thrombocytopenia** (Table 12–3)

   a. **Autoimmune thrombocytopenia: immune thrombocytopenic purpura (ITP).** In the patient with autoimmune thrombocytopenia, autoantibodies (antibodies against self) are directed and bound to platelet antigens, such as platelet GPs and glycolipids. Antibody-bound platelets are removed by binding to the crystallizable fragment (Fc) receptors on monocytes and macrophages in the reticuloendothelial system of the liver and spleen. The mechanism of antibody clearance of immunoglobulin G (IgG) coated platelets is similar to that seen with antibody-coated red blood cells. Thrombocytopenia, which can occur in either of two forms, ensues.

      (1) **Acute ITP** is most often seen in **children.** It is often preceded by viral illness. The thrombocytopenia and clinical symptoms of bleeding may be severe, but the disorder is generally self-limited.

      (2) **Chronic ITP** is usually seen in **adults.** It often presents in women between 20 and 40 years of age. Spontaneous remissions are infrequent. Patients present with a variable degree of platelet-type bleeding symptoms and do not have splenomegaly.

      (3) The bone marrow is normal in both acute and chronic ITP. Therefore, it is a diagnosis of exclusion.

      (4) **Secondary ITP** may be seen in association with systemic lupus erythematosus, chronic lymphocytic leukemia, autoimmune thyroiditis, and lymphoma.

   b. **Alloimmune thrombocytopenia.** In alloimmune thrombocytopenia, the patient's serum contains antibodies to antigens not present on the patient's own platelets.

      (1) **Posttransfusion purpura** is a rare disorder that begins approximately 1 week after blood or platelet transfusion. The pathogenesis of the disorder is not completely known.

         (a) The patient's serum contains a high-titer specific alloantibody (i.e., antibody against an antigen not present on the patient's own platelets).

         (b) In most cases, the patient is $Pl^{>A1}$ negative and has been immunized previously by exposure to Pl^{A1}-positive platelets through pregnancy or transfusion.

         (c) The patient's own platelets are destroyed in an immune reaction that occurs when challenged by the presence of small numbers of Pl^{A1}-positive platelets from a Pl^{A1}-positive blood transfusion.

TABLE 12–3 • Immmune-Mediated Thrombocytopenia

Autoimmune thrombocytopenia
   Immune thrombocytopenic purpura (acute and chronic)
Alloimmune thrombocytopenia
   Posttransfusion purpura
   Neonatal isoimmune thrombocytopenia
Drug-induced immune thrombocytopenia
Heparin-induced thrombocytopenia

(2) **Neonatal isoimmune thrombocytopenia** is a life-threatening transient immune-mediated disorder that occurs in 1 in 200 newborns. It occurs by passive transfer of maternal IgG alloantibodies across the placenta, resulting in premature destruction of the infant's platelets. Typically, the mother is Pl^{A1} negative and has developed Pl^{A1} antibodies by exposure to blood transfusions from Pl^{A1}-positive donors or from prior pregnancy with a Pl^{A1}-positive baby. In neonatal isoimmune thrombocytopenia, the affected infant is Pl^{A1} positive.

c. **Drug-induced immune thrombocytopenia.** Many drugs may cause idiosyncratic immune-mediated platelet destruction (Table 12–4).

(1) In some cases, the antibody-binding fragment (Fab) portion of the autoantibody IgG molecule recognizes a neoepitope created by the binding of the offending drug to a platelet surface glycoprotein (GP). The antibody-coated platelet is cleared by the spleen.

(2) In other instances, the drug and antibody form an immune complex that binds to the platelet's Fc receptor.

(3) Thrombocytopenia will improve only if the offending drug is discontinued.

(4) **Heparin-induced thrombosis–thrombocytopenia syndrome.** Heparin can cause two clinically distinct syndromes.

(a) The first form of heparin-induced thrombocytopenia is associated with mild thrombocytopenia (rarely < 100,000/μL) and thought to be caused directly by heparin interaction with platelets. Generally, the thrombocytopenia is of no clinical consequence and resolves once the medication is discontinued.

(b) The second form of heparin-induced thrombocytopenia is associated with increasingly severe thrombocytopenia in the setting of thromboembolic phenomena. The thrombocytopenia is caused by an antibody that leads to platelet activation in the presence of heparin. The antibody is directed to a complex of heparin and PF$_4$. This antibody–heparin–PF$_4$ complex binds to platelet FcγRII receptor, causing platelet activation, degranulation, and platelet thrombi formation (Fig. 12–4).

TABLE 12–4 • Drugs Associated with Immune Thrombocytopenia

Methyldopa
Amrinone
Chlorothiazide
Phenytoin
Valproic acid
Sulfonamides
Penicillins and β-lactam antibiotics
Gold salts
Heparin
Furosemide
Cocaine
Procainamide
Quinidine
Quinine

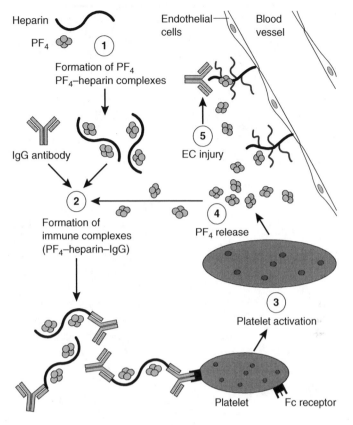

FIGURE 12–4. Mechanism of heparin-induced thrombocytopenia. The presence of (*1*) a complex between heparin and platelet factor 4 (*PF₄*) results in (*2*) the formation of immune complexes (PF₄-heparin-IgG). This antibody (*3*) by its Fc portion binds to the platelet FcγRII receptor, resulting in platelet activation that leads to thrombocytopenia. The activated platelets release more PF₄ that forms more immune complexes or binds to heparin-like molecules on the membrane of endothelial cells (*EC*), (*5*) allowing antibody to bind and induce endothelial cell injury. The platelet activation that arises through this mechanism results in a spectrum of disease from mild thrombocytopenia to an acute, prothrombotic state resulting in limb ischemia, myocardial infarction, and stroke. (Reprinted with permission from Aster RA. Heparin-induced thrombocytopenia and thrombosis. *N Engl J Med* 1995;332:1375.)

3. **Thrombocytopenia caused by increased destruction: non–immune-mediated thrombocytopenia** (Table 12–5)
   a. **Disseminated intravascular coagulation (DIC)** is associated with an increased turnover and consumption of platelets that may exceed the capacity for bone marrow megakaryocytes to produce platelets. In DIC, an excess of thrombin is generated throughout the vasculature, resulting in increased consumption of clotting factors, formation of fibrin, and platelet activation. The degree of thrombocytopenia in DIC varies.
   b. **Thrombotic thrombocytopenic purpura (TTP) and hemolytic uremic syndrome (HUS)** are characterized by a pentad of fever, mental status changes, renal insufficiency, microangiopathic hemolytic anemia, and thrombocytopenia.
      (1) TTP is more common in adults. In TTP, endothelial damage or perturbation by a variety of mechanisms (e.g., infection, immune complexes, cytotoxic antibodies, HIV, pregnancy, cancer) leads to abnormal release of unusually large vWF molecules from storage sites. These multimers presumably participate in increased adhesion and aggregation of platelets in susceptible individuals who are missing a vWF processing enzyme (a metalloprotease called ADAMTS13, a disintegrin and metalloprotease with a thrombospondin-1-like domain [TSP]) because of a deficiency or an antibody that interferes with its action. There is little generation of fibrin clot or consumption of coagulation factors. Multiorgan failure occurs from diffuse platelet plugs of small

TABLE 12–5 • Differential Diagnosis of Acquired Destructive Thrombocytopenias

	PT	aPTT	Platelet Count	Schistocytes
DIC	Increased	Increased	Decreased	Sometimes present
ITP	Normal	Normal	Decreased	None
TTP	Normal	Normal	Decreased	Present
HUS	Normal	Normal	Decreased	Present

aPTT, activated partial thromboplastin time; DIC, disseminated intravascular coagulation; HUS, hemolytic uremic syndrome; ITP, immune thrombocytopenic purpura; PT, prothrombin time; TTP, thrombotic thrombocytopenic purpura.

arterioles. Hence, the prothrombin time, activated partial thromboplastin time, and fibrinogen levels are normal. Only the platelet count and hemoglobin are decreased (Table 12–5).

    (2) HUS is seen more frequently in children than in adults. It usually presents with frank renal failure, unlike TTP. The pathophysiology of HUS is thought to be similar to the pathophysiology of TTP [see V.A.3.b.(1)].

  4. Thrombocytopenia caused by sequestration

    a. Splenic enlargement results in increased pooling of blood within a pathologically enlarged spleen (**hypersplenism**).

    b. Platelet survival within the spleen is shortened by the longer exposure time to splenic phagocytic cells.

    c. Hypersplenism may be secondary to:

      (1) Congestive splenomegaly caused by portal hypertension from cirrhosis of the liver or congestive heart failure

      (2) Infectious disorders, particularly infectious mononucleosis

      (3) Myeloproliferative and lymphoproliferative disorders

      (4) Other hematologic neoplasms and storage disorders, such as agnogenic myeloid metaplasia

B. Thrombocytosis (Table 12–6)

  1. Primary (autonomous) thrombocytosis. Production of platelets and growth of hematopoietic progenitor cells in primary thrombocytosis is independent of growth factors. The platelets may not function normally, and a variety of morphologic, metabolic, and membrane abnormalities are found. The patient may have bleeding with normal platelet counts or more frequently, arterial and venous occlusions.

TABLE 12–6 • Causes of Thrombocytosis

Primary or autonomous production
  Essential thrombocytosis
  Polycythemia vera
  Chronic myelogenous leukemia
  Myelodysplastic syndrome
Secondary or reactive thrombocytosis
  Iron deficiency
  Malignancy
  Postsplenectomy
  Inflammatory disorders

2. **Secondary (reactive) thrombocytosis.** Secondary thrombocytosis accounts for 80% of platelet counts greater than 700,000/μL. Patients with reactive thrombocytosis rarely have symptoms of thrombosis. The most common cause of reactive thrombocytosis is iron deficiency.

VI. QUALITATIVE PLATELET DISORDERS

A. **General features**
  1. Qualitative platelet disorders are characterized by abnormalities in platelet function. The platelet count is usually normal, but the bleeding time is prolonged.
  2. Clinical features vary. However, most patients have mucocutaneous bleeding.
  3. Qualitative platelet disorders may be congenital or acquired. Acquired platelet function defects are more common.
B. **Congenital platelet disorders** (Table 12–7)
  1. **Disorders of adhesion**
      a. **Von Willebrand disease (vWD)** (see Chapter 10, IX) is an autosomal dominant disorder of a plasma protein important in the adhesion of platelets to injured vascular subendothelium. In vWD, vWF binding to GPIb-IX-V is reduced. Pseudo-vWD is a disorder that mimics type IIB vWD, a subtype in which the defective vWF multimers bind spontaneously to GPIb-V-IX. In pseudo-vWD, the platelet GPIb-IX-V complex receptor has increased affinity for vWF, which consequently binds spontaneously to the receptor and causes platelet agglutination independent of ristocetin.
      b. **Bernard-Soulier syndrome** is a rare autosomal recessive disorder. In the homozygous state, the bleeding time is prolonged and thrombocytopenia with giant platelets is found on the peripheral blood smear. The heterozygous state is clinically silent except for the finding of occasional large platelets on the peripheral blood smear. Platelet aggregation tests show loss of response to ristocetin. Thrombin aggregation is also somewhat reduced, but aggregation to ADP, epinephrine, and collagen is normal. Bernard-Soulier platelets show impaired adhesion. The molecular defect is a decrease in the presence or expression of the platelet GPIb-IX-V receptor.

TABLE 12–7 • Congenital Platelet Disorders

Disorders of adhesion
  Von Willebrand disease
  Pseudo–von Willebrand disease
  Bernard-Soulier syndrome
Disorders of aggregation
  Afibrinogenemia
  Glanzmann thrombasthenia
Disorders of activation (secretion)
  Storage pool deficiency
  Heterogenous deficiency or defects in platelet
    stimulus–response coupling pathways
Disorders of platelet procoagulant activities
  Scott syndrome
  Platelet factor V Quebec

---

  2. **Disorders of aggregation**
     a. **Afibrinogenemia** is a rare disorder. Patients with afibrinogenemia have platelet-type, mucosal, and cutaneous bleeding and deep muscle hematomas. Fibrinogen levels in the plasma and platelets are extremely low. Consequently, fibrinogen is not available for binding to platelets during aggregation. Abnormalities of platelet aggregation mirror those of Glanzmann thrombasthenia (see VI B 2 b), although they are far less severe in afibrinogenemia.
     b. **Glanzmann thrombasthenia** is a rare autosomal recessive entity that causes serious platelet-type bleeding problems. Platelets adhere but have absent or defective GPIIb-IIIa. Platelets do not aggregate to ADP, epinephrine, collagen, or thrombin; neither primary nor secondary wave aggregation is observed. The GPIb-IX-V receptor is intact, so platelets respond to ristocetin. Glanzmann thrombasthenia is a lifelong bleeding disorder characterized by petechiae and easy bruising.
  3. **Disorders of activation (secretion)**
     a. **Overview.** Platelet adhesion and the initial events of aggregation are followed by platelet secretion. There are two main categories of platelet secretion defects.
        (1) In the first category of defects, platelets are unable to undergo the release reaction because they lack the normal storage granules.
        (2) In the second category of defects, the granules are present but cannot be mobilized to release because of abnormalities in a metabolic pathway, such as impaired thromboxane A_2 synthesis, as seen in aspirin-induced platelet aggregation defects.
     b. **Storage pool deficiency (SPD)** is a heterogenous group of disorders of secretion in which there is a deficiency of either dense granules (δ-SPD) or α-granules (α-SPD). A deficiency of α-granules is also known as gray platelet syndrome and is characterized by platelets and megakaryocytes that are deficient in α-granule proteins (e.g., PF_4, β-thromboglobulin, platelet-derived growth factor, vWF, thrombospondin). SPD can be congenital; however, it may be acquired in chronic platelet activation states (e.g., immune thrombocytopenia). SPD can also be acquired when platelets pass across abnormal vascular surfaces (e.g., cardiopulmonary bypass apparatus), leading to partial degranulated and spent platelets.
     c. **Defects in platelet stimulus–response coupling pathways** (primary secretion defects) concern the signal transduction pathways into which the surface receptors are locked and are the most common platelet function defects. Platelets may have defects in cyclooxygenase, defects in G-coupled proteins (e.g., $G\alpha_q$ deficiency), or an abnormality in the translocation of or response to intracellular calcium. The platelets have normal granules but generate abnormal amounts of thromboxane A_2.
  4. **Disorders of platelet procoagulant activities**
     a. **Scott syndrome** is a rare defect in expression of acidic phospholipids on the platelet-activated surface. It is characterized by decreased factor Xa binding, hence decreased prothrombin activation.
     b. **Platelet factor V Quebec** is a platelet multimerin defect associated with a defect in platelet α-granule proteins and procoagulant activity.
C. **Acquired platelet disorders** (Table 12–8)
  1. **Uremia** (renal failure) produces highly variable and unpredictable results of platelet aggregation tests. The bleeding time is prolonged, and patients are

---

TABLE 12–8 • Acquired Platelet Disorders

Uremia
Myeloproliferative disorders
Myelodysplastic disorders
Acute leukemia
Dysproteinemias (e.g., myeloma, macroglobulinemia)
Cardiopulmonary bypass
Antiplatelet antibodies
Liver disease
Drugs (e.g., penicillins, cephalosporins, ibuprofen, aspirin,
    GPIIb-IIIa antagonists, dextran, heparin, thienopyridines)

---

quite sensitive to the effects of aspirin. Abnormalities in vascular and platelet prostaglandin metabolism may account for some of the bleeding problems. Other possible causes include abnormalities in vWF induced by uremia and decreased red blood cell–promoted platelet–vessel wall collisions due to anemia. Uremic bleeding can be partially corrected by dialysis and the administration of cryoprecipitate, estrogens, or 1-deamino-8-D-arginine vasopressin (DDAVP).

2. **Myeloproliferative disorders,** such as polycythemia vera, myelofibrosis, and essential thrombocytosis, cause variable degrees of thrombotic and/or hemorrhagic symptoms. Stroke, Budd-Chiari syndrome, and portal vein thrombosis are characteristic of myeloproliferative disorders. Multiple defects in aggregation have been described, but the most characteristic is loss of the first and second wave of aggregation with epinephrine.

3. **Myelodysplastic disorders and acute leukemias** are clonal disorders in which all cell lines are abnormal morphologically and metabolically. A variety of abnormalities in platelet function can be found.

4. **Dysproteinemias** are characterized by increased amounts of plasma immunoglobulin that increase plasma viscosity and interfere with fibrin polymerization. Paraproteins may nonspecifically coat platelets and interfere with the binding of agonists to their receptors, impairing platelet adhesion and aggregation.

5. **Cardiopulmonary bypass** is associated with platelet dysfunction. Platelets adhere to artificial surfaces during bypass and partially activate, releasing granule constituents. When recirculated, these platelets may have receptors occupied by fibrin or other molecules and may be less responsive to endogenous hemostatic stimuli when needed. In addition, platelet counts after the bypass are typically lower than before the bypass because of hemodilution from transfusion and loss of fully aggregated or adherent platelets on bypass tubing.

6. **Antiplatelet antibodies** may cause platelet dysfunction by binding to receptors and inducing partial platelet activation. Antiplatelet antibodies may also stereochemically interfere with the binding of vWF or fibrinogen to platelet receptors.

7. **Liver disease** produces variable platelet aggregation results. The increased levels of fibrin degradation products seen in cirrhosis because the liver cannot clear these products may result in interference in binding of fibrinogen to its platelet receptor. Liver disease is also frequently associated with hypersplenism and thrombocytopenia.

8. **Various drugs** can affect platelet function in a variety of ways (Table 12–8).

VII.   PLATELET RECEPTORS IN CLINICAL PRACTICE

A. **Overview.** Platelet receptor inhibitors are widely used in the treatment of unstable angina and acute myocardial infarction and during angioplasty procedures. Platelet activation occurs through multiple pathways in the platelet (e.g., thrombin, collagen receptors, ADP, etc.) (Fig. 12–5). Regardless of the pathway, the platelet–platelet interaction and thrombus formation are regulated ultimately through the GPIIb-IIIa receptor complex (integrin $\alpha_{IIb \beta3}$) (Fig. 12–5). Agonists of platelet activation facilitate the conformational change necessary for the GPIIb-

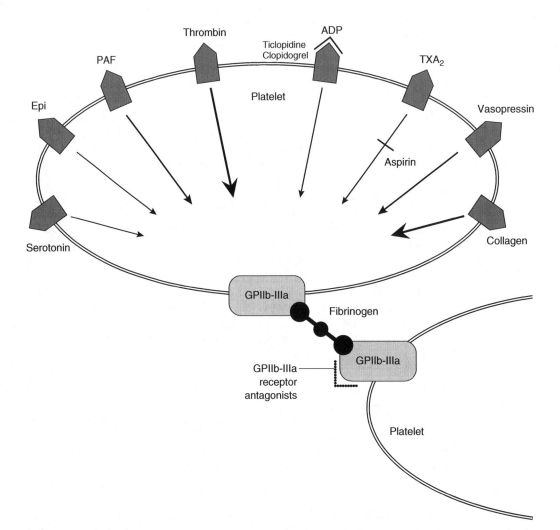

FIGURE 12–5. Platelet receptor inhibitors in clinical practice. Various platelet receptors have become targets for the development of antiplatelet agents approved for use in arterial thrombotic states (e.g., acute coronary syndromes, strokes). Present-day agents that target the platelet glycoprotein IIb–IIIa (*GPIIb–IIIa*) receptor (integrin $\alpha_{IIb} \beta_3$) include abciximab (a chimeric human–mouse monoclonal antibody), eptifibatide (a cyclic peptide), and tirofiban (a nonpeptide mimetic). The adenosine diphosphate (*ADP*) receptor involved in platelet aggregation (P2Y$_{12}$) is targeted by two competitive antagonists: ticlopidine and clopidogrel. Aspirin inhibits cyclooxygenase I and II, which target the thromboxane A$_2$ receptor TXA$_2$ downstream. *Epi*, epinephrine; *PAF*, platelet-activating factor; *TXA$_2$*, thromboxane A$_2$. This figure is adapted from Vorchheimer DA, Badimon JJ, Fuster V. Platelet glycoprotein IIb/IIIa receptor antagonists in cardiovascular disease. *JAMA* 1999;281:1408.

IIIa receptor to become receptive to fibrinogen, vWF, thrombospondin, or vitronectin binding. All of these receptor ligands contain the identical peptide sequence—arginine, glycine, aspartic acid.

B. **Cyclooxygenase inhibitors**
   1. **Aspirin** inhibits aggregation by irreversibly binding to platelet cyclooxygenase I, inhibiting the thromboxane A_2 pathway of platelet aggregation and release. It is recommended for treatment of unstable angina, acute myocardial infarction, and pretransluminal and posttransluminal angioplasty.
   2. **Sulfinpyrazone** is a uricosuric agent related to phenylbutazone. It has an incomplete and reversible inhibition of cyclooxygenase activity at highest dose.
   3. **Nonsteroidal anti-inflammatory drugs** also have a reversible inhibition of cyclooxygenase.

C. **Adenosine diphosphate receptor inhibitors**
   1. **Ticlopidine hydrochloride** (Ticlid) and **clopidogrel bisulfate** (Plavix) are thienopyridine derivatives with potent antiplatelet activity. They selectively inhibit the binding of ADP to its receptor and therefore block ADP-dependent aggregation.
   2. There are three ADP receptors on platelets.
      a. The ADP receptor involved in platelet–platelet aggregation is a $P2Y_{12}$ purinergic receptor.
      b. The two other ADP receptors on platelets are the $P2Y_1$ purinergic receptor that is involved in platelet shape change and the $P2X_1$ receptor that is an ion gate channel for calcium.

D. **GPIIb-IIIa receptor antagonists**
   1. Because platelet aggregation depends on the binding of fibrinogen to GPIIb-IIIa (integrin $\alpha_{IIb} \beta_3$), blocking this interaction is critical in preventing activated platelets from aggregating.
   2. A variety of drugs competitively inhibit the binding of fibrinogen to GPIIb-IIIa in clinical practice.
      a. **Abciximab** is a chimeric human–mouse monoclonal antibody to the GPIIb-IIIa receptor that interferes with fibrinogen binding.
      b. **Eptifibatide** is a cyclic peptide inhibitor of GPIIb-IIIa.
      c. **Tirofiban** are nonpeptide receptor antagonists of GPIIb-IIIa.

VIII. SUMMARY

Platelet disorders encompass a variety of hereditary and acquired diseases that can be divided into disorders of number and function. Some overlap exists between these two major categories. Understanding the basic roles of the platelet, bone marrow, spleen, and immune system in normal conditions and in specific diseases will aid the clinician in determining the cause of an abnormal platelet count. A fundamental knowledge of the mechanisms involved in platelet adhesion and aggregation allows for better understanding of platelet functional disorders and the role of platelets in diseases such as atherosclerosis and thrombosis.

SUGGESTED READING

Buchanan GR. Quantitative and qualitative platelet disorders. *Clin Lab Med* 1999;19:71–86.

Cines DB, Blanchette VS. Immune thrombocytopenia purpura. *N Engl J Med* 2002;346:995–1008.

Drews RE, Weinberger SE. Thrombocytopenic disorders in critically ill patients. *Am J Respir Crit Care Med* 2000;162:347–351.

Fausett B, Silver RM. Congenital disorders of platelet function. *Clin Obstet Gynecol* 1999;42:390–405.

George JN. Platelets. *Lancet* 2000;355:1531–1539.

Horrell CJ, Rothman J. Establishing the etiology of thrombocytopenia. *Nurse Pract* 2000;25:68, 71–72, 74–77.

Lankford KV, Hillyer CD. Thrombotic thrombocytopenic purpura: new insights in disease pathogenesis and therapy. *Transfus Med Revs* 2000;12:244–257.

Loscalzo J, Schafer AI. *Thrombosis and Hemorrhage.* Baltimore: Williams & Wilkins, 1998.

Mhawech P, Saleem A. Inherited giant platelet disorders. *Am J Clin Pathol* 2000;113:176–190.

Peck-Radosavljevic M. Hypersplenism. *Eur J Gastroenterol Hepatol* 2001;13:317–323.

Rao AK, Gabbeta J. Congenital disorders of platelet signal transduction. *Arterioscler Thromb Vasc Biol* 2000;20:285–289.

Rodgers GM. Overview of platelet physiology and laboratory evaluation of platelet function. *Clin Obstet Gynecol* 1999;42:349–359.

Shapiro AD. Platelet function disorders. *Haemophilia* 2000;6(Suppl 1):120–7.

Tullu MS, Dixit PS, Nair SB, et al. Glanzmann's thrombasthenia. *Indian J Pediatr* 2001;68:563–566.

CHAPTER 13

Evaluation of Thrombosis

- ALVIN H. SCHMAIER

I. INTRODUCTION

Thrombosis is the most common cause of death in the world. In the United States, acute coronary syndromes and stroke, both arterial thrombotic conditions, are the number one and three killers, respectively. In the world, acute coronary syndromes and stroke are the number one and two killers, respectively.

II. OVERVIEW

A. **Key concepts**
1. Thrombosis (arterial and venous) is produced by a shift in the balance between procoagulant and profibrinolytic systems (i.e., between thrombin-generating mechanisms and clot-lysing or plasmin-generating mechanisms).
2. The genesis of thrombosis can be defects in vascular structure, tissue, cells, or plasma proteins.
3. Molecular causes of thrombosis are recognized in 20%–40% of patients, depending on the population.
4. Therapy for thrombosis focuses on prevention of future clots and lysis of existing clots.

B. **Pathogenic features.** Most individuals who present with thrombosis have one or more of the following features at the time of presentation:
1. Vessel damage
2. Stasis of blood
3. Platelet, leukocyte, and endothelial cell dysfunction
4. Excessive activation of coagulation and/or reduced activation of fibrinolytic proteins

C. **Red (fibrin) versus white (platelet) clots.** The structure of a thrombus varies with the vessel in which it is located.
1. In a high-flow arterial vessel, platelet thrombi are seen. These macroscopic aggregates of platelets have a white appearance.
2. In low-flow vessels (e.g., veins), the initial platelet plug, which may have started the thrombus, is often not detected. These clots result from the accumulation of red blood cells in fibrin strands and are called red thrombi.

D. **Response after acute vessel injury.** Four phases can be used to characterize repair of a vessel injury.
1. **Initial phase:** platelet thrombus formation
2. **Acute phase:** active fibrin clot formation, initiation of the inflammatory response

3. **Intermediate phase:** thrombus limitation, inflammatory response
4. **Chronic phase:** readsorption and recanalization of the clot

III.   ARTERIAL THROMBOSIS

A. **Overview.** Arterial thrombosis can range from large vessel occlusions that result in myocardial infarction, stroke, peripheral arterial vessel occlusion, and ischemic bowel syndrome to small vessels that result in digital ischemia or vasculitis.

B. **Etiology**
   1. Arterial thrombosis is most often associated with ongoing vascular disease as seen with diabetes mellitus, hyperlipidemias, and hypercholesterolemia or with vasculitis due to connective tissue disorders or antiphospholipid antibody syndrome.
   2. Hematologic conditions associated with arterial thrombosis include heparin-induced thrombocytopenia and thrombosis syndrome (HITTS), thrombotic thrombocytopenic purpura (TTP), hemolytic uremic syndrome (HUS), purpura fulminans due to homozygous protein C or S deficiency, and myeloproliferative disorders.

C. **Risk factors.** Elevation of certain proteins or amino acids is associated with arterial thrombosis. These proteins include factor VII, fibrinogen, lipoprotein(a), and homocysteine.
   1. **Lipoprotein(a), or Lp(a),** consists of low-density lipoprotein (LDL) and apolipoprotein(a). Apolipoprotein(a) has 98% sequence homology to one region on plasminogen (kringle IV). Lp(a) is atherogenic, targeting LDL away from its clearance receptor. Lp(a) is also prothrombotic. It prevents plasminogen from binding to cells or fibrin, which inhibits plasminogen activation from initiating fibrinolysis. Thus, increased levels of Lp(a) increase the risk of thrombosis by reducing fibrinolysis and increasing atherogenesis.
   2. **Elevation of plasma homocysteine is a risk factor for both arterial and venous thrombosis** (Figure 13–1).
      a. Elevation of homocysteine arises from defects in two enzymes: N^5, N^{10}-methylenetetrahydrofolate reductase or cystathionine β-synthase. Homocysteine levels also rise in vitamin B_6, vitamin B_{12}, and folate deficiency. N^5,N^{10}-methylenetetrahydrofolate reductase is present in vessel walls. Mutations in this enzyme are common (C677T) and may exist in 35% of the population in the United States. However, these mutations do not correlate with vascular disease or thrombosis.
      b. Elevation of plasma homocysteine results in endothelial cell dysfunction. The normal anticoagulant surface of endothelial cells is converted to a prothrombotic surface, which is manifested by increased factor V expression, reduced protein C activation as a result of reduced thrombomodulin (a receptor protein for protein C on endothelium) expression, reduced tissue plasminogen activator (t-PA) activation of plasminogen, and enhanced Lp(a) binding to fibrin.

D. **Treatment of arterial thrombosis**
   1. Arterial thrombosis associated with elevated homocysteine ($\geq 11\,\mu M$) should be treated with folate.
   2. Arterial thrombosis associated with acute coronary syndrome, stroke, or stent placement is treated with a combination of antiplatelet and antifibrin-generating anticoagulants.
      a. **Antiplatelet agents**

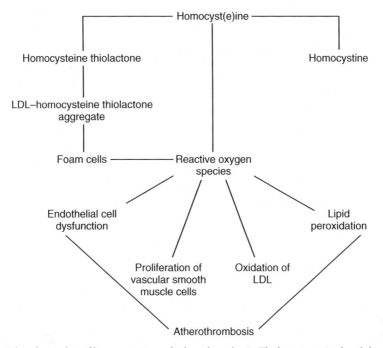

FIGURE 13–1. The relationship of homocysteine and atherothrombosis. The homocysteine breakdown product, homocysteine thiolactone, results in oxidative modification of low-density lipoprotein (*LDL*). LDL promotes the formation of foam cells, which in turn yield a reactive oxygen species. Homocysteine itself can be a direct source of a reactive oxygen species. These reactive oxygen species result in endothelial cell dysfunction, proliferation of subendothelial vascular smooth muscle cells, lipid peroxidation, and oxidation of LDL, which together contribute to atherothrombosis. (Adapted with permission from Welch GN, Loscalzo J. Homocysteine and atherothrombosis. *N Engl J Med* 1998;338:1042–1050.)

       (1) Aspirin (platelet cyclooxygenase inhibitor)
       (2) Thienopyridines (ticlopidine, clopidogrel): inhibitors of $P2Y_{12}$ adenosine diphosphate receptor
       (3) Glycoprotein IIb/IIIa ($\alpha_{IIb}\beta_3$ Integrin) antagonists, including:
          (a) Abciximab, a chimeric mouse-human monoclonal antibody
          (b) Tirofiban, a nonpeptide mimetic
          (c) Eptifibatide, a cyclic peptide inhibitor
    b. Antifibrin-generating agents
       (1) Standard heparin
       (2) Low-molecular-weight heparins
       (3) Hirulog

IV. VENOUS THROMBOSIS

    A. Overview. Venous thrombosis occurs in low-flow situations. After vessel injury, venous thrombi propagate proximally to occlude a vessel. One experimental model to create a venous thrombosis required the following: vessel injury, reduced blood flow, inhibition of an anticoagulant system, and induction of an inflammatory response. Although venous thrombi are gelatinous, venous thrombosis has an inflammatory component.
    B. Causes of venous thrombosis
       1. Protein defects (Figure 13–2)
          a. Factor V Leiden (20%–40%). Factor V Leiden is a G to A mutation at base

COAGULATION   **FIBRINOLYSIS**

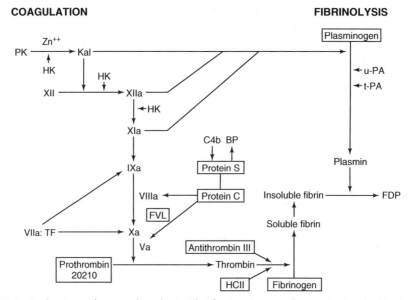

FIGURE 13–2. Biochemistry of venous thrombosis. This figure juxtaposes the proteins involved in the coagulation and fibrinolytic systems. The proteins that are inscribed in *boxes* represent recognized defects associated with thrombosis. Coagulation factors XII, XI, IX, X, VII, and V are represented by their Roman numeral alone. An *a* after the Roman numeral indicates an activated protein. *C4b BP*, C4b binding product; *FDP*, fibrin degradation product; *FVL*, factor V Leiden; *HCII*, heparin cofactor II; *HK*, high-molecular-weight kininogen; *Kal*, plasma kallikrein; *PK*, prekallikrein; *TF*, tissue factor; *t-PA*, tissue plasminogen activator; *u-PA*, urokinase plasminogen activator.

pair 1691 of coagulation factor V that results in a Q^{506} amino acid instead of an R^{506} amino acid. Because it cleaves after arginine^{506}, factor V Leiden is resistant to inactivation by activated protein C (APC), resulting in increased factor Va and thus increased thrombin formation. This polymorphism in factor V is a common defect in the Near East and Europe. By itself, it is a relatively low risk factor for thrombosis; however, when combined with other risk factors (e.g., pregnancy, smoking, other protein defects) the potential for thrombosis increases.

   b. **Homocysteine (10%)** (see section III.C.2.)
   c. **Prothrombin 20210 (6%).** Prothrombin 20210 is a single base pair mutation at position 20210 (G to A) in the distal 3' area of the untranslated region of the prothrombin gene (factor II). This polymorphism results in an elevation of normal prothrombin. It is the third most common defect associated with thrombosis. By itself, it is a relatively low risk for thrombosis. It may have a predilection for coexpression with factor V Leiden.
   d. **Protein C (4%).** Protein C is the zymogen of the major anticoagulant system in the body. APC is a vitamin K–dependent enzyme whose function is to inactivate factors Va and VIIIa and stimulate fibrinolysis (see Fig. 8–6). In the absence of APC inactivation of factors Va and VIIIa, thrombin formation is increased. Deficiencies or defects in protein C are a serious risk factor for thrombosis. A number of clinical syndromes are associated with protein C deficiency, including:
   (1) Venous thrombosis (heterozygous defect)
   (2) Coumadin skin necrosis (heterozygous defect)

          (3) Neonatal purpura fulminans (homozygous defect)

     e. **Protein S (3%–4%).** Protein S is a vitamin K–dependent protein that is not an enzyme. Free protein S serves as a cofactor (i.e., binding site) for APC to localize to cell surfaces. It is regulated by a complement protein, C4b binding protein. Thus, in inflammatory states, free protein S can be reduced as a result of binding to C4b binding protein. Pregnancy and estrogens reduce protein S. A deficiency or defect in protein S is a serious risk factor for thrombosis.

     f. **Dysfibrinogenemia (3%).** Some dysfibrinogenemias are abnormal fibrinogen molecules that have a propensity for accelerated clotting.

     g. **Antithrombin (1%).** Antithrombin is a serpin (serine protease inhibitor) that inhibits each of the coagulation system enzymes. Antithrombin allows heparin to function as an anticoagulant. It was the first protein defect recognized to be associated with venous thrombosis. All patients are heterozygous for the deficiency; homozygous antithrombin deficiency is not compatible with life. It is a severe prothrombotic defect that requires anticoagulation therapy for life.

     h. **Dysplasminogenemia (< 1%).** Dysplasminogenemia is caused by an abnormal plasminogen molecule that has reduced ability to form plasmin; thus, these molecules have a reduced ability to lyse clots.

     i. **Reduced heparin cofactor II (incidence unknown).** Reduced levels of heparin cofactor II, a serpin directed to thrombin, have been associated with venous thrombosis in some patients.

     j. **Elevation of plasminogen activator inhibitor-1 (incidence unknown)**

     k. **Elevation of factors XI, VII, IX, VIII, X, and II.** In the individual patient, the predictive value of a single elevation is not known.

  2. **Hematologic diseases**

     a. **Disseminated intravascular coagulation (see Chapter 11)**

     b. **HITTS (see Chapter 12)**

     c. **Antiphospholipid antibody syndrome.** Antiphospholipid antibodies bind to endothelium and interfere with its constitutive anticoagulant nature by interfering with the anticoagulant properties of annexin V. Paradoxically, some of these patients have lupus anticoagulants, additional antibodies that interfere with the clot-based prothrombin time and activated partial thromboplastin time assays. Although these assays are prolonged, the patients have prothrombotic states.

     d. **TTP (see Chapter 12)**

     e. **HUS (see Chapter 12)**

     f. **Myeloproliferative disorders (e.g., polycythemia vera, essential thrombocythemia)**

C. **Risk factors for venous thrombosis**

  1. **Age.** After 2 weeks of bed rest, the likelihood of venous thrombosis is 20% for a 20-year-old individual and 60% for a 60-year-old individual.

  2. **Prolonged immobility.** An immobilized individual is more likely to develop venous thrombosis than an individual who is physically active.

  3. **Obesity.** Obese individuals are more sedentary and are at greater risk for venous thrombosis than individuals who are not obese. Obesity is the most common risk factor associated with venous thrombosis.

  4. **Neurologic disease.** Many individuals who have strokes have thrombosis in the paretic limb but not in the limb that is functioning.

5. **Cardiac disease.** An uncomplicated myocardial infarction carries a low risk of thrombosis. However, a patient with heart failure associated with a myocardial infarction has a 25% risk for deep venous thrombosis (DVT), and 25% of these patients have a pulmonary embolus.

6. **Pregnancy and the postpartum period.** Pregnancy and the postpartum period are associated with an increased risk of thrombosis.

7. **Oral contraceptives.** Oral contraceptives are associated with an increased risk of thrombosis. If the patient has the factor V Leiden mutation (see Section IV. B.1.a.). the risk is increased 28-fold.

8. **Surgery.** Surgery is a well-recognized risk factor for thrombosis. The degree of risk depends on the nature of the surgery and the amount of time the patient is under anesthesia. For example, orthopedic surgery (hip, knee) is associated with actual flexing and occlusion of the femoral and popliteal veins, respectively. The incidence of DVT is 35%–40% and 50%, respectively. The risk of DVT in other surgeries follows accordingly:

   a. Abdominothoracic surgery, 14%–35%

   b. Urologic surgery: transurethral resection, 7%; suprapubic prostatectomy, 35%

   c. Gynecologic surgery: vaginal hysterectomy, 7%; total abdominal hysterectomy, 27%

9. **Malignancy and thrombosis.** The incidence of occult malignancy in patients with idiopathic thrombosis is only 0.5%–5.8%. However, patients with idiopathic DVT or pulmonary embolism have a three-fold higher than normal likelihood of presenting with occult malignancy within 3 years of presentation of the clot. Furthermore, if a patient has a malignancy, there is a 20% likelihood that thrombosis will develop at some time during the course of the illness.

D. **Treatment of venous thrombosis.** Venous thrombosis presents as DVT or a pulmonary embolus. It can lead to stroke by a paradoxical embolus as a result of a patent foramen ovale. Treatment is usually with antifibrin-generating agents.

1. **Treatment principles**

   a. Prevention is the method of choice for immobile high-risk patients.

   b. Once a thrombus has been recognized, the goal of treatment is to prevent recurrence, propagation, and embolism.

   c. Anticoagulant treatment to prevent recurrence, propagation, or embolism is with standard heparin, low-molecular-weight heparin, hirudin, or argatroban acutely followed by oral anticoagulation with warfarin (a vitamin K antagonist).

2. Lysis of clots occurs with thrombolytic therapy (e.g., t-PA, streptokinase, urokinase).

V. SUMMARY

Thrombosis is a medical situation for which the physician must have a high index of suspicion. Unlike bleeding states, thrombosis has no diagnostic screening tests. Appreciating the disorders and conditions listed in this chapter will serve the physician well in diagnosing and treating these conditions.

SUGGESTED READING

Bauer KA. Inherited and acquired hypercoagulable states. In: Loscalzo J, Schafer A, eds. *Thrombosis &* *Hemorrhage,* 2nd ed. Baltimore: Williams & Wilkins; 1998:863–900.

Myeloid Cell Physiology and Disorders

- LILLI M. PETRUZZELLI

I. INTRODUCTION

Myeloid cells are a subset of white blood cells (WBCs), or leukocytes. This subset includes neutrophils, eosinophils, monocytes, and basophils. These cells mediate host defense against infection and modulate the immune response. All of these cells, along with erythrocytes and platelets, are derived from a common myeloid stem cell precursor (see Figure 2–6).

II. LABORATORY STUDIES

A. An automated cell counter is used to determine the number of WBCs in each microliter (μL) or cubic millimeter (mm^3) of blood.

B. The cells are further analyzed to determine the percentage of each subtype, or the **relative proportion** of each type of cell.

C. The **absolute number** of each circulating component of WBCs is determined by multiplying the percentage of each type of cell by the total number of WBCs.

D. Table 14–1 defines the terms used to describe variations in the WBC differential.

E. Tables 14–2 and 14–3 show typical WBC counts and the relative proportion of each type of cell in various clinical situations.

III. SUBSETS OF MYELOID CELLS

A. **Neutrophils** play a central role in host defense against infection. They are normally the major component of circulating WBCs. Neutrophils act by ingesting (i.e., phagocytizing) offending organisms and releasing toxic oxygen metabolites into the surrounding tissue. Neutrophils are needed continuously, and turnover is constant. These cells mature in the bone marrow for approximately 12 days, then enter the circulation, where they remain for approximately 12 hours. Finally, they are recruited to the tissue, where they perform their specified function for approximately 12 hours. Blood cells develop in the bone marrow, and the earliest cells (stem cells) become committed to a specific type of blood cell. As they develop, the blood cells become restricted in their ability to differentiate; this occurs at various points for the different WBC types. Commitment begins in the bone marrow at the myeloblast stage, and proliferation occurs through the promyelocyte and myelocyte stages. Metamyelocytes, band forms, and mature neutro-

TABLE 14–1 • Terms to Describe Variations of the WBC Differential

Term	Definition	Example
Absolute	Actual number of specific type of WBC/mm³ or μL of blood	ANC (number/mm³) = total WBC count × % neutrophils in differential; if WBC count is 5000/mm³ and neutrophils are 20%, ANC is 1000/mm³
Relative	Relation of number of specific type of WBC to total WBC count (percentage shown in WBC differential)	If WBC count is 5000/mm³ and differential shows 90% of these cells to be neutrophils, neutrophils are described as relatively increased (relative neutrophilia); "normal" or reference neutrophil % is 50%–80%
-Philia, -cytosis	Indicate increased levels in blood: -philia is used for granulocytes; -cytosis is used for lymphocytes and monocytes	Neutrophilia, eosinophilia, monocytosis, lymphocytosis
-Penia	Suffix indicating decreased levels in blood; applicable to any WBC, platelets, many nonhematologic substances normally in blood	Neutropenia, thrombocytopenia

ANC, absolute neutrophil count; WBC, white blood cell.

phils no longer divide. Proliferation and maturation depend on the presence of colony-stimulating factors (CSF), such as granulocyte CSF (G-CSF) and granulocyte–macrophage CSF (GM-CSF), in combination with other factors. Each stage is defined by characteristic granules. Classes of granules include primary (azurophilic), secondary (specific), and tertiary. All three classes of granules have specific enzymes and different staining characteristics on blood smears (Figure 14–1).

B. **Eosinophils** are distinguished from neutrophils at the early myelocyte stage. They contain bright-staining orange-red granules that are composed of major basic protein (MBP), peroxidase, and other lysosomal enzymes. After these cells spend approximately 9 days maturing in the bone marrow and 3–8 days in the circulation, they cross the endothelial barrier in the lymph nodes. These cells contain immunoglobulin E receptors on their surface. These receptors, which are not found in neutrophils, play a role in killing parasites. In nonallergic people, the eosinophil count is usually less than 400 cells/μL and averages 120 cells/μL.

TABLE 14–2 • Representative White Blood Cell Counts

Age	WBCs (μL)	PMN (%)	Band (%)	Lympho-cytes (%)	Monocytes (%)	Eosinophils (%)	Basophils (%)
Birth	22,000	60	2	30	5	2	1
1 to 4 years	11,000	35	3	55	5	3	1
6 years to teens	9000	50	3	40	4	2	1
Adult	8000	70	2	20	5	2	1

WBC, white blood cell; PMN, polymorphonuclear.

TABLE 14–3 • White Blood Cell Counts in Disease States

Condition	WBCs (μL)	PMN (%)	Band (%)	Lympho-cytes (%)	Monocytes (%)	Eosinophils (%)	Basophils (%)
Bacterial infection	16,000	78	8	9	3	1	1
Viral infection	3500	50	1	41	5	2	1
Chemotherapy	2800	65	0	20	12	2	1
Steroid therapy[a]	12,000	78	4	14	2	0	0
Splenectomy[b]	13,000	50	2	40	5	2	1

WBC, white blood cell; PMN, polymorphonuclear.
[a]WBC counts also reveal 2% metamyelocytes.
[b]Nucleated red blood cells and target cells are also seen after splenectomy.

C. **Basophils and mast cells** are the two populations of cells containing prominent cytoplasmic granules that exhibit intense dark purple histochemical staining. Basophils are easily identified in the peripheral blood by their dark, dense granularity on Wright-Giemsa stain. Basophils last approximately 7 days in the circulation. In contrast, mast cells have a longer life and reside in connective tissue. Both types of cells are believed to play a critical role in host defense against parasites.

D. **Monocytes.** Once in the tissue, monocytes differentiate into macrophages and remove microorganisms and noxious agents (see Chapter 2, VI B). Like neutrophils, these cells phagocytize pathogens. They also generate toxic oxygen metabolites that have a role in killing microorganisms. Finally, monocytes play an essential role in the presentation of antigen to T lymphocytes.

IV. NEUTROPHIL DISORDERS

A. **Overview.** Neutrophil disorders may be acquired or inherited. They may occur in production, in the maturation of granules, in the expression of proteins that are necessary for critical function, or in the recruitment of cells from the circulation.

B. **Disorders in the number of circulating neutrophils.** Evaluation of these disorders includes a complete blood count and determination of the percentage of each class of WBC. Because underlying diseases and medications may affect the neutrophil count, this information must be linked to the clinical evaluation. **Normal**

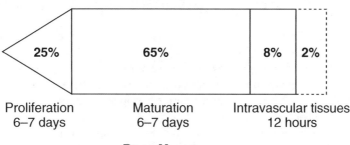

| 25% | 65% | 8% | 2% |
| Proliferation 6–7 days | Maturation 6–7 days | Intravascular tissues 12 hours | |

Bone Marrow

FIGURE 14–1. Time frame of neutrophil proliferation and maturation. Beginning with the myeloblast (the earliest precursor cell that can be detected by eye), cells mature and proliferate. Once cells reach the myelocyte stage, they no longer proliferate but continue to mature until they reach the neutrophil or polymorphonuclear cell stage. At this point, they leave the bone marrow for the circulation and can be recruited to the tissue for host defense.

values for neutrophil counts vary with age, sex, and race. For example, the lower limit of the normal neutrophil count is $1500/\mu L$ in most populations and ranges to $7,700/\mu L$; African Americans have a lower neutrophil limit, approximately $1000/\mu L$.

1. **Neutrophilia** is present when the neutrophil count exceeds the upper limit of the normal range by two standard deviations from the mean value for normal individuals. The value is higher in children than in adults. Neutrophilia is caused by both chronic and acute conditions.
   a. **Chronic stimulation and expansion** of the number of neutrophils occurs in a number of conditions, including:
      (1) Infection
      (2) Cancer (breast, gastric, lung)
      (3) Myeloproliferative disorders
      (4) Pregnancy and lactation
      (5) Eclampsia
      (6) Chronic acidosis
      (7) Anxiety
      (8) Down syndrome
      (9) Heavy metal poisoning
      (10) Metastatic infiltration of bone marrow
      (11) Proliferation of immature circulating forms (e.g., leukemia)
      (12) Recovery of the bone marrow from a toxic incident
   b. An **acute rise** in the neutrophil count may occur when neutrophils shift from the marginating pool (i.e., neutrophils mobilized at the endothelial cell wall) to the circulating pool. These shifts occur:
      (1) During exercise
      (2) During epinephrine administration
      (3) During episodes of hypoxia and stress
      (4) In response to steroid administration
2. **Neutropenia** is present if the neutrophil count is less than $1500/\mu L$. Mild neutropenia is present when the neutrophil count is $1000–1500/\mu L$; complications rarely develop in this situation. A neutrophil count of $500–1000/\mu L$ is associated with increased risk of infection. When the neutrophil count is $500/\mu L$, the patient has considerable susceptibility to infection with endogenous organisms in the skin, oropharynx, and intestine. Infections with gram-positive cocci, especially *Staphylococcus aureus,* are common in these patients. Neutropenia is caused by decreased production or increased use of neutrophils or by a shift of cells from the circulating pool to the marginating pool.
   a. **Conditions that cause decreased production of neutrophils result in neutropenia.**
      (1) **Medication** is the major cause of neutropenia. G-CSF is used to stimulate neutrophil production, particularly in patients undergoing chemotherapy. Drugs associated with neutropenia include:
         (a) Chemotherapeutic agents
         (b) Anti-inflammatory agents (e.g., sulindac [Clinoril])
         (c) Antibiotics (e.g., sulfonamides, high-dose penicillins)
         (d) Phenothiazines
         (e) Antithyroid drugs (e.g., methimazole, propylthiouracil)
      (2) **Autoimmune diseases** (e.g., rheumatoid arthritis, Sjögren syndrome, Felty syndrome, systemic lupus erythematosus, idiopathic thrombocy-

topenic purpura, hemolytic anemia) are also associated with neutropenia.

(3) Neutropenia may also be a component of **lymphoid diseases** (e.g., Hodgkin disease, non-Hodgkin lymphoma, chronic lymphocytic leukemia) and **viral illnesses** (e.g., Epstein-Barr virus, human immunodeficiency virus, hepatitis). In addition to decreased neutrophil production in the bone marrow, antibodies directed against neutrophils may be associated with lymphoid diseases and viral illnesses.

b. **Enhanced removal of neutrophils from the circulation** occurs when neutrophils move into the marginating pool. This is seen with:

(1) Hemodialysis

(2) Cardiopulmonary bypass

(3) Endotoxin release associated with overwhelming bacterial sepsis

c. Neutropenia is a major clinical feature of **idiopathic chronic neutropenia** and **adult-onset cyclic neutropenia.** In cyclic neutropenia, neutrophils disappear from the circulation at regular 3-week intervals. Levels of other blood components can also fluctuate. This condition has a number of rare forms, one of which is congenital neutropenia that is associated with a number of other defects and is usually fatal during childhood.

C. **Structural and functional defects in neutrophils.** Chemotactic agents are peptides and proteins that diffuse from the site of tissue injury, bind to specific receptors on the cell surface, and stimulate neutrophils to attach and migrate through the blood vessel wall (Figure 14–2). After neutrophils move from the circulation and cross the endothelial cell barrier, they phagocytize invading organisms and destroy them with the help of granules. Disorders of neutrophil function impair the ability of neutrophils to move from the circulation, phagocytize particles, or degranulate. The net result is varying degrees of impaired neutrophil function. Several inherited disorders have been defined at the molecular level as causes of structural and functional neutrophil defects (Table 14–4).

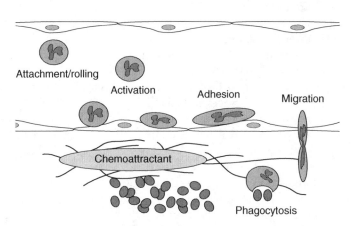

FIGURE 14–2. Recruitment of white blood cells from the circulation. The diagram shows a neutrophil; however, other members of the myeloid series are recruited from the circulation by a similar scheme. Neutrophils are normally freely circulating and do not adhere to the blood vessel wall. In response to tissue injury by either an invading organism or damage to the endothelium, the selectins are up-regulated and the neutrophil rolls along the vessel wall through the interaction of its receptor with the selectin. Integrins activated by chemokines released at the site of tissue damage enable the neutrophil to adhere tightly to the blood vessel wall. The neutrophil subsequently migrates through the endothelial cell layer, where it carries out its functions of host defense (e.g., phagocytosis of bacteria, elaboration of activated oxygen species).

TABLE 14–4 • Structural and Functional Defects in Neutrophils

Step	Disease	Molecular Defect
Rolling	LAD-2	Sialyl Lewis^x carbohydrate
Tight adhesion	LAD-1	β_2 Integrin expression
Migration	Specific granule deficiency	
	Chediak-Higashi syndrome	Vacuolar sorting protein
Oxidative burst	CGD	NADPH oxidase
	Myeloperoxidase deficiency	HOCl production
Phagocytosis	LAD-1	β_2-Integrin expression
Degranulation	Specific granule deficiency	
	Chediak-Higashi syndrome	Vacuolar sorting protein

CGD, chronic granulomatous disease; HOCl, hypochlorite; LAD, leukocyte adhesion deficiency; NADPH, reduced nicotinamide adenine dinucleotide phosphate.

1. **Leukocyte adhesion deficiency (LAD)** is a group of rare diseases that have led to the understanding that recruitment across the endothelial cell barrier occurs as a result of specific protein–protein and protein–carbohydrate interactions. These disorders are characterized by recurrent bacterial and fungal infections and neutrophilia. The neutrophil count is often 20,000–30,000/μL. Two types are recognized: LAD-1 and LAD-2.
   a. **LAD-1** is caused by a defect in the cell surface expression of the β_2-integrin family of proteins. Patients who lack this protein expression have markedly decreased or absent neutrophils at the site of inflammation because the cells cannot adhere to the endothelial cell wall.
      (1) The severity of the disease is related to the level of expression.
      (2) Infections include delayed separation of the umbilical cord in infants, skin infections, chronic leg ulcers, and gingivitis. *Staphylococcus aureus*, gram-negative organisms (e.g., *Escherichia coli*), and fungal agents are usually responsible.
      (3) Diagnosis is made by flow cytometry with an antibody to the β_2-integrin subunit.
      (4) Treatment includes antibiotics if the condition is mild and bone marrow transplant if severe.
   b. **LAD-2** is a complex disease associated with leukocyte adhesion defects, neurologic defects, craniofacial defects, and the Bombay (hh) erythrocyte phenotype. These patients have an impaired ability to form fucosylated carbohydrate structures on neutrophils and other cells. When this structure is absent, neutrophils do not roll along the endothelial cell wall, which is the initial step in the recruitment of neutrophils from the circulation. If rolling does not occur, neutrophils do not cross the endothelium and cannot travel to the site of infection.
2. **Chronic granulomatous disease** (CGD) is a rare disease characterized by recurrent life-threatening bacterial and fungal infections. Infections occur because of an impaired ability to kill bacteria after they are phagocytized. Several proteins have been cloned and are known to be defective in association with CGD. These proteins are distinct components of the enzyme nicotinamide adenine dinucleotide phosphate (NADPH) oxidase in phagocytes, which is responsible for the production of superoxides that play a key role in bacterial killing.

    a. Catalase-positive bacteria and fungi pose a major risk of infection in patients with CGD.

      (1) Ingested bacteria are contained in the phagosome, and myeloperoxidase is delivered by degranulation.

      (2) Hydrogen peroxide (H_2O_2) is produced in the neutrophil and converted to oxygen species that kill microorganisms by NADPH oxidase.

      (3) Normal neutrophils produce sufficient H_2O_2 to overcome the H_2O_2 that is catabolized by the catalase produced by bacteria. In CGD, because of the defects in the subunits of NADPH, little or no H_2O_2 is formed.

      (4) Therefore, the catalase that is produced by the microorganism overcomes any residual H_2O_2.

      (5) In this situation, *S. aureus, Serratia, Salmonella, Candida,* and *Aspergillus* pose a risk of infection.

    b. Clinically, the disease varies in severity and time of presentation (childhood to adulthood). Microabscesses and granulomas point to the diagnosis.

    c. The diagnosis can be made by examining the colorless to blue-black change of the dye nitroblue tetrazolium (NBT) once it is intraphagosomal. Patients with CGD have markedly diminished conversion of the dye to the blue-black color.

3. Specific granule deficiency is a rare autosomal recessive inherited disorder. These patients have a relative deficiency of specific granules that contain the enzymes necessary for the migration and delivery of receptors to the cell surface. These receptors are needed for complete neutrophil function. As a result, patients with this disease have impaired migration of neutrophils and recurrent infections of the skin, sinuses, and lungs.

4. Chédiak-Higashi syndrome (CHS) is a rare autosomal recessive disorder associated with immune deficiency.

    a. Neutrophils from patients with CHS show a defect in the formation of granules. Defects in lysosomes and vesicular structures are also seen in other cells throughout the body.

    b. The underlying defect is believed to be caused by abnormal sorting during a specific stage of granule formation. This abnormality results in a deficiency in the incorporation of cathepsin G and elastase in granules. This defect results in impaired chemotaxis and killing of microorganisms.

    c. Patients with CHS are susceptible to infection, bleeding, and lymphoproliferative disorders. These patients also have oculocutaneous albinism and peripheral neuropathy.

5. Hereditary myeloperoxidase syndrome affects approximately 1 in 4000 people and is usually found incidentally on morphologic examination of neutrophils. The major finding is intact phagocytosis of bacteria and fungi but impaired ability to kill fungi (e.g., *Candida, Aspergillus*). Some patients have recurrent visceral fungal infections.

V. EOSINOPHIL DISORDERS

A. Eosinopenia is less well characterized than neutropenia. The average eosinophil count is 200 cells/μL and can range from 0–400 cells/μL. The eosinophil count can decrease as a result of infection or administration of steroids, prostaglandins, or epinephrine. However, unlike neutropenia, this condition is usually transient and is not associated with a significant risk of infection.

B. **Eosinophilia** is characterized by an absolute eosinophil count greater than 400/μL. Causes include:

1. Allergic reaction to certain drugs (e.g., aspirin, sulfonamides, penicillins, nitrofurantoin) or to iodide-containing substances (most common causes)
2. Allergy to environmental agents (e.g., grass, trees, dust)
3. Asthma
4. Dermatitis (e.g., eczema, psoriasis)
5. Vasculitis
6. Ulcerative colitis
7. Malignancy (e.g., Hodgkin disease, lymphoma, brain and skin tumors, acute leukemia)
8. Serum sickness
9. Infection with parasites, both protozoan (e.g., pneumonocytis, toxoplasmosis, malaria) and metazoan (e.g., ascariasis, trichinosis, schistosomiasis)

C. **Idiopathic hypereosinophilia** is associated with an elevation of the circulating eosinophil count and may result in dysfunction of the heart, central nervous system, kidneys, lungs, gastrointestinal tract, or skin. Most eosinophil function is associated with degranulation and release of MBP. MBP kills parasites but is also toxic to the skin, intestine, tracheal epithelial cells, and other mononuclear cells. Treatment is usually instituted when the eosinophil count exceeds 5000/μL.

VI. BASOPHIL DISORDERS

A. A low basophil count is associated with glucocorticoid treatment and hypersensitivity reactions.

B. The basophil count is increased in patients with allergic conditions, infection, endocrinopathies, and myeloproliferative disorders (e.g., chronic myelogenous leukemia, polycythemia vera, myeloid metaplasia, essential thrombocytosis). Mast cell infiltration of the skin or other organs also occurs. The symptoms of mast cell infiltration, which are caused by excess histamine, include urticaria and dizziness. The malignant form of mast cell infiltration is systemic mastocytosis.

VII. MONOCYTE DISORDERS

A. Monocyte disorders parallel those seen with neutrophils. The average circulating monocyte count is 300/μL and can range from 0–800 cells/μL.

B. **Monocytopenia** occurs in response to stress and after glucocorticoid administration.

C. **Monocytosis** is present when the absolute monocyte count exceeds 800/μL. It occurs in:

1. Myelodysplastic syndrome
2. Neutropenic states (e.g., cyclic neutropenia)
3. The recovery phase of agranulocytosis
4. Exacerbations of lymphoma
5. Patients who have undergone splenectomy
6. Subtypes of leukemia
7. Response to infection (e.g., cytomegalovirus, tuberculosis, subacute bacterial endocarditis, syphilis)
8. Patients with underlying inflammatory disease

VIII. SUMMARY

Each of the members of the myeloid series—neutrophils, eosinophils, basophils, and monocytes—plays a critical role in host defense against pathogenic organisms. Some of the roles overlap and others are unique to each class of cells. The members of this series exhibit variations in number in response to disease or infection. An understanding of the regulation of their blood levels and functions aids in understanding the clinical picture of a patient. Although the list appears exhaustive, a considerable amount about the function of each of these cells has yet to be uncovered.

Hematopoietic Differentiation and the Development of Neoplastic Diseases

- LLOYD M. STOOLMAN

I. INTRODUCTION

A. A neoplastic transformation occurs when acquired genetic alterations release the affected cell from the normal controls on cell division and survival. When this occurs, the cell proliferates, accumulates, and displaces normal cells with replicas of itself (i.e., clones). The cells that accumulate are called a **neoplasm.**
  1. Neoplasms that do not metastasize (i.e., spread to distant organs) are referred to as **benign,** although they may still compromise function in the host organ or tissue.
  2. Neoplasms that metastasize are referred to as **malignant.**
B. Neoplastic disorders of the hematopoietic system include **myeloproliferative syndromes, myelodysplastic syndromes,** and **malignant neoplasms.** Neoplastic disorders arise at multiple stages of hematopoietic differentiation. Although current laboratory techniques (e.g., cytogenetics and molecular genetics) sometimes identify specific lesions associated with these diseases, in most cases a precise genetic basis cannot be determined. The most clinically useful schemes for classification of the hematopoietic neoplasms are based on morphologic (size, shape, nuclear and cytoplasmic features), biochemical, cytogenetic, and antigenic profiles of the abnormal cells and the patterns they form in the involved tissues (histopathology).
C. This chapter describes hematopoietic differentiation from its origins in the bone marrow through primary and secondary lymphoid organs and into the bloodstream. The consequences of neoplastic transformations at different stages of normal development are highlighted using selected diseases.

II. THE HEMATOPOIETIC SYSTEM

A. The hematopoietic system is made up of **dispersed organs connected by the bloodstream and lymphatics.**
B. Three features distinguish the hematopoietic system from all other systems.
  1. Its functional units are individual highly motile cells rather than multicellular tissues designed to function in one location.

2. In the course of normal differentiation, immature cells are constantly moving (trafficking) through the bloodstream from one site or organ in the hemato-poietic system to another.

3. Normal host defense involves the constant trafficking of mature leukocytes (e.g., granulocytes, monocytes, lymphocytes) from their site of production through the bloodstream to all tissues, organs, and fluids in the body.

C. Clonal hematopoietic diseases in this system frequently involve multiple sites from the outset, produce changes visible in the bloodstream, and in the case of malignancy, disseminate (metastasize) early via the bloodstream.

III.   HEMATOPOIESIS AND LYMPHOCYTE DIFFERENTIATION

A. After birth, normal hematopoiesis begins with **hematopoietic stem cells (HSCs)** in the bone marrow (Fig. 15–1) (see Chapter 2, III).

1. HSCs normally circulate in the bloodstream in small numbers ($<0.5\%$).

2. Neoplastic disorders that arise from HSCs generally come to medical atten-tion because of symptoms and signs that result from widespread involvement of the bone marrow. In contrast, neoplastic transformation in other tissues and organs generally presents as a mass (tumor) of clonal neoplastic cells at the site of transformation.

B. Normal **red blood cells (RBCs)**, **platelets**, and **white blood cells (WBCs)**, with the exception of lymphocytes, are at or near full maturity when released from the bone marrow into the peripheral blood (Fig. 15–1).

C. **Lymphocyte differentiation** involves the **bone marrow, thymus,** and **secondary lymphoid organs** throughout the body.

1. After branching off from pluripotent stem cells, T- and B-lymphocyte prog-enitors must develop the clonal diversity that distinguishes the adaptive from the innate immune system.

a. In humans, B-lymphocyte progenitors (i.e., pre–B cells) undergo re-arrangement of the antigen (Ag) combining regions of both the heavy- and light-chain genes, culminating in the expression of multiple immunoglob-ulin M (IgM) molecules on the cell surface. The IgM molecules on indi-vidual cells contain either a κ- or λ-light chain, express identical amino acid sequences, and constitute the first Ag receptors for the cell. In humans, these events probably occur in the bone marrow.

(1) B cells with Ag-receptors on their surface that have not encountered Ag are referred to as naïve B cells.

(2) Naïve B cells leave the bone marrow and traffic via the bloodstream and lymphatics through secondary lymphoid organs and tissues until they encounter the appropriate Ag (see III.C.2.).

b. In contrast to B cells, human T-cell progenitors (pre–T cells) must traffic through the bloodstream to the **thymus** before acquiring functional T-cell Ag receptors.

(1) The thymus is fully developed and populated by pre–T cells at the time of birth. However, continued trafficking of pre–T cells from the bone marrow to the thymus occurs after birth.

(2) Under the influence of cortical epithelial cells and thymic dendritic cells in the thymus, pre–T cells develop into Ag-responsive α/β and γ/δ T cells. This process entails rearrangement of the T-cell Ag-receptor genes, expression of the Ag receptors on the cell surface, acquisition of sur-face receptors required for recognition of the major histocompati-bility complex (MHC) associated peptides (i.e., CD4 or CD8), and

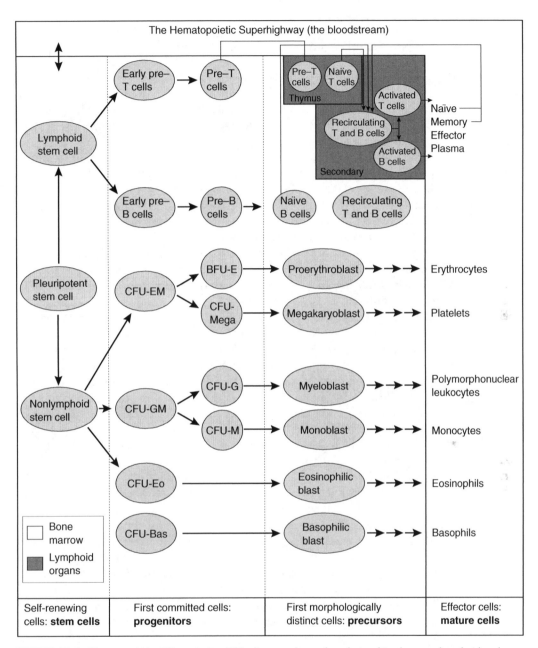

FIGURE 15–1. Hematopoietic differentiation. This diagram shows the relationships between lymphoid and non-lymphoid cells and the stages at which maturing cells enter the bloodstream. Stem cells are the least differentiated forms in the bone marrow. The progenitors are named according to the precursors they produce in culture. The precursors are designated by the least mature form (the blast) in each lineage. Pre–T cells and pre–B cells are lymphocytes before antigen (Ag) receptor expression. Naïve T and B cells are lymphocytes that express Ag receptors but have not responded to Ag. Activated T and B cells are differentiating in response to antigenic stimulation. Recirculating T and B cells represent the naïve and memory cells that are in constant motion through lymphoid organs as part of immune surveillance. The names of individual cell types are illustrative and less important than the developmental stage they represent. The various stem and progenitor cells depicted are inferred from experimental systems. *BFU-E,* burst-forming unit, erythrocytes; *CFU-Bas,* colony-forming unit, basophils; *CFU-EM,* colony-forming unit, erythrocytes and megakaryocytes; *CFU-Eo,* colony-forming unit, eosinophils; *CFU-G,* colony-forming unit, granulocytes; *CFU-GM,* colony-forming unit, granulocytes and macrophages; *CFU-M,* colony-forming unit, macrophages; *CFU-Mega,* colony-forming unit, megakaryocytes.

acquisition of surface receptors required for signal transduction through the Ag receptor (i.e., CD3).

   (3) The receptors involved in Ag recognition and signal transduction drive both positive and negative selection within the thymus. Positive selection preserves cells that recognize self-MHC molecules. Negative selection eliminates T cells that react with many autoantigens (self-Ags).

   (4) If all goes well, the naïve T cells that emerge from the thymus into the circulation show minimal reactivity with autoantigens and respond best when foreign antigenic peptides are complexed with self-MHC molecules.

2. Naïve T and B cells complete their development to effector cells in **secondary lymphoid organs.** Secondary lymphoid organs include the lymph nodes, spleen, and specialized collections of organized lymphoid tissues associated with mucosal surfaces of the upper airway (e.g., nasal passages, tonsils, adenoids), gastrointestinal tract (e.g., Peyer patches, gut-associated lymphoid tissues), and bronchi (e.g., bronchus-associated lymphoid tissues). In addition, most organs can transiently develop organized lymphoid collections reminiscent of lymph nodes when chronically stimulated. For example, in the synovium of joints in patients with rheumatoid arthritis, the thyroid parenchyma in Hashimoto thyroiditis, and the bone marrow of aging individuals, organized lymphoid tissues (lymphoid follicles) frequently develop. Secondary lymphoid organs promote interactions between antigen-presenting cells (APCs) and recirculating lymphocytes. In addition, they provide a phagocytic filter for particulates and a repository for antibody-secreting plasma cells.

  a. T- and B-cell proliferation occurs in different regions in secondary lymphoid organs.

   (1) B cells form nodular (rounded, follicular) collections that develop germinal centers during immunologic responses. The size and number of B-cell follicles with germinal centers is a measure of immunologic activity in the organ.

   (2) The B cells in germinal centers contain enlarged nuclei with irregular contours, nucleoli, and abundant cytoplasm. These cytologic features indicate B-cell or T-cell proliferative activity.

   (3) At the edge of the germinal center is a rim of small lymphocytes that are indistinguishable from those in the bloodstream. These cells have small, round nuclei with condensed patches of chromatin and very little cytoplasm. These cytologic features characterize the inactive (resting) lymphocytes that make up most of the recirculating pool.

   (4) T-cell proliferation occurs in the areas between and deep to the B-cell follicles. In lymph nodes, this area is referred to as the diffuse cortex; in the spleen it is known as the periarteriolar sheath. Lymphocytes with features of both inactive and active cells can normally be found here.

   (5) Channels (sinusoids) lined by fenestrated endothelium and phagocytic cells criss-cross lymph nodes. The sinusoids are joined to both the afferent (incoming) and efferent (outgoing) lymph. These channels deliver APCs, T cells, and B cells from interstitial fluids into the substance of the lymph node. They also carry the naïve, memory, and effector cells generated in the lymph nodes down the chain and back into the bloodstream.

  b. The perpetual movement of naïve (and some memory) lymphocytes from the bloodstream into secondary lymphoid organs and back into the bloodstream is referred to as **lymphocyte recirculation.** This process maximizes the exposure of lymphocytes to optimally processed Ag; thus, it is an essential part of immune surveillance. Specialized vascular adhesion receptors, chemokine receptors, and chemokines are required for recirculation through lymph nodes.

(1) A receptor on lymphocytes known as L selectin binds to glycoproteins expressed on specialized venules found primarily in lymph nodes (i.e., high endothelial venules).

(2) This adhesive interaction causes lymphocytes to roll along the endothelial surface of high endothelial venules, where they interact with one of several chemokines synthesized in the lymph node.

(3) The chemokines trigger a second series of adhesive interactions involving members of the integrin and immunoglobulin supergene families.

(4) These adhesive interactions arrest the rolling motion of lymphocytes on the endothelial surface and promote their migration through the blood vessel wall into the cortex of the lymph node.

(5) The recirculating lymphocytes collide with APCs and activated lymphocytes in the lymph node. Contact with APCs carrying the appropriate self-MHC peptide complex triggers proliferation and differentiation into memory or effector cells.

(6) Unstimulated lymphocytes along with newly minted memory and effector cells exit the lymphoid organ via lymphatics (except in the spleen), percolate through additional lymphoid organs along the chain, and ultimately return to the bloodstream for either continued recirculation or delivery to immune responses in tissues.

c. In contrast to naïve and recirculating memory lymphocytes, **effector cells** acquire new targeting receptors (i.e., vascular adhesion and chemokine receptors) that direct them away from organized lymphoid organs and into **inflamed or injured tissues.**

(1) Because foreign Ags generally originate in inflamed or injured tissues, vascular adhesion and chemokine receptors promote the recruitment of circulating effector cells into the sites where immunologic responses are under way. For example, T cytotoxic cells generated in cervical lymph nodes draining virally infected pharyngeal epithelium use their newly acquired receptors to bind and traverse the inflamed blood vessels at the site of infection.

(2) Recruitment of effector cells is independent of Ag; all effector cells with the appropriate targeting receptors can enter active immunologic lesions.

(3) However, the retention and survival of cells that enter tissues is Ag dependent. In the previous example [see III.C.2.c.(1)], the subsequent interaction of effector cells with virally infected epithelium results in their retention and survival; other effector cells either reenter the lymphatic system or die through apoptosis.

d. The dispersion of lymphoid organs throughout the body and the constant trafficking of lymphoid cells through them help explain several confusing aspects of the neoplastic diseases affecting lymphocytes.

(1) Neoplastic diseases can arise in any organ normally visited by lymphocytes or their progenitors, including the secondary lymphoid organs, bone marrow, thymus, and nonlymphoid sites.

(2) Malignancies of lymphocytes may retain the cell surface receptors that

control the trafficking behavior of the parent cell; thus, they are frequently as motile as the cells from which they arise. Consequently, these malignancies metastasize relatively early through the bloodstream, showing particular affinity for the organs involved in lymphocyte development and differentiation.

(3) The stage of lymphocyte differentiation at which a neoplastic transformation occurs influences the site where the malignant cells first appear and their subsequent metastatic behavior.

    (a) For example, neoplasms of pre–B cells and pre–T cells frequently present in the bone marrow or thymus with visible blood involvement at the onset of disease.

    (b) In contrast, neoplasms of Ag-responsive B lymphocytes frequently present as masses in one or more lymph nodes (lymphadenopathy) with visible blood and bone marrow involvement later in their course.

IV. LABORATORY EVALUATION OF THE BONE MARROW

A. The bone marrow is a fibrofatty gelatinous matrix occupying the spaces between boney trabeculae. Blood vessels, nerves, and hematopoietic cells at all stages of differentiation are suspended in this fluid culture system. These cells are bathed in growth factors that mediate hematopoietic differentiation or maturation.

B. The most undifferentiated hematopoietic cells, the HSCs and progenitors, make up a small percentage of nucleated cells in the bone marrow (< 1%–2%). Differentiating hematopoietic precursors are the most numerous cells in the bone marrow (Fig 15–1).

1. The HSCs and progenitors can both self-renew (i.e., make copies with the same developmental potential) and differentiate (i.e., progress toward a single lineage). The HSCs self-renew primarily and retain the broadest developmental potential. The progenitors show less self-renewal and greater development toward specific lineages.

2. The early stages of hematopoietic differentiation cannot be readily distinguished from one another on cytologic (appearance), antigenic, or biochemical grounds.

3. Once an immature hematopoietic cell acquires recognizable cytologic, antigenic, or biochemical features indicative of a single lineage, it is referred to as a precursor.

C. The clonal hematopoietic diseases that arise in the bone marrow have profound effects on the appearance and distribution of hematopoietic precursors.

1. The earliest precursors (blast forms) have high nuclear to cytoplasmic ratios, nuclei with fine chromatin, nucleoli, and little evidence of lineage-specific differentiation in the microscope. Marker antigens (e.g., CD13 or CD33 for granulocytes, CD14 for monocytes, CD1 or CD2 for pre–T cells, CD19 or CD20 for pre–B cells) and cytoplasmic enzymes (e.g., myeloperoxidase for granulocytes, α-naphthylbutyrate esterase for monocytes) indicative of a specific lineage appear at this point.

2. As differentiation progresses, lineage-specific cytoplasmic and nuclear changes occur. These changes are sufficiently distinctive that trained observers can identify the stages of maturity of WBCs, RBCs, and megakaryocytes on stained bone marrow smears.

a. The precursors of polymorphonuclear granulocytes contain reddish azurophilic cytoplasmic granules and nuclei that condense and segment during maturation.

   b. RBC precursors show progressive cytoplasmic hemoglobinization (i.e., change from purple to red), nuclear condensation, and eventual nuclear karyorrhexis as the cells approach maturity.

   c. Megakaryocytes are large multinucleate cells with cytoplasm that looks like the platelets that bud from their plasma membranes.

   d. Monocytes have ribbon-like nuclei with abundant, frequently vacuolated cytoplasm containing few granules.

   e. Resting lymphocytes are small cells with condensed patches of nuclear chromatin forming a soccer ball pattern and a thin rim of agranular cytoplasm.

D. Laboratory evaluation of the bone marrow involves two procedures: aspiration and biopsy. These procedures generate specimens that can be used for a variety of clinical tests, including microscopic examination, microbial culture, Ag analysis (e.g., flow cytometry), enzyme analysis (e.g., cytochemistry), cytogenetics (e.g., karyotyping), and molecular genetics (e.g., fluorescence in situ hybridization or polymerase chain reaction analysis for detection of clonal gene rearrangements).

  1. Bone marrow aspiration

   a. The aspirate is obtained by inserting a large-bore needle (affixed to a syringe containing anticoagulant) into the marrow cavity after anesthetizing the overlying skin and periosteum then drawing the plunger back. A drop of bone marrow is carefully smeared onto a glass slide or cover slip, fixed in methanol, and stained with Wright-Giemsa stain before microscopic evaluation. Occasionally, pathologic changes in the bone marrow (e.g., fibrosis, marrow packed with immature cells) inhibit aspiration, resulting in a dry tap.

   b. Examination of the stained bone marrow smear is the best way to assess the structural characteristics of individual cells. Based on the cytologic appearances of precursors, it is possible to estimate the myeloid to erythroid ratio and conduct a bone marrow leukocyte differential count.

   (1) The myeloid to erythroid ratio is the ratio of all WBCs to all nucleated RBCs. It provides an estimate of the relative proliferative activities in the two most numerous groups of nucleated cells in the bone marrow.

   (2) The bone marrow leukocyte differential count provides the frequency distribution for the major recognizable stages of leukocyte differentiation (i.e., blast forms, promyelocytes, myelocytes, metamyelocytes, band forms, segmented neutrophils, eosinophils, basophils, lymphocytes, and monocytes).

  2. Bone marrow biopsy

   a. Bone marrow biopsies are obtained with a specialized needle that removes a core of the marrow without disturbing its architecture. It is then fixed, embedded in paraffin, sectioned in 1- to 5-micron slices, stained with hematoxylin and eosin, and examined under the microscope.

   b. Examination of a bone marrow biopsy section is the best way to assess the overall cellularity of the marrow and to detect architectural alterations.

   (1) Normally, hematopoietic cells form islands within the fibrofatty marrow stroma. The percentage of the marrow cavity occupied by hematopoietic cells normally declines during life. As a general rule, the percentage occupied by fat cells is approximately equal to an individual's age in years. In neonates, hematopoietic cells occupy all of the cavity. In a 50-year-old person, approximately 50% of the marrow consists of hematopoietic cells and 50% consists of fat. However, primary and secondary diseases that alter the production of normal hematopoietic cells (e.g., aplastic anemia) or increase the production of abnormal hematopoietic cells (e.g., hematopoietic neoplasms) will affect the cellularity.

(2) Space-occupying lesions (e.g., metastatic malignancies, granulomas, abscesses, fibrosis) can also be detected on the biopsy. The bone marrow is a frequent site of metastasis for some cancers (e.g., breast, prostate, lymphoma). Consequently, bone marrow biopsies are frequently performed to help determine whether systemic metastases have occurred from the primary malignancy. This procedure, referred to as staging, helps determine prognosis and therapy.

V.   LABORATORY EVALUATION OF THE PERIPHERAL BLOOD

A. The bloodstream receives undifferentiated and differentiated hematopoietic cells from the bone marrow and the primary and secondary lymphoid organs. Consequently, it provides a window on events occurring in these organs.

B. Because blood is easier to obtain than tissue biopsies, quantitative analysis and microscopic examination of a peripheral blood smear is the first step in the laboratory evaluation of suspected hematopoietic diseases.

1. The clinical laboratory uses high-speed cell counters to perform the complete blood count (CBC). Generally, the results are reported as the number of cells per microliter or cubic millimeter. The complete blood count includes absolute counts of WBCs, RBCs, and platelets.

2. The frequency distribution for WBC types (i.e., the differential count) is performed either by machine or by microscopic examination of stained blood smears. Typically, 100–200 consecutive cells are examined, each is assigned to a lineage, and the final count in each category is converted to a percentage.

   a. Machine counts are inaccurate when abnormal blood cells (e.g., reactive, dysplastic, neoplastic) are present in the bloodstream.

   b. Microscopic examination of circulating abnormal cells is frequently essential for establishing a diagnosis.

   c. Therefore, a microscopic examination of the peripheral blood should be performed on all patients with abnormal total cell counts or suspected hematologic disease.

   d. B cells and T cells look similar under the microscope, except for plasma cells. Consequently, Ag analysis (e.g. flow cytometry or immunocytochemistry) is needed to distinguish between these cell types.

C. An increase in the absolute number of one or more WBC types is generically referred to as **leukocytosis**. Increases involving a single lineage may be further specified (e.g., lymphocytosis, granulocytosis, monocytosis, eosinophilia, basophilia). Increases in RBC and platelet numbers are referred to as erythrocytosis and thrombocytosis, respectively. Leukocytosis may be caused by:

1. Normal inflammatory and immunologic responses
2. Autoimmune diseases
3. Myeloproliferative disorders
4. Hematopoietic malignancies

D. A decrease in the absolute number of one or more WBC types is generically referred to as **leukopenia**. Decreases involving individual lineages (e.g., neutropenia, lymphopenia) may by singled out. RBC and platelet deficiencies are referred to as anemia and thrombocytopenia, respectively. Leukopenias may be caused by:

1. Increased peripheral use (e.g., some infections), sequestration (e.g., spleno-megaly), or destruction (e.g., autoimmune disorders)
2. Hematopoietic production disorders (e.g., drug suppression, radiation treatment, aplastic anemia)
3. Primary or secondary cellular immune deficiencies (e.g., DiGeorge syndrome, severe combined immunodeficiency, HIV infection)
4. Hematopoietic dysplasias
5. Hematopoietic malignancies

E. Hematopoietic neoplasms may insert cytologically abnormal cells into the bloodstream. When abnormal cells exceed approximately 1% of the circulating population, they can be detected by visual inspection of a peripheral blood smear. In some cases, the abnormal cells make up a substantial percentage of the circulating pool, allowing a definitive diagnosis without more invasive procedures (e.g., bone marrow or organ biopsy).

VI. BONE MARROW DISEASES

A. **Overview.** Diseases affecting the bone marrow can be organized into three broad classes: **systemic diseases** that secondarily affect the bone marrow (e.g., infections, autoimmune disorders, endocrine and metabolic dysfunction), primary disorders of **hematopoietic production or function** that result from causes other than neoplastic transformations, and the **clonal hematopoietic disorders** (e.g., hematopoietic neoplasms). The remainder of this section focuses on the clonal hematopoietic disorders that arise in the bone marrow.

B. **Clonal hematopoietic disorders**

1. Three groups of clonal hematopoietic disorders are distinguished by their clinical and laboratory features: **chronic myeloproliferative disorders, myelodysplastic syndromes,** and **acute leukemias.** All arise from hematopoietic cells at early stages of differentiation in the bone marrow (i.e., stem cells, progenitors, early precursors). Consequently, all clonal hematopoietic disorders present with clinical and laboratory evidence of bone marrow dysfunction with or without concomitant involvement of the peripheral blood. Figures 15–2 to 15–4 illustrate the points at which clonal transformations may occur and the influence of the events on subsequent hematopoietic differentiation.

2. **Chronic myeloproliferative disorders** (see Chapter 16)

   a. The myeloproliferative disorders arise when acquired genetic alterations at the stem cell level result in overproduction of one or more nonlymphoid elements in the bone marrow (Fig. 15–2). The initial defect increases production along the affected lineages but does not prevent maturation. Precursors and mature cells accumulate in the marrow and peripheral bloodstream. In addition, the clonal stem cells seed the spleen, resulting in variable degrees of **splenomegaly.**

   b. Four major categories are recognized according to their lineages and clinical presentation:

      (1) **Chronic myelogenous leukemia (CML)** (granulocytes and monocytes)

      (2) **Polycythemia vera** (erythrocytes)

      (3) **Essential thrombocytosis** (megakaryocytes and platelets)

      (4) **Myelofibrosis with myeloid metaplasia (MMM)** (megakaryocytes and marrow fibrosis)

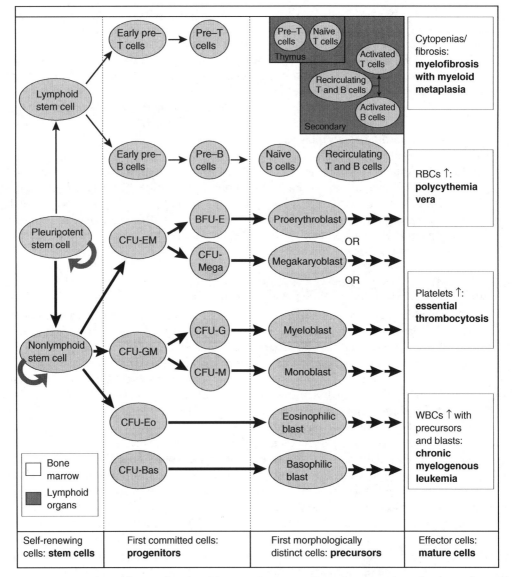

FIGURE 15–2. Myeloproliferative disorders. The curved arrows indicate the point where clonal transformation most likely occurs. The heavy lines and arrows indicate which cells are affected by the clonal transformation. The boxed text at the right details the major finding in the peripheral blood for each of the disorders. *BFU-E,* burst-forming unit, erythrocytes; *CFU-Bas,* colony-forming unit, basophils; *CFU-EM,* colony-forming unit, erythrocytes and megakaryocytes; *CFU-Eo,* colony-forming unit, eosinophils; *CFU-G,* colony-forming unit, granulocytes; *CFU-GM,* colony-forming unit, granulocytes and macrophages; *CFU-M,* colony-forming unit, macrophages; *CFU-Mega,* colony-forming unit, megakaryocytes; *RBCs,* red blood cells; *WBCs,* white blood cells.

    c. All myeloproliferative disorders can progress to **acute leukemia.** The risk of progression is greatest (approaching 100%) in CML.

    d. The myeloproliferative disorders can also progress to a spent phase, when marrow fibrosis and extensive extramedullary hematopoiesis are the primary features. In patients with MMM, myelofibrosis and extramedullary hematopoiesis are the presenting features.

    e. The genetic basis for CML (chronic phase) is known and provides the basis for its diagnosis and a target for new therapies.

(1) CML develops when a reciprocal translocation between chromosomes 9 and 22 creates a truncated chromosome 22 carrying a functional *bcr-abl* transgene.

(2) Routine karyotyping detects the truncated chromosome 22 (Philadelphia chromosome) in approximately 90% of patients. In the remainder of patients, fluorescent in situ hybridization or reverse transcriptase polymerase chain reaction must be used to detect the *bcr-abl* fusion gene at the molecular level.

(3) The *bcr-abl* fusion gene encodes functional tyrosine kinase that produces a disease resembling human CML when expressed in murine hematopoietic cells.

(4) A recently released tyrosine kinase inhibitor dramatically reduces the cell count in CML patients, confirming a causal link between the neoenzyme and chronic–phase disease.

3. **Myelodysplastic syndromes** (See Chapter 16)

a. The myelodysplastic syndromes arise when acquired defects at the stem cell level produce severe structural abnormalities during maturation and premature cell destruction (Fig. 15–3).

b. Consequently, patients have peripheral cytopenias, hypercellular bone marrow, and cytologically abnormal cells at all stages of differentiation in the bone marrow and peripheral blood. Abnormal granulocytes with two lobes (pseudo–Pelger-Huëet cells), giant platelets, and a variety of dysmorphic RBCs may be visible in the peripheral blood.

c. A variety of clonal cytogenetic abnormalities are associated with myelodysplastic syndromes, but the molecular genetic causes of the disorders are unknown.

d. Patients may die of complications resulting from thrombocytopenia (bleeding) or neutropenia (infections).

e. As in the myeloproliferative disorders, progression to **acute leukemia** occurs in a substantial number of patients, particularly those with treatment-related myelodysplastic syndromes (i.e., myelodysplastic syndromes that occur after therapy with myelosuppressive drugs or radiation).

4. **Acute leukemias** (See Chapter 17)

a. Acute leukemia develops when acquired defects result in clonal expansion without significant maturation beyond the earliest stages of precursor development (Fig. 15–4).

b. Blast forms rapidly accumulate in the bone marrow and frequently but not always enter the bloodstream in large numbers.

c. The rapidity of clonal expansion compromises the normal bone marrow, producing signs and symptoms of bone marrow failure (bruising, fatigue, infections resulting from cytopenia). Patients generally present with peripheral cytopenia, variable (sometimes massive) numbers of blast forms in the bloodstream, and hypercellular marrow infiltrated with the malignant blast forms. The malignant blasts must account for more than 20% of the bone marrow or peripheral blood leukocytes for a diagnosis of acute leukemia. Lesser numbers of blast forms are seen in myeloproliferative and myelodysplastic disorders.

d. Acute leukemias are divided into two broad groups based on lineage, as defined by their cytologic, antigenic, and biochemical features (Fig. 15–4).

(1) **Acute lymphoblastic leukemias (ALL)** consist of blast forms with the antigenic characteristics of pre–B cells, pre–T cells and (rarely) naive B-cells

(2) **Acute myelogenous leukemias (AML)** consist of blast forms with the

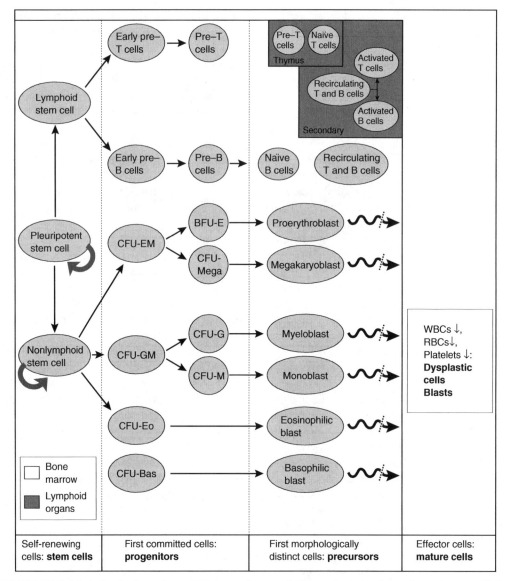

FIGURE 15–3. Myelodysplastic syndromes. The curved arrows indicate where clonal transformation most likely occurs. The wavy lines with dotted slashes indicate the lineages that develop structural abnormalities and die prematurely. The boxed text at the right details the major finding in the peripheral blood for these disorders. *BFU-E,* burst-forming unit, erythrocytes; *CFU-Bas,* colony-forming unit, basophils; *CFU-EM,* colony-forming unit, erythrocytes and megakaryocytes; *CFU-Eo,* colony-forming unit, eosinophils; *CFU-G,* colony-forming unit, granulocytes; *CFU-GM,* colony-forming unit, granulocytes and macrophages; *CFU-M,* colony-forming unit, macrophages; *CFU-Mega,* colony-forming unit, megakaryocytes; *RBCs,* red blood cells; *WBCs,* white blood cells.

antigenic and/or enzymatic characteristics of one or more nonlymphoid precursors (most often granulocytic or monocytic precursors).

VII. LYMPHOMAS

A. Overview. The term *lymphoma* is applied to a variety of lymphoid malignancies that generally arise outside of the bone marrow and present with tissue infiltrates.

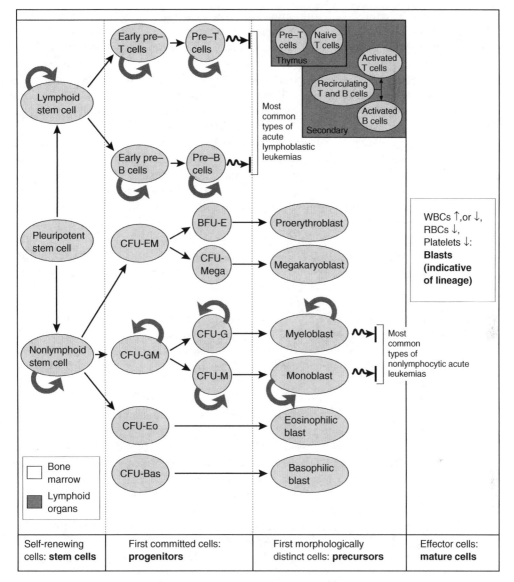

FIGURE 15–4. Acute leukemias. The curved arrows indicate potential transformation points for the acute pre–T cell, acute pre–B cell, and some acute myelogenous leukemias. The wavy lines with solid slashes indicate where transformation limits further differentiation, resulting in accumulation of early precursors. The boxed text at the right details the major findings in the peripheral blood. *BFU-E*, burst-forming unit, erythrocytes; *CFU-Bas*, colony-forming unit, basophils; *CFU-EM*, colony-forming unit, erythrocytes and megakaryocytes; *CFU-Eo*, colony-forming unit, eosinophils; *CFU-G*, colony-forming unit, granulocytes; *CFU-GM*, colony-forming unit, granulocytes and macrophages; *CFU-M*, colony-forming unit, macrophages; *CFU-Mega*, colony-forming unit, megakaryocytes; *RBCs*, red blood cells; *WBCs*, white blood cells.

The neoplasms of nonlymphoid hematopoietic cells generally present with bone marrow involvement because most stages of normal differentiation occur in this organ. However, neoplasms of lymphoid cells may present in the bone marrow, the peripheral lymphoid organs, or nonlymphoid organs because normal differentiation and trafficking involves all of these sites. Furthermore, the functional attributes of the parent cell are frequently retained after neoplastic transformation. For example, malignancies that arise from plasma cells (e.g., **multiple myeloma, Waldenström macroglobulinemia**) (see Chapter 20) generally secrete large quantities of monoclonal immunoglobulin, producing monoclonal gammopathy. Also, malignancies that arise from lymphocytes found in secondary lymphoid organs (e.g., **non-Hodgkin lymphomas**) may retain the adhesion and chemokine receptors responsible for recirculation through lymph nodes. Consequently, non-Hodgkin lymphomas may spread through the bloodstream to multiple noncontiguous lymph nodes early in the course of disease.

B. **Clinical presentation of lymphomas.** The lymphoid malignancies that arise outside of the bone marrow generally present as a tumor (mass) of clonal cells. The lymph nodes, spleen, skin, gut-associated lymphoid tissues, bone marrow, thymus, and many nonlymphoid organs may be involved initially, reflecting the functional diversity within this group of neoplasms (Fig. 15–5). The lymphomas that arise from lymphocytes found in lymph nodes generally present with lymph node enlargement (**lymphadenopathy**) involving one or more frequently noncontiguous chains. Involvement of the spleen may occur alone or in concert with other sites, producing **splenomegaly**. However, lymphadenopathy and splenomegaly are nonspecific signs. Normal and pathologic immune reactions, metabolic storage diseases, metastatic cancers of any type, and hemodynamic alterations in the spleen (e.g., portal hypertension) can also produce these signs.

C. **Diagnosis and classification of lymphomas.** Lymphomas are diagnosed and classified according to the cytologic characteristics of the malignant cells, the histopathology of their tissue infiltrates, and the antigenic or genetic profiles of the neoplastic cells.

1. **Diagnosis of lymphomas.** To establish a diagnosis of lymphoma it is necessary to obtain a biopsy of tissues infiltrated by the malignant cells.

   a. The major clinical question facing the practitioner is when to perform a biopsy. Lymphadenopathy is most commonly secondary to a local or systemic nonneoplastic disorder. However, lymphadenopathy that is massive, involves multiple noncontinuous chains, progresses, or cannot be attributed to a known local or systemic disease should prompt a biopsy.

   b. The pathologist generally processes the specimen for multiple studies depending on its size and the clinical differential diagnosis. A portion is fixed and stained for microscopic examination, another portion is processed for Ag or genetic analysis, and a portion may be cultured if infection is a consideration.

2. **Classification of lymphomas** (see Chapter 18)

   a. The lymphomas are a diverse group of malignancies that from a clinical perspective include the non-Hodgkin lymphomas, Hodgkin disease, and a variety of other lymphoid malignancies that may produce tissue infiltrates outside the bone marrow.

   b. Several lymphomas are biologically and clinically related to lymphoid leukemia. These neoplasms arise at the stages of lymphocyte development when trafficking between organs and tissues normally occurs.

      (1) **Acute lymphoblastic leukemia** (pre–T-cell type) and **lymphoblastic lymphoma** both arise from pre–T cells (Fig. 15–5). The malignant cells look the same and have identical antigenic profiles. The management, treatment, and overall prognosis are the same.

         (a) Acute lymphoblastic leukemia (pre–T-cell type) is diagnosed if the patient primarily manifests bone marrow and peripheral blood involvement.

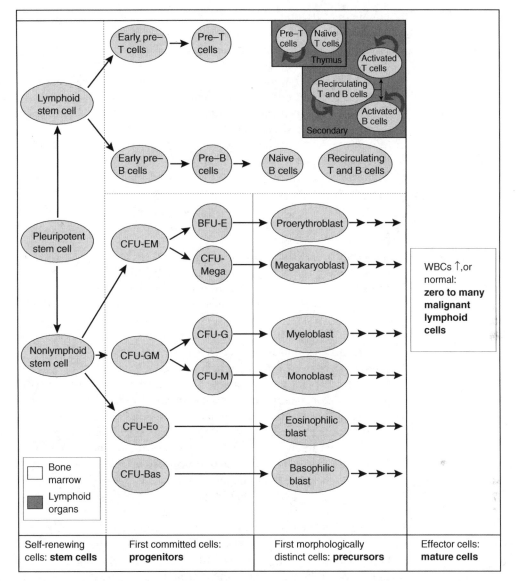

FIGURE 15–5. Non-Hodgkin lymphomas. The curved arrows show several points where clonal transformation results in the development of lymphomas. The boxed text at the right details the major finding in the peripheral blood. *BFU-E,* burst-forming unit, erythrocytes; *CFU-Bas,* colony-forming unit, basophils; *CFU-EM,* colony-forming unit, erythrocytes and megakaryocytes; *CFU-Eo,* colony-forming unit, eosinophils; *CFU-G,* colony-forming unit, granulocytes; *CFU-GM,* colony-forming unit, granulocytes and macrophages; *CFU-M,* colony-forming unit, macrophages; *CFU-Mega,* colony-forming unit, megakaryocytes; *WBCs,* white blood cells.

    (b) Lymphoblastic lymphoma is diagnosed if thymic enlargement is the principle feature at presentation.

  (2) Chronic lymphocytic leukemia and **small lymphocytic lymphoma** arise from small, inactive-appearing lymphocytes that readily circulate through the bone marrow, spleen, and lymph nodes (Fig. 15–5). In some cases, patients mainly have bone marrow, peripheral blood, and splenic involvement. In other cases, lymphadenopathy with minimal peripheral blood and bone marrow involvement occurs initially. The malignant cells look the same and share antigenic profiles. The diseases also pursue similar clinical courses.

(3) **Non-Hodgkin lymphomas** retain the trafficking behavior of normal lymphocytes; thus, they can spread through both the bloodstream and lymphatics. In addition, non-Hodgkin lymphomas may develop a leukemic phase, when large numbers of malignant cells enter the peripheral blood. This complication generally reflects a progression in the disease that increases the risk of widespread hematogenous metastases.

c. The confusing relationships between the various types of lymphoid neoplasms prompted revision of the classification system in 1994.

(1) The new system, the Revised European–American classification of Lymphoid Neoplasms (REAL), divides lymphoid neoplasms into four categories based on morphologic and antigenic characteristics:

(a) Precursor B-cell neoplasms

(b) Precursor T-cell neoplasms

(c) Peripheral B-cell neoplasms

(d) Peripheral T-cell and natural killer cell neoplasms

(2) These categories are further subdivided based on the clinical, morphologic, immunophenotypic, and genotypic differences among the lymphoid neoplasms.

(a) Disease names in common use are retained. For example, **follicular, diffuse,** and **mantle cell** designations for three types of B-cell lymphomas are retained and combined with a variety of other neoplasms of mature B cells in the peripheral B-cell neoplasm group.

(b) In addition, neoplasms that are antigenically identical but capable of presenting as either leukemia or lymphoma are combined under a single diagnostic category. For example, T-cell acute lymphoblastic leukemia and lymphoblastic lymphoma are combined as **precursor T lymphoblastic leukemia/lymphoma** in the precursor T-cell neoplasm group. Chronic lymphocytic leukemia and small lymphocytic lymphoma are combined as **chronic lymphocytic leukemia/small lymphocytic lymphoma** in the peripheral B-cell neoplasm group.

(3) The REAL system provides an inclusive framework for all lymphoid neoplasms except Hodgkin disease. The distinctive pattern of spread for Hodgkin disease (i.e., through contiguous lymph nodes and lymph node chains, generally before dissemination) and some uncertainty regarding the lineage of the malignant cell in Hodgkin disease warrant a separate classification system at present (see Chapter 19).

VIII. SUMMARY

The hematopoietic neoplasms are a diverse and complex group of diseases. However, a clear understanding of normal hematopoietic differentiation and leukocyte trafficking behavior will help the student remember the origins, interrelationships, and clinical presentations of these clonal disorders.

SUGGESTED READING

Cotran RS, Kumar V, Collins T, eds. *Robbin's Pathologic Basis of Disease.* 6th ed. Philadelphia: Saunders, 1999.

Janeway CA, Travers P, Walport M, Capra JB. Immunobiology-The Immune System in Health and Disease. 4th ed. London: Elsevier Science Ltd/Garland Publishing, 1999

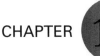

CHAPTER 16

Myeloid Stem Cell Disorders

• HARRY P. ERBA

I. INTRODUCTION

Granulocytes, erythrocytes, and platelets all differentiate from a primitive myeloid stem cell. Disorders of the myeloid stem cell proliferation and differentiation may therefore cause four abnormalities in the quantity and/or quality of these differentiated blood cells. Decreased number of stem cells will lead to aplastic anemia and decreased numbers of cells in each lineage (cytopenias). The cells present will retain normal function. On the other hand, dysplastic maturation of the myeloid stem cell as seen in the myelodysplastic syndromes typically causes both cytopenia and abnormal function of the mature blood cells. Finally, uncontrolled hyperplastic proliferation and differentiation of the myeloid stem cells defines the myeloproliferative disorders. These disorders cause increased numbers of the mature blood elements (-cytosis).

II. APLASTIC ANEMIA

A. **Overview.** Aplastic anemia (AA) is defined as peripheral blood **pancytopenia** with **bone marrow hypocellularity** (i.e., < 25% cellular). Severe AA is defined by an absolute neutrophil count less than $500/\mu L$, a platelet count less than $20,000/\mu L$, and an absolute reticulocyte count less than $50,000/\mu L$.

B. **Pathophysiology.** There is evidence that the normal development of the hematopoietic stem cell (HSC) may be suppressed by the immune system in AA. Spontaneous remission of idiopathic AA after failed bone marrow transplantation led to the hypothesis that the immunosuppressive conditioning regimen allowed return of normal hematopoiesis. These observations spawned successful clinical trials of immunosuppressive agents in patients with AA (see II.F.3.). Therefore, in many cases AA is a form of **autoimmune disease.**

C. **Etiology.** The causes of AA can be classified as idiopathic, secondary, or inherited (Table 16–1).

1. Approximately 50% of AA cases are idiopathic.

2. Secondary causes of AA should be excluded by appropriate history and laboratory investigation.

3. Other physical anomalies may suggest an inherited cause of AA. For example, café au lait spots, short stature, thumb abnormalities, and renal malformations are frequent findings in patients with Fanconi anemia. The diagnosis of

TABLE 16–1 • Classification of Aplastic Anemia

Idiopathic aplastic anemia
Secondary aplastic anemia
    Ionizing radiation
    Cytotoxic chemotherapy
    Benzene
    Idiosyncratic drug reactions
        Chloramphenicol
        Sulfonamides
        Nonsteroidal anti-inflammatory drugs
        Gold salts
        Arsenic
        Carbonic anhydrase inhibitors
        Antiepileptics (e.g., diphenylhydantoin)
    Viruses
        Epstein-Barr virus
        Hepatitis viruses
    Pregnancy
    Immune-mediated diseases
        Transfusion-associated graft versus host disease
    Eosinophilic fasciitis
    Thymoma
    Paroxysmal nocturnal hemoglobinuria
Inherited aplastic anemia
    Fanconi anemia

Fanconi anemia is confirmed by demonstrating increased rates of sister chromatid exchange in peripheral blood lymphocytes in response to agents such as diepoxybutane and bleomycin.

D. **Clinical presentation.** Patients with AA usually present with symptoms and signs of **bone marrow failure.**

1. Anemia leads to pallor, weakness, fatigue, dyspnea on exertion, palpitations, exertional chest pain, headache, and pounding tinnitus.

2. Thrombocytopenic hemorrhage may take the form of easy bruising, petechiae (especially in dependent areas or in tissues with increased hydrostatic pressure), gingival bleeding, epistaxis, and menorrhagia.

3. Neutropenic infections occur but typically are not the reason for seeking medical attention.

4. Constitutional symptoms, adenopathy, and splenomegaly should all suggest alternative causes of pancytopenia.

E. **Differential diagnosis: laboratory evaluation of pancytopenia.** Pancytopenia may be caused by a number of intrinsic defects of bone marrow function or extramedullary diseases (Table 16–2).

1. History and physical examination can usually exclude extramedullary causes of pancytopenia (e.g., sepsis, hypersplenism, systemic lupus erythematosus).

2. Megaloblastic changes seen on the peripheral blood smear may suggest deficiency of cobalamin or folic acid, which can be confirmed by serum assays for these vitamins.

3. Patients receiving cytotoxic chemotherapy or ionizing radiation therapy have predictable, reversible pancytopenia that does not require further investigation.

TABLE 16–2 • Causes of Pancytopenia

Aplastic anemia
   Idiopathic
   Secondary
   Inherited
Myelodysplastic syndromes
Bone marrow infiltration
   Leukemia
   Lymphoma
   Myeloma
   Carcinoma
   Granulomatous diseases (e.g., sarcoidosis)
   Fibrosis
   Congenital storage disorders (e.g., Gaucher disease)
Nutritional deficiencies
   Vitamin B_{12} deficiency
   Folic acid deficiency
Bone marrow toxins
   Alcohol
Hypersplenism
Sepsis
Systemic disorders

---

4. Examination of a bone marrow core biopsy (Fig. 16–1) with aspirate is required for the diagnosis of AA and the exclusion of myelodysplastic syndromes and bone marrow infiltrative disorders. Hypocellular variants of acute leukemia or myelodysplastic syndromes can be distinguished from AA by bone marrow morphology and the presence of clonal cytogenetic abnormalities in both acute leukemia and myelodysplastic syndromes.

F. **Treatment.** Supportive care, allogeneic HSC transplantation, and immunosuppressive therapy all play a role in the treatment of AA.

1. **Supportive care**

   a. Many practices have been advocated for the prevention of infection in neutropenic patients, including avoidance of fresh flowers, abstinence from fresh fruits and vegetables, isolation in laminar airflow rooms, and oral administration of nonabsorbable antibiotics to sterilize the intestinal tract. None of these preventive measures have been shown to be superior to adequate **handwashing** alone.

   b. **Antibiotics** are the mainstay of therapy for patients with neutropenic infections. The risk of infection increases with the duration of neutropenia, the severity of neutropenia (absolute neutrophil count $< 1000/\mu L$ associated with increased risk and $< 100/\mu L$ associated with highest risk), and the presence of indwelling IV catheters. Neutropenic patients are at greatest risk for bacterial and fungal infections.

   c. **Granulocyte colony-stimulating factor (G-CSF) and granulocyte-macrophage colony-stimulating factor (GM-CSF)** can lead to improvement of the neutrophil count, especially when given in high doses. Unfortunately, response rates are lowest in AA patients with the most severe neutropenia. Granulocyte transfusions are sometimes prescribed in desperate situations (e.g., sepsis unresponsive to antibiotics). Patients treated with

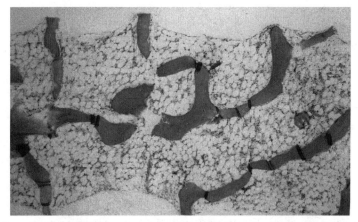

FIGURE 16–1. Posterior iliac crest bone marrow core biopsy from patient with severe aplastic anemia. Normal hematopoietic cells are virtually absent. Most of the marrow cellularity is composed of adipose cells.

granulocyte transfusions may develop adult respiratory distress syndrome, febrile reactions, and cytomegalovirus infection.

d. The trigger for **red blood cell (RBC) transfusion** depends on the physiologic status of the patient. For example, patients with cardiovascular disease should be maintained at higher hemoglobin (Hb) levels. Each unit of packed RBCs contains 200–250 mg of iron that will accumulate in the body; therefore, transfusion-related hemochromatosis can cause cirrhosis with hepatic failure, cardiomyopathy, arthritis, and endocrinopathies (e.g., diabetes mellitus, hypopituitarism). Iron chelation therapy with desferrioxamine mesylate should be considered for patients who have received more than 25–50 units RBC transfusion and are expected to have an extended survival.

e. **Androgens** can stimulate erythropoiesis in AA patients, but these drugs can cause virilization and hepatotoxicity.

f. The value of **prophylactic platelet transfusion** for prevention of life-threatening hemorrhage or increased survival has never been proved. If prophylactic platelet transfusion is used, it is reasonable to maintain the platelet count above $5000/\mu L$. Patients become refractory to repeated platelet transfusion. The development of anti–human leukocyte antigen (HLA) antibodies (alloimmunization) in AA patients leads to decreased platelet survival. Analgesics that cause a qualitative platelet defect (e.g., aspirin, nonsteroidal antiinflammatory drugs) should be avoided in the thrombocytopenic patient.

2. **Allogeneic hematopoietic stem cell transplantation**

a. Normal hematopoiesis can be reconstituted in AA patients by transplantation of HLA-matched HSCs. Recent studies have reported an 80% survival rate for AA patients undergoing allogeneic HSC transplantation.

b. Patients receive an immunosuppressive conditioning regimen, such as high-dose cyclophosphamide, antithymocyte globulin (ATG), and total body irradiation, before allogeneic HSC infusion to allow donor cell engraftment. Even an identical twin donor (syngeneic donor) requires significant immunosuppression to prevent graft failure.

c. Most patients do not have an HLA-identical family member donor available. Unrelated donors are available through the National Marrow Donor

Program, but the risk of significant posttransplant complications (including death) is higher.

d. Late complications of allogeneic HSC transplantation include graft failure, acute and chronic graft versus host disease (GVHD), and second malignancies. Because the risk of graft rejection rises with the number of pretransplant transfusions, transfusions should be limited in patients who are potential candidates for HSC transplant.

3. **Immunosuppressive therapy**

a. Infusion of **ATG or antilymphocyte globulin (ALG)** can result in restoration of normal hematopoiesis. These products are heterologous sera from horses or rabbits that have been immunized with human thymocytes or lymphocytes. Hematologic improvement occurs in approximately 50% of AA patients; however, remission can take 1–3 months (significantly longer than with allogeneic HSC transplantation). The major toxicity of ATG and ALG is serum sickness characterized by fever, chills, rash, and arthritis. Corticosteroids are typically administered with ATG and ALG to decrease the risk of allergic reaction.

b. **Cyclosporine** can lead to hematologic remissions in 50% of AA patients. The toxicities of cyclosporine include hypertension, hirsutism, renal insufficiency, tremors, opportunistic infections, and thrombotic thrombocytopenic purpura. The combination of cyclosporine with ATG or ALG produces higher response rates (i.e., 70%–80%) than ATG or ALG alone.

c. Immunosuppressive therapy is associated with a number of late complications that are not seen after allogeneic HSC transplantation. **Relapse** occurs in 30%–90% of initial responders to immunosuppressive therapy, depending on the study and length of follow-up. A minority of patients develop **clonal HSC disorders,** such as myelodysplastic syndrome, acute myelocytic leukemia (AML), or paroxysmal nocturnal hemoglobinuria.

d. The choice between allogeneic HSC transplantation and immunosuppressive therapy for AA patients depends on a number of factors. Age above 40 years, active infection, and extensive prior transfusion are risk factors for serious morbidity and mortality after allogeneic HSC transplantation. Donor availability, cost, and patient preference are other considerations. In the past 10 years, survival of AA patients treated with bone marrow transplantation or immunosuppressive therapy is the same (i.e., approximately 80% at 5 years).

III. CLONAL MYELOID STEM CELL DISORDERS

A. **Overview.** Two broad classes of clonal myeloid stem cell disorders are the **myelodysplastic syndromes (MDS)** and the **myeloproliferative diseases (MPD),** such as chronic myelocytic leukemia (CML), polycythemia vera (PCV), essential thrombocythemia (ET), and myelofibrosis with myeloid metaplasia (MMM).

1. Patients with MDS usually present with cytopenias. Patients with MPD tend to present with an elevated blood count and splenomegaly. Some patients have features of both MDS and MPD. All patients with MDS and MPD have a finite risk of developing **AML.**

2. Unlike most cases of AA, MDS and MPD are clonal stem cell diseases. Clonality can be detected by any of several assays. Glucose-6-phosphate dehydrogenase is an X-encoded enzyme with many polymorphic isoforms that has been used for determination of clonality in MPD and MDS. Cytogenetic

analysis of bone marrow hematopoietic progenitor cells from patients with MDS and MPD may also demonstrate a structural or numeric alteration of the normal diploid karyotype. All cells derived from the same clonal event inherit the same cytogenetic abnormality. The absence of a cytogenetic abnormality does not necessarily rule out a clonal myeloid stem cell process.

B. **Myelodysplastic syndromes**

1. **Overview.** MDS refers to a heterogeneous group of acquired **bone marrow failure** disorders. MDS has been given various names over the years, including refractory anemia, dysmyelopoietic syndrome, oligoclonal leukemia, smoldering leukemia, and preleukemia. Many of the old terms reflect the tendency of MDS to progress to AML. Historically, this group of disorders was recognized as a cause of peripheral blood cytopenias not caused by nutritional deficiencies. MDS is characterized by peripheral blood cytopenias with morphologic evidence of dysplasia in the bone marrow progenitor cells. The bone marrow is typically hypercellular, which indicates ineffective hematopoiesis. The incidence of MDS increases with age. Although the overall annual incidence of MDS is 6–10 in 100,000 people, the incidence in individuals over 80 years of age is 89 in 100,000 people.

2. **Pathogenesis.** The pathogenesis of MDS remains incompletely understood.

   a. Abnormal differentiation of the HSC in MDS may be a result of **genetic mutation.** Depending on the patient population and the sensitivity of the analysis, 30%–70% of patients with MDS have cytogenetic abnormalities. Deletions of the long arm of chromosomes 5 and 7 are frequently found in MDS. Although a number of genes important for hematopoietic maturation map to chromosome 5q, no candidate gene has been identified. Only a minority of MDS patients have a mutation of a known oncogene (e.g., *ras*) or tumor suppressor gene (e.g., p53, Rb).

   b. Other factors have also been implicated in the pathogenesis of MDS. Accelerated apoptosis is characteristic of myelodysplastic bone marrow. Neoangiogenesis has been associated with progression of MDS. As in idiopathic AA, evidence suggests that immunologic suppression of normal hematopoiesis occurs in MDS.

3. **Natural history and prognosis.** MDS may progress to AML with more than 20% myeloblasts in the peripheral blood or bone marrow. Alternatively, patients with MDS may succumb to the complications of cytopenias (e.g., neutropenic infection, thrombocytopenic hemorrhage). Because MDS is a disease of the elderly, patients may also die of unrelated causes. Patients with MDS have a wide variation in both survival and risk of transformation to AML.

   a. The French-American-British (FAB) working group first attempted to address this heterogeneity by subcategorizing MDS. The FAB classification scheme uses percentage of peripheral blood and bone marrow blasts, the presence of ringed sideroblasts and Auer rods, and the absolute number of circulating monocytes. Five subgroups of MDS are thereby described: refractory anemia (RA), refractory anemia with ringed sideroblasts (RArs), refractory anemia with excess blasts (RAEB), refractory anemia with excess blasts in transformation (RAEBT), and chronic myelomonocytic leukemia (CMML). Survival and risk of transformation to AML are related to the FAB classification, with RAEB and RAEBT carrying the worst prognosis (Fig. 16–2).

   b. Recently, the International MDS Risk Analysis Workshop developed the International Prognostic Scoring System (IPSS). Researchers analyzed data from patients with *de novo* MDS who had received only hematopoietic

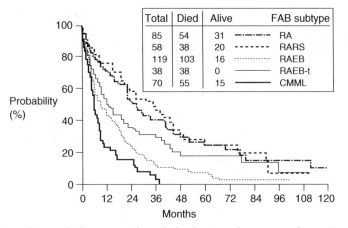

Total	Died	Alive	FAB subtype
85	54	31	RA
58	38	20	RARS
119	103	16	RAEB
38	38	0	RAEB-t
70	55	15	CMML

FIGURE 16–2. Overall survival of patients with myelodysplastic syndromes according to French-American-British (FAB) classification. *CMML*, chronic myelomonocytic leukemia; *RA*, refractory anemia; *RAEB*, refractory anemia with excess blasts; *RAEBT*, refractory anemia with excess blasts in transformation; *RArs*, refractory anemia with ringed sideroblasts. (Reprinted with permission from Sanz GF et al. Two regression models and a scoring system for predicting survival and planning treatment in myelodysplastic syndromes: a multivariate analysis of prognostic factors in 370 patients. *Blood* 1989;74:395–408.)

growth factors or supportive care. The IPSS uses the number of cytopenias, percentage of bone marrow blasts, and cytogenetic risk group to define four risk groups in MDS (Table 16–3). The time to progression to AML and overall survival are related to the prognostic risk group. Patients with treatment-related MDS have an especially poor prognosis.

4. **Etiology.** The cause of MDS in an individual patient is not usually apparent. However, it can be the result of either inherited disorders or acquired following exposure to marrow-toxic agents.

   a. Young patients with MDS often have a **familial hematologic disorder** or a **congenital defect in DNA repair** (e.g., Fanconi anemia).

   b. **Benzene** may cause MDS as well as AA and AML.

   c. MDS may be a complication of **chemotherapy** or **ionizing radiation** exposure. Of the cytotoxic chemotherapy drugs, **alkylating agents** (e.g., nitrogen mustard, chlorambucil, melphalan, cyclophosphamide) are the most likely to induce MDS. MDS usually occurs more than a year after exposure

TABLE 16–3 • International Prognostic Scoring System for Patients with Myelodysplastic Syndromes

Cytopenia	Marrow Blasts (%)	Cytogenetics[a]	Score
0–1	< 5	Good	0.0
2–3	5–10	Intermediate	0.5
		Poor	1.0
	11–20		1.5
	21–30		2.0

Risk groups: low, 0; intermediate 1, 0.5–1; intermediate 2, 1.5–2; high, ≥ 2.5.
[a]The bone marrow karyotypes with a relatively good prognosis are normal diploid, del(5q) alone, del(20q), and −Y. The poor-risk cytogenetic group includes patients with complex karyotypes (i.e., more than three abnormalities) and chromosome 7 abnormalities.

to chemotherapy. The incidence of treatment-related MDS peaks 4–5 years after cytotoxic drug exposure.

d. Treatment-related MDS may also be a late complication of **autologous HSC transplantation** for non-Hodgkin lymphoma in more than 15% of patients.

5. **Clinical presentation.** Patients with MDS have symptoms related to **peripheral blood cytopenias.** However, the diagnosis may be made in the asymptomatic patient after a routine complete blood count. Patients with MDS may have single-lineage cytopenias, bicytopenia, or pancytopenia. The presence of **adenopathy** and **splenomegaly** is more common in MDS than AA.

6. **Laboratory evaluation.** The diagnosis of MDS is made by careful morphologic examination of a **peripheral blood smear** and **bone marrow aspirate.**

   a. Peripheral blood erythrocytes may display anisocytosis, poikilocytosis, teardrop forms, nucleated cells, and macrocytosis. Dyserythropoietic features of the bone marrow include **megaloblastic maturation** and **abnormalities of the erythroblast nuclei** (e.g., budding, fragmentation, internuclear bridging). Ringed sideroblasts are erythroblasts with Prussian blue–positive granules surrounding the cell nucleus (Fig. 16–3A). These granules are iron-laden mitochondria.

   b. Cytoplasmic hypogranulation of neutrophils and granulocytic precursors as well as nuclear hyposegmentation or hypersegmentation of neutrophils are hallmarks of dysplastic maturation (Fig. 16–3B). Myeloblasts may account for up to 30% of marrow nucleated cells according to the FAB classification system or for up to 20% of marrow cells according to WHO classification. Auer rods, which are linear aggregates of primary granules, can at times be identified in these cells.

   c. Patients with MDS may have giant hypogranular platelets and exhibit prolonged bleeding time. Dysplastic megakaryocytes may be small (micromegakaryocytes) or contain multiple separate nuclei (pawn ball nuclei).

   d. Further laboratory tests may be needed to exclude other causes of peripheral blood cytopenias. Specifically, megaloblastic anemias caused by deficiency of folic acid or cobalamin can be difficult to distinguish from MDS by morphologic examination alone. Measurement of folic acid and cobalamin levels and/or response to replacement therapy allows one to distinguish the disorders. Certain viral infections, especially HIV, can cause dysplastic bone marrow changes that are not clonal.

7. **Treatment.** The only potentially curative treatment of MDS is **allogeneic HSC transplantation;** no other intervention has been shown to extend survival of MDS patients.

   a. After allogeneic HSC transplantation for MDS, disease-free survival of MDS patients is 40%–45%. However, a number of factors, including advanced age, high IPSS risk group, treatment-related MDS, increasing disease duration, advanced FAB subtype, and certain cytogenetic abnormalities, adversely affect survival and relapse rates. Most MDS patients are not suitable candidates for allogeneic HSC transplantation; supportive care alone remains the standard of care for these patients (see II.F.1.).

   b. Hematopoietic growth factors have also been used in patients with MDS.

      (1) **GM-CSF** and **G-CSF** increase the neutrophil count in approximately 80% of MDS patients. There does not appear to be an increased risk of transformation to AML. GM-CSF may decrease the risk of major infection in neutropenic MDS patients.

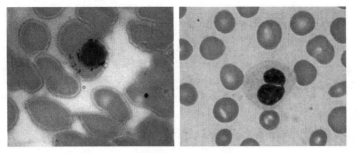

FIGURE 16–3. Morphologic features of peripheral blood and bone marrow cells in myelodysplastic syndromes. **A.** Prussian blue stain demonstrating a ringed sideroblast. **B.** Hypogranular neutrophil with a bilobed nucleus (Pelger-Huët nuclear anomaly).

        (2) High doses of **erythropoietin (EPO)** may lead to improvement of the Hb and hematocrit (Hct). The response rate depends on the patient's pretreatment endogenous EPO level; EPO levels less than 0.5 mU/mL are associated with a greater chance of response.

    c. A variety of therapeutic approaches have been taken in MDS.

        (1) A number of agents, such as **cytarabine** and **azacitidine**, induce HSC differentiation in MDS patients.

        (2) Patients with hypoplastic MDS may respond to immunosuppressive regimens, including **ATG** or **cyclosporine.**

        (3) **Intensive chemotherapy** similar to that used for AML induction therapy may result in complete remission of MDS. However, the period of marrow aplasia is prolonged in these patients, and mortality is increased by neutropenic infections, and the duration of complete remission is typically short.

C. **Myeloproliferative disorders**

  1. **Chronic myelocytic leukemia**

    a. **Overview.** CML is a clonal stem cell disorder. The annual incidence of CML is 1 in 100,000 people, accounting for 15%–20% of all leukemia. There is no significant geographic or racial variation, but the disease is slightly more common in men than women (1.4:1). The peak incidence is 40 to 60 years of age.

    b. **Pathogenesis.** All myeloid elements (i.e., granulocytic, megakaryocytic, erythroid, and monocytic elements) are involved in CML. B cells are variably involved, and T cells are only rarely involved. The implication of this observation is that the transformation event in CML occurs in an early HSC capable of both myeloid and lymphoid differentiation. In contrast to MDS, granulocytic and erythroid progeny of CML stem cells mature normally, have normal life spans, and function normally. Occasionally, there is a mild qualitative platelet defect.

        (1) In 1960, Nowell and Hungerford identified an unusually short autosome, later named the **Philadelphia (Ph) chromosome,** in the white blood cells (WBCs) of CML patients. The Ph chromosome was the first genetic event associated with a malignancy. In 1973, Janet Rowley demonstrated that the Ph chromosome was the result of a reciprocal translocation involving the long arms of chromosomes 9 and 22, that is, t(9;22)(q34;q11). A decade later, Heisterkamp and colleagues reported that the Ph chromosome breakpoints were in the c-*abl* (abelson

leukemia) gene on chromosome 9 and the *bcr* (breakpoint cluster region) gene on chromosome 22, resulting in an abnormal 210-kd protein with enhanced tyrosine kinase (TK) activity. Murine HSCs transfected with the *bcr-abl* fusion gene and transplanted into lethally irradiated mice produce a syndrome closely resembling human CML; therefore, the *bcr-abl* fusion gene is necessary and sufficient to cause CML.

(2) The *abl* protooncogene is encoded on the long arm of chromosome 9 and is composed of nine exons that are homologous to v-*abl*. The translation product of c-*abl* mRNA is 145 kd and has TK activity. The *bcr* gene is on chromosome 22, contains more than 20 exons, and spans more than 100 kilobase (kb) of DNA. Two *bcr* proteins (130 and 160 kd) are widely expressed in normal tissues, but their function is not understood. The major breakpoint cluster region (M-bcr) of the *bcr* gene spans 5.8 kb and includes five exons. The Ph chromosome results from translocation between chromosomes 9 and 22 (Fig. 16–4).

(3) An 8.5-kb mRNA is produced after splicing out all introns as well as exons 1b and 1a of *abl*. The protein product is 210 kd (p210) and has enhanced TK activity. The transforming activity of *bcr-abl* depends on its TK activity. The *bcr-abl* fusion protein inhibits apoptosis, affects adhesion of hematopoietic progenitors to the marrow stromal cells, and alters normal differentiation of HSCs.

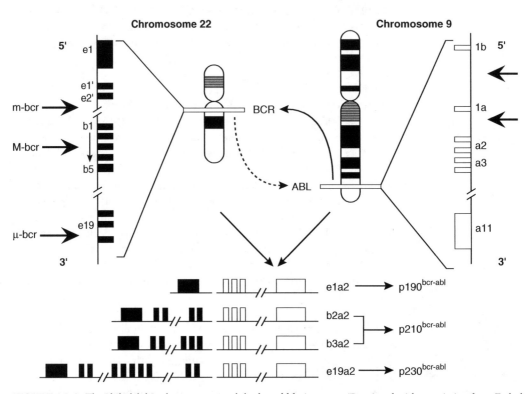

FIGURE 16–4. The Philadelphia chromosome and the *bcr-abl* fusion gene. (Reprinted with permission from Faderl S, Kantarjian H, Talpaz M. Chronic myelogenous leukemia: update on biology and treatment. *Oncology* 1999;13: 169–180. Fig. 1, p 171.)

c. **Natural history and prognosis.** The natural history of CML is divided into three phases (i.e., **chronic** or **stable phase, accelerated phase,** and **blast crisis**) that can be used to determine the prognosis.

   (1) Although most patients present in the stable phase, some present in blast crisis. CML often progresses through an accelerated phase before blast crisis and is less responsive to standard therapy during both of these phases. Blast crisis is usually the terminal event in the natural history of CML and is characterized by fever, sweats, weight loss, and bone pain. The strict definition of blast crisis is the appearance of more than 30% blasts in the peripheral blood or bone marrow. Although most patients accumulate blasts with a myeloid phenotype, one third develop a lymphoblastic crisis.

   (2) The length of the stable phase determines survival, because few patients die of disease-related complications during the stable phase. The risk of blast crisis is 10%–15% in each of the first 2 years after diagnosis of stable phase CML and increases to 25% each year thereafter.

   (3) The prognosis of CML patients who do not undergo allogeneic HSC transplantation has been well documented; the median survival of patients with hydroxyurea- or busulfan-treated CML is 3.5 years. Several continuous variables predict survival in patients who do not undergo allogeneic HSC transplantation, including percentage of peripheral blood blasts, spleen size, age, platelet count, and basophil count.

d. **Etiology. Ionizing radiation** is the only known causative agent.

e. **Clinical presentation.** Approximately 50% of CML patients are asymptomatic at presentation and are diagnosed only after routine physical examination and complete blood count. Common presenting complaints include fatigue, weight loss, abdominal fullness or pain, and easy bruising or bleeding. Most patients have splenomegaly at diagnosis; 50% have hepatomegaly. Fever and adenopathy each occur in only 10% of CML patients at diagnosis.

f. **Laboratory evaluation.** Peripheral blood smear, bone marrow aspiration, and bone marrow core biopsy are used in the diagnosis of CML.

   (1) In CML, the **peripheral blood smear** strongly suggests the disease (Fig. 16–5). Patients present with **leukocytosis;** 30% of patients have a WBC count greater than $100,000/\mu L$. Two thirds of CML patients are anemic at diagnosis. Either thrombocytopenia (10%) or thrombocytosis (50%) is present. Granulocytic precursors circulate in the peripheral blood (i.e., a left shift or shift to immaturity). Most of the granulocytes are neutrophils and myelocytes. Absolute basophilia is also characteristic of CML. Circulating nucleated normoblasts, some with dysmorphic features, and fragments of megakaryocytes are also seen on the peripheral blood smear.

   (2) The **bone marrow aspirate** and **core biopsy** are **hypercellular** in CML, with a myeloid–erythroid ratio often exceeding 20:1. There is megakaryocytic hyperplasia with frequent dwarf megakaryocytes (micromegakaryocytes). There may be mild reticulin fibrosis. Increased numbers of histiocytes (i.e., pseudo–Gaucher cells and sea-blue histiocytes) are observed, reflecting increased intramedullary cell turnover.

   (3) **Both CML and leukemoid reactions cause leukocytosis with a left shift.** A leukemoid reaction is a benign bone marrow response to a systemic inflammatory stimulus (e.g., abscess, metastatic carcinoma). Occasionally,

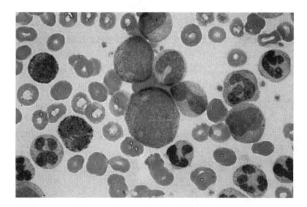

FIGURE 16–5. Peripheral blood smear of patient with chronic phase of chronic myelocytic leukemia showing a shift to immaturity (left shift) with band forms, metamyelocytes, neutrophilic myelocytes, and progranulocytes. There is also a basophil.

patients with metastatic cancer develop a leukemoid reaction before diagnosis. Several features can be used to distinguish these two processes. Patients with CML have splenomegaly and basophilia, whereas patients with leukemoid reactions do not. Leukocyte alkaline phosphatase activity is typically low in CML but elevated in leukemoid reactions.

(4) **Diagnosis of CML** (and distinction from a leukemoid reaction) **is confirmed by demonstration of the *bcr-abl* fusion gene.** Classic karyotypic analysis demonstrates the Ph chromosome in at least 90% of patients with CML. However, another 5% of CML patients have variant or complex chromosomal translocations that still result in fusion of the *bcr* and *abl* genes. The remaining CML patients do not have any evidence of the Ph chromosome by classic cytogenetics. Fluorescence *in situ* hybridization and reverse transcriptase polymerase chain reaction (RT-PCR) confirm the presence of the *bcr-abl* fusion gene in the majority of the remaining CML patients.

g. **Treatment.** Treatment methods are based on the phase of CML (i.e., chronic phase or blast crisis).

(1) **Treatment of the chronic phase**

(a) **Observation.** If the patient is asymptomatic and without significant splenomegaly, leukocytosis, or cytopenia, close observation is an option. Observation may be particularly appropriate for elderly and pregnant CML patients.

(b) **Pheresis.** Physical removal of WBCs or platelets may be necessary for treatment of CML patients. Patients with central nervous system or pulmonary symptoms or signs related to extreme leukocytosis may respond promptly to leukapheresis. Likewise, platelet-pheresis may be necessary for the treatment of severe thrombocytosis complicated by thrombosis. Cytopheresis may also be useful in the routine management of the pregnant CML patient.

(c) **Cytotoxic chemotherapy.** Standard cytotoxic chemotherapy is used to obtain hematologic remission (i.e., absence of disease-related symptoms, resolution of splenomegaly, and normalization of blood counts). However, these agents do not delay or prevent blast crisis. **Busulfan** is an orally administered DNA alkylating agent that was introduced almost 40 years ago for the treatment of stable-phase CML. This drug has a number of undesirable toxicities, including infertility, unpredictable and irreversible marrow aplasia, pneumonitis, pulmonary fibrosis, and addisonian crisis. **Hydroxyurea** is a ribonucleotide reductase inhibitor often used for control of stable-phase CML. It is administered daily by mouth. The major toxicities of hydroxyurea include reversible myelosuppression, megaloblastosis, rash, and mucocutaneous ulceration (rare). Hydroxyurea must be administered chronically for maintenance of hematologic response.

(d) **Interferon-α (IFN-α).** Treatment with IFN-α, a protein drug administered daily by subcutaneous injection, also results in a complete hematologic response in 80% of stable-phase CML patients. However, IFN-α, unlike hydroxyurea, suppresses the CML clone and delays progression to blast crisis in some patients. Cytogenetic analysis may show a decrease in the percentage of Ph chromosome–positive cells. Only 5%–25% of early stable-phase CML patients have a complete cytogenetic remission (i.e., 0% Ph chromosome–positive cells) with IFN-α therapy. Two large randomized control trials demonstrated improved survival of stable-phase CML patients treated with IFN-α compared with hydroxyurea or busulfan. Patients who attain a major cytogenetic response (< 35% Ph chromosome–positive cells) with IFN-α therapy have the greatest benefit. The addition of **cytarabine** to IFN-α increases the cytogenetic remission rate and overall survival of stable-phase CML patients compared with IFN-α alone. Toxicities of IFN-α include flu-like syndrome (fever, chills, myalgias, malaise), anorexia, cytopenias, neuropathy, depression, liver function test abnormalities, hypothyroidism, vitiligo, porphyria cutanea tarda, and immune-mediated toxicities (e.g., polymyositis, Raynaud phenomenon). Compliance with prolonged daily administration of IFN-α is difficult to maintain.

(e) **Allogeneic HSC transplantation.** Allogeneic HSC transplantation is the **only known curative therapy for stable-phase CML.** Patients receive high-dose cyclophosphamide together with busulfan or fractionated total body irradiation. Patients are then rescued by IV infusion of bone marrow or peripheral blood HSCs from an HLA-compatible donor. Several clinical observations indicate that the donor cells also have a graft versus leukemia effect. For example, the relapse rate after allogeneic HSC transplantation is increased in T-cell depletion of the donor graft, with absence of acute or chronic GVHD, and after syngeneic (identical twin donor) HSC transplantation. The relapse-free survival after allogeneic HSC transplantation for stable-phase CML is 60%; overall survival is 80%. Survival of stable-phase CML patients after allogeneic HSC transplantation is best if the procedure is performed within 1 year of diagnosis and before evidence of the accelerated phase. Sensitive assays for the CML clone (e.g., RT-PCR for *bcr-abl*) may continue to be positive for 6 months after allogeneic HSC transplantation in patients who are ultimately cured of their disease. Most patients who have a relapse of stable-phase CML can enter remission with immunotherapy. Withdrawal of immunosuppressive therapy with or without infusion of donor lymphocytes can induce a graft versus leukemia effect and lead to a second complete remission of the disease. Unfortunately, this procedure may be complicated by GVHD or bone marrow aplasia.

(f) **Inhibitor of the *bcr-abl* TK.** The enhanced TK activity of the *bcr-abl* p210 fusion protein is necessary for the development of CML (see III.C.1.b.). Therefore, it seems reasonable to target this protein pharmacologically. Imatinib mesylate (Gleevec) occupies the adenosine triphosphate–binding site of *abl* and prevents its TK activity. Phase I and II trials of imatinib mesylate in IFN-refractory stable-phase CML patients have shown high rates of response. The hematologic complete remission rate is 90%; the complete and major cytogenetic remission rates are 30% and 50%, respectively. Imatinib mesylate has now been shown to be superior to IFN-α as initial therapy of chronic phase CML in terms of both cytogenetic response and toxicity. The major toxicities of imatinib mesylate are nausea and vomiting (especially if it is not taken with food), edema, effusions, myalgias, and liver function test abnormalities.

(2) **Treatment of blast crisis**

(a) Although remissions can be attained in some patients with **intensive induction chemotherapy,** the remission is typically short. Myeloid blast crisis tends to resist standard AML induction therapy. Some 60% of patients with lymphoid blast crisis enter complete remission with a standard acute lymphocytic leukemia induction regimen (**anthracycline, vincristine,** and **prednisone**), but median overall survival remains short (< 6 months). **Imatinib mesylate** can induce remissions in patients with CML blast crisis, but the remissions are not durable.

(b) Event-free survival after allogeneic HSC transplantation is 35% for accelerated-phase CML and 10%–15% for blast crisis. The lower survival rate after allogeneic HSC transplantation for advanced phases of CML is due to a higher relapse rate when the transplant is performed in accelerated-phase CML or blast crisis.

2. **Polycythemia vera**

a. **Overview.** Polycythemia and erythrocytosis are synonymous, both indicating an elevation of the **Hb** and **Hct above normal.** However, PCV is only one cause of polycythemia. In fact, PCV is often a diagnosis of exclusion.

(1) True polycythemia (see III.C.2.c.) must first be distinguished from relative polycythemia caused by contraction of the plasma volume. Relative polycythemia is usually caused by dehydration from excessive gastrointestinal fluid or insensible fluid loss. Gaisböck syndrome is a chronic cause of relative polycythemia.

(2) The Polycythemia Vera Study Group developed criteria for the diagnosis of PCV to ensure the uniformity of patients treated on multicenter clinical trials. Major criteria for the diagnosis of PCV are elevated RBC mass, normal arterial oxygen saturation, and splenomegaly. Minor criteria are thrombocytosis, leukocytosis, elevated leukocyte alkaline phosphatase, and elevated vitamin B_{12} level or vitamin B_{12} binding capacity. To be diagnosed with PCV, patients must have either all three major criteria or the first two major criteria with any two of the minor criteria.

b. **Natural history.** PCV may progress over years to a **spent phase,** also known as postpolycythemic myelofibrosis.

(1) Within 15 years of diagnosis, 50% of PCV patients enter the spent phase. These patients become progressively more anemic and develop massive splenomegaly. In addition, their bone marrow becomes fibrotic.

(2) The risk of AML in PCV patients maintained with phlebotomy alone is 1%–2%. However, the risk of progression to AML increases once the disease enters the spent phase. The risk is also increased by agents used to treat PCV, including chlorambucil, radioactive phosphorus, and hydroxyurea. Nonetheless, with adequate control of the disease, patients with PCV have a life expectancy similar to that of age-matched controls.

(3) Thrombotic complications and major hemorrhage are significant causes of morbidity and mortality in 30%–40% of PCV patients.

c. **Etiology.** Causes of true polycythemia may be classified as either primary or secondary. Primary polycythemia is due to erythropoietin-independent red blood cell production (PCV). Secondary polycythemia may be either physiologically appropriate or pathologic production of **excessive EPO.**

(1) Any cause of **tissue hypoxia** results in increased EPO secretion and stimulation of erythropoiesis. Tissue hypoxia may be caused by decreased arterial oxygen tension (e.g., high altitude, pulmonary diseases, hypoventilation, sleep apnea, right-to-left cardiac shunts), decreased Hb oxygen-carrying capacity (e.g., methemoglobinemia, elevated carboxyhemoglobin), and decreased oxygen delivery (e.g., high-affinity Hb variants).

(2) Alternatively, unregulated autonomous EPO secretion may result in polycythemia. Some **tumors,** including renal cell carcinoma, hepatocellular carcinoma, cerebellar hemangioblastomas, and uterine fibroids, can secrete EPO. Excessive EPO production has also been documented in **benign renal disorders** (e.g., hydronephrosis, polycystic kidney disease, renal artery stenosis) and after **renal transplantation.** In addition, excessive autonomous production of EPO may be due to **inherited mutations.**

(3) Administration of exogenous EPO may cause polycythemia. In addition, physiologic increases in androgen production (male puberty) and administration of pharmacologic doses of androgens will also stimulate erythropoiesis.

d. **Clinical presentation.** Patients with PCV may present either with symptoms related directly to erythrocytosis or with sequelae of splenomegaly.

(1) Untreated PCV patients often have a ruddy complexion and conjunctival plethora.

(2) Left upper quadrant abdominal pain due to splenomegaly and splenic infarcts may also be a presenting complaint.

(3) PCV patients may have symptoms of **hyperviscosity** due to the elevated Hct. Patients may have headache, vertigo, visual changes, or mental confusion. In fact, the goal of PCV therapy is to maintain the Hct at less than 45%; above this level blood viscosity increases dramatically and cerebral blood flow slows.

(4) Arterial and venous thromboses are a major cause of morbidity and mortality in 30%–40% of PCV patients.

(a) Major thrombotic events, such as cerebrovascular accidents, myocardial infarction, deep venous thrombosis, and Budd-Chiari syndrome, are common complications (30%–40% of patients) of erythrocytosis and thrombocytosis.

(b) **Erythromelalgia** (painful erythema of the hands or feet) is a result of thrombosis of the arterial microvasculature.

(c) Digital ischemia with ulceration may also be seen in patients with PCV.

(5) Conversely, patients with PCV may have hemorrhagic complications.

(6) Patients with PCV may have iron deficiency caused by chronic occult gastrointestinal bleeding. The nature of their illness may be obvious only after iron supplementation.

(7) Pruritus, especially after bathing, is a common complaint of PCV patients. The cause of the pruritus is unclear.

e. **Laboratory evaluation.** The goal of the laboratory evaluation is to distinguish PCV from secondary polycythemia.

(1) The RBC mass assay is used to distinguish relative from true polycythemia only. Any cause of true polycythemia, including PCV, will **elevate the RBC mass.** In PCV, the RBC mass should be greater than 36 mL/kg body weight in men and greater than 32 mL/kg body weight in women.

(2) Many patients with PCV also have **leukocytosis** or **thrombocytosis.** In fact, although it is not necessary for diagnosing PCV, the bone marrow will show hyperplasia of all three myeloid lineages.

(3) Cytogenetic analysis of a bone marrow aspirate may demonstrate **clonal abnormalities** (e.g., deletion of the long arm of chromosome 20, trisomy 8, trisomy 9) in 20% of patients with untreated PCV. The frequency of cytogenetic changes increases with therapy or progression to AML.

(4) The endogenous serum **EPO level should be low in patients with PCV.** Almost all other causes of true polycythemia should result from an elevated EPO level. A normal EPO level in the setting of polycythemia is inappropriately elevated. Furthermore, some causes of secondary polycythemia elevate the EPO level only temporarily (e.g., sleep apnea). Patients with PCV may also have a low normal EPO level. Therefore, an endogenous EPO level above normal indicates secondary polycythemia, but a normal EPO level is less helpful.

f. **Treatment.** The best treatment approach in PCV remains controversial.

(1) **Periodic phlebotomy** alone to maintain the Hct less than 45% is considered adequate treatment. However, the risk of thrombotic complications is increased in the first 2–3 years of phlebotomy compared with PCV patients treated with myelosuppressive agents. Furthermore, chronic phlebotomy ultimately leads to iron deficiency and reactive thrombocytosis. Thrombocytosis may contribute to the thrombotic and hemorrhagic complications of the disease.

(2) **Hydroxyurea** is the myelosuppressive agent usually chosen for control of PCV. Other myelosuppressive agents (e.g., chlorambucil, radioactive phosphorus) are associated with a greater risk of transformation to AML. Although **IFN-α** may also control the disease, compliance with maintenance therapy is difficult because of the toxicities of this agent. Anagrelide may be used to treat the associated thrombocytosis (see III.C.3.e.2.).

3. **Essential thrombocythemia**

a. **Overview.** The diagnosis of ET requires exclusion of all causes of reactive thrombocytosis and other MPD. The median age at diagnosis is 50–60 years, and incidence in men and women is similar. However, a second peak incidence occurs at 30 years of age, with a predominance of female patients. Rare familial cases have been described. Progression to myelofibrosis and AML is less common than in PCV.

b. **Etiology.** Thrombocytosis may be caused by any **MPD** or may be secondary to a number of **nonmyeloid disorders.**

   (1) Thrombocytosis may be due to iron deficiency.

   (2) Any chronic inflammatory disease, including malignancy and chronic infection, may cause reactive thrombocytosis.

   (3) Splenectomy, congenital asplenia, or complete splenic infarction can result in thrombocytosis.

   (4) The platelet count may rise above normal after recovery from a myelosuppressive agent, such as alcohol or chemotherapy (rebound thrombocytosis).

   (5) The vinca alkaloids and epinephrine may also cause thrombocytosis.

   (6) Thrombocytosis may be associated with acute hemorrhage or chronic hemolysis.

c. **Clinical presentation.** Although patients with ET may be asymptomatic at diagnosis, they may have **thrombotic complications, hemorrhagic sequelae,** or both.

   (1) The thrombotic complications of ET are similar to those of PCV (erythromelalgia, digital ischemia, myocardial infarction, stroke, deep venous thrombosis, Budd-Chiari syndrome). Pregnancy may terminate prematurely in 45% of cases as a result of placental thrombi and infarcts.

   (2) Hemorrhagic complications are thought to be a result of the many qualitative defects of platelet function in ET. One in five young patients may have these serious complications.

   (3) **Splenomegaly** is present in 30%–50% of patients.

d. **Laboratory evaluation.** The diagnostic criteria for ET include a platelet count greater than 600,000/μL, exclusion of all causes of reactive thrombocytosis, normal RBC mass, stainable iron in the marrow, less than one third of marrow core biopsy with collagen fibrosis, and absence of the Ph chromosome. Most (but not all) patients with reactive thrombocytosis have a platelet count less than 1 million/μL.

e. **Treatment.** Not all patients with ET require therapy. The difficulty is identifying which patients are at risk for major thrombotic or hemorrhagic complications. Hemorrhage has been associated with aspirin, nonsteroidal antiinflammatory drugs, and platelet counts greater than 2 million/μL. Thrombotic complications have been associated with history of thrombosis, risk factors for atherosclerotic disease, and advanced age. Both hemorrhagic and thrombotic complications are more common in the perioperative setting if the disease is poorly controlled. If the patient is asymptomatic, observation alone may be reasonable. However, patients who have a history of thrombosis, who have risk factors for atherosclerotic disease, or who are awaiting surgery should begin therapy.

   (1) Both **hydroxyurea** and IFN-α have been used successfully to control ET in most patients.

   (2) **Anagrelide,** a nonmyelosuppressive agent, controls the thrombocytosis of ET in more than 90% of patients within 1–2 weeks. The agent, which

is administered orally, appears to block megakaryocytic maturation. There has been no associated increase in the risk of transformation to AML. The major adverse reactions of anagrelide include palpitations, headache, anemia, fluid retention, diarrhea, and dizziness.

(3) **Plateletpheresis** can physically lower the platelet count temporarily. It should be considered for management of acute events (e.g., cerebrovascular accidents) but is not indicated for chronic management.

(4) Pregnant patients may be managed with observation alone, antiplatelet agents, IFN-α, and/or platelet pheresis.

4. **Myelofibrosis with myeloid metaplasia**

a. **Overview.** Myeloid metaplasia is synonymous with **extramedullary hematopoiesis,** which occurs primarily in the **liver and spleen;** however, extramedullary hematopoiesis may be seen in almost any organ. Splenic hematopoiesis may substantially increase portal blood flow. Portal hypertension with its complications may result from the increased portal blood flow as well as thrombosis of small portal veins. Splenic infarction is another consequence of splenic hematopoiesis. Hematopoiesis of serosal surfaces can result in large pleural effusions, pericardial effusions, or ascites. When hematopoiesis occurs in the epidural space, dramatic neurologic consequences may ensue. Myeloid metaplasia may also be seen in the course of PCV and ET. The median age at diagnosis is approximately 65 years (only 20% of patients are younger than 50 years).

b. **Prognosis.** The median survival of patients with myelofibrosis is 3–5 years; however, there is a wide range. Negative prognostic factors include advanced age, anemia, hypercatabolic symptoms, cytogenetic abnormalities, leukocytosis, leukopenia, and thrombocytopenia. Young patients without anemia, hypercatabolic symptoms, and cytogenetic abnormalities may have a life expectancy of more than 10 years.

c. **Clinical presentation.** The most common symptoms at presentation are weight loss, low-grade fever, night sweats, fatigue, and left upper quadrant abdominal pain. More than 90% of patients have **splenomegaly;** 50% have **hepatomegaly.** Most patients are **anemic** at diagnosis; 20% have an Hb less than 8 g/dL.

d. **Laboratory evaluation.** The diagnosis of MMM is suggested by the examination of a **peripheral blood smear.**

(1) **Myelophthisis** and **leukoerythroblastosis** are used interchangeably to describe the characteristic peripheral blood findings. Immature granulocytic precursors (predominantly myelocytes but also progranulocytes and myeloblasts) and nucleated RBCs (erythroblasts) are found on examination of a blood smear. The RBCs will also display a teardrop shape (dacrocyte). Large platelets are seen. The WBC and platelet counts may be elevated, normal, or low. Because other disorders that infiltrate the bone marrow lead to identical changes (e.g., metastatic carcinoma, lymphoma, Hodgkin disease, myeloma, CML, MDS), examination of a bone marrow core biopsy is necessary for establishing the diagnosis of MMM.

(2) The bone marrow often cannot be aspirated in cases of MMM. A **bone marrow core biopsy** will have increased collagen **and reticulin fibers.** The fibroblasts that produce the myelofibrosis are not part of the clonal process. Platelet-derived growth factor and transforming

growth factor-β released from clonal megakaryocytes and monocytes–histiocytes stimulate fibroblast proliferation.

e. **Treatment.** Drug therapy is inadequate for myelofibrosis.

   (1) **Hydroxyurea** is used for control of organomegaly, leukocytosis, and thrombocytosis. **Androgens** and **low-dose prednisone** may lead to improvement of anemia in the minority of patients. **IFN-α** has also been used.

   (2) **Splenectomy** is indicated for symptomatic splenomegaly, portal hypertension, transfusion-dependent anemia, and severe thrombocytopenia. Patients with thrombocytopenia have the least benefit. The procedure can be complicated by both hemorrhage and thrombosis, with a 10% operative mortality rate. Median survival after splenectomy is 2 years. Acute leukemia, accelerated hepatomegaly, and severe thrombocytosis occurs in approximately 20% of splenectomized patients. Splenic irradiation is an alternative therapy but can be complicated by severe cytopenias.

   (3) Both **autologous** and **allogeneic HSC transplantation** have been performed in patients with myelofibrosis. Successful engraftment after allogeneic HSC transplantation has resulted in reversal of the bone marrow fibrosis and return of normal bone marrow histology. Young patients with good performance status are usually considered the best candidates for these intensive therapies.

IV. SUMMARY

The myeloproliferative and myelodysplastic syndromes are clonal myeloid stem cell disorders unlike aplastic anemia. However, any of these myeloid stem cell disorders may progress to acute myelocytic leukemia.

SUGGESTED READING

Tefferi A. Myelofibrosis with myeloid metaplasia.
  N Engl J Med 2000;342:1255–1265.

CHAPTER 17

Acute Leukemia

- HARRY P. ERBA

I. INTRODUCTION

Acute leukemia is defined as the malignant accumulation of transformed hematopoietic progenitor cells. Leukemic blast cells retain the capability of self-renewal, but unlike normal hematopoietic stem cells (HSCs), they have limited or no potential for terminal differentiation. Leukemic infiltration of the marrow space ultimately leads to bone marrow failure, so most patients present with consequences of cytopenias. The acute leukemias can be classified by morphology, histochemical staining, and immunophenotype into two broad categories: acute myelocytic leukemia (AML) and acute lymphocytic leukemia (ALL). The distinction between the two acute leukemias is clinically important because the treatments and prognoses are different.

II. EPIDEMIOLOGY OF ACUTE LEUKEMIA

A. The annual incidence of AML in the United States is 2–3 in 100,000 people. The incidence increases with age; fewer than 1 in 100,000 people under age 30 years contract the disease, but 15 in 100,000 people over age 80 years contract the disease. The annual incidence of ALL is 1 in 60,000 people, with 75% of patients less than 15 years old.

B. The median age of patients with AML is approximately 65 years. In contrast, the peak incidence of ALL is 3–5 years. AML accounts for 80% of adult acute leukemia but only 15%–20% of childhood acute leukemia.

C. Both AML and ALL have a slight male predominance.

D. Siblings of patients with ALL have a fourfold risk of developing ALL. The monozygotic twin of a patient with ALL has a 20% risk of developing ALL.

III. ETIOLOGY OF ACUTE LEUKEMIA

A. A number of environmental factors and clinical conditions are associated with acute leukemia.

    1. **Ionizing radiation** is a known leukemogen. Survivors of the atomic bomb explosions over Japan during World War II are at increased risk for developing acute leukemia if exposed to more than 100 cGy of radiation. Also, patients treated with spinal radiation therapy for ankylosing spondylitis between 1935 and 1954 had a fivefold increased risk of developing AML.

    2. **Benzene** is known to cause AML, myelodysplastic syndrome, and aplastic anemia.

3. Patients with **Down syndrome** (trisomy 21) and **chromosome breakage disorders** (e.g., Fanconi anemia, Bloom syndrome) are at increased risk for developing acute leukemia.

4. The **myeloproliferative disorders** and **myelodysplastic syndromes** may progress to AML.

5. **Chemotherapy** can cause treatment-related AML.

B. In most patients with acute leukemia, no predisposing condition or agent can be identified.

IV. CLINICAL PRESENTATION OF ACUTE LEUKEMIA

A. **Bone marrow failure.** Patients with acute leukemia most often present with constitutional symptoms and signs of bone marrow failure.

1. Fatigue and weakness are due to both symptomatic anemia and a hypermetabolic state. However, some patients are not anemic at presentation because of the explosive onset of acute leukemia and the relatively long survival of red blood cells (RBCs).

2. Thrombocytopenic hemorrhage most often manifests as petechiae and atraumatic ecchymoses.

3. Neutropenic infections are potentially life-threatening complications of acute leukemia. Typically, patients present with pneumonia, cellulitis, or sepsis. The most common causative agents are staphylococcal, streptococcal, and enteric gram-negative bacteria and a variety of fungal species.

4. Bone marrow infiltration may result in severe bone pain.

B. **Leukostasis.** Although a minority of patients are leukopenic at presentation and may not have significant numbers of circulating malignant blasts, most patients with acute leukemia present with **leukocytosis.**

1. Stasis of blood flow may occur in the cerebral and pulmonary vasculature when the blast count is above $50,000/\mu L$.

   a. Patients with **cerebral leukostasis** complain of headache, confusion, and visual disturbance. These patients may progress quickly to coma or a variety of stroke syndromes.

   b. **Pulmonary leukostasis** can cause dyspnea at rest, tachypnea, inspiratory rales, and pulmonary infiltrates.

2. Leukostasis is more common in AML than ALL. This is most likely due to the larger size of the blasts and the expression of adhesion proteins in AML.

C. **Coagulopathy.** Both **disseminated intravascular coagulation (DIC)** and **primary fibrinolysis** contribute to the hemorrhagic diathesis of acute leukemia.

1. Induction chemotherapy for any acute leukemia can precipitate DIC.

2. DIC is more common in patients with AML, especially those with acute progranulocytic and monocytic leukemias. Patients with acute progranulocytic leukemia (APL) may present with DIC or fibrinolysis that can result in either intracranial or gastrointestinal hemorrhage before treatment.

3. In DIC, the prothrombin and activated partial thromboplastin times are elevated and the fibrinogen level is low. In fibrinolysis, it is possible that only the fibrin degradation products or D-dimer will be elevated.

D. **Extramedullary acute leukemia.** Leukemic blasts can infiltrate any organ.

1. Patients with ALL are likely to present with adenopathy and splenomegaly due to infiltration of these lymphoid organs.

2. AML with monocytic differentiation is most often associated with extramedullary disease.

3. Cutaneous infiltration (i.e., leukemia cutis) and gingival hypertrophy are frequently seen in patients with acute monoblastic leukemias. Leukemic involvement of the skin usually appears as nontender violaceous subcutaneous nodules or plaques. However, leukemia cutis must be distinguished from hematomas, cutaneous infections (e.g., ecthyma gangrenosum), and Sweet syndrome (a noninfectious acute febrile neutrophilic dermatosis).

4. Leukemic meningitis is unusual at the time of presentation of AML and ALL. However, it is common during the later course of disease in patients with ALL, especially if prophylactic central nervous system therapy is not administered.

5. Rarely, patients with AML may develop extramedullary disease without involvement of the peripheral blood or bone marrow. These solid tumors of leukemic myeloblasts are known as chloromas, granulocytic sarcomas, or myeloblastomas, and they may be mistaken for non-Hodgkin lymphoma without a careful pathologic examination. Extramedullary AML is very responsive to local radiation therapy. However, without systemic therapy, these patients usually develop medullary disease within weeks to months.

E. **Metabolic abnormalities.** A number of metabolic abnormalities are found in patients with acute leukemia at presentation.

1. Tumor lysis syndrome may be present before therapy, especially in ALL. Patients with tumor lysis syndrome may develop life-threatening hyperkalemia. However, many patients with AML are actually hypokalemic at presentation, possibly as a result of renal tubular injury by lysozyme released from blasts.

2. Hyperuricemia and hyperphosphatemia can lead to renal insufficiency due to urate nephropathy and nephrocalcinosis.

3. Elevation of serum hepatic transaminases is common.

4. The serum lactate dehydrogenase may be elevated, especially in patients with ALL.

5. Artifactual hypoglycemia or hypoxia may result from the *in vitro* metabolic activity of the leukemic blasts after phlebotomy.

V. DIAGNOSIS AND CLASSIFICATION OF ACUTE LEUKEMIA

A. **Classification guidelines.** Accurate diagnosis and classification of acute leukemia is important for selection of the appropriate therapy. According to the French-American-British (FAB) classification system, **blasts must account for more than 30% of the nucleated cells** in the peripheral blood or bone marrow aspirate to make a diagnosis of acute leukemia. More recently, the World Health Organization suggested that the threshold for diagnosis of AML be lowered to 20% blasts.

B. **Morphology.** Eight morphologic subtypes of AML and three morphologic subtypes of ALL are distinguished according to the FAB classification system based on the morphologic features of the blasts.

1. Blasts are large, immature hematopoietic progenitor cells with open chromatin and single to multiple nucleoli. Differentiation of myeloblasts from lymphoblasts by morphology alone can be difficult.

   a. Myeloblasts tend to have more abundant cytoplasm and may contain cytoplasmic granules. Auer rods, which are linear aggregates of primary cytoplasmic granules, are found only in myeloblasts (Fig. 17–1).

   b. Lymphoblasts often have a high nuclear cytoplasmic ratio and less conspicuous nucleoli (Fig. 17–2).

2. AML is divided into subtypes by the FAB classification system based on apparent level of differentiation: undifferentiated (M0), granulocytic (M1–M2),

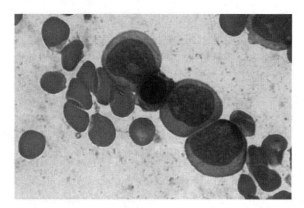

FIGURE 17–1. Three myeloblasts with a baso-philic erythroblast. Note the Auer rod in the cy-toplasm of one of the myeloblasts.

progranulocytic (M3), monoblastic (M4–M5), erythroblastic (M6), and mega-karyoblastic (M7). APL (M3) is the most important subtype of AML to rec-ognize because it requires unique therapy (see VIII C).

3. Likewise, the biology, prognosis, and treatment of the L3 subtype of ALL are distinct from the L1 and L2 subtypes. The L3 blasts are characteristically larger than L1 and L2 blasts and have deeply basophilic cytoplasm and cyto-plasmic vacuolization.

C. **Histochemical stains.** Morphologic details of blasts on Wright-Giemsa–stained bone marrow or peripheral blood smears may not be sufficient to distinguish AML from ALL. Identification of certain lineage-specific enzyme markers can help in the differential diagnosis of acute leukemia.

1. Myeloperoxidase is a cytoplasmic enzyme found in the primary granules of granulocytic precursors. It can be detected in AML blasts using cytochemical stains.

2. Expression of lysozyme indicates myeloid differentiation.

3. Detection of nonspecific esterase helps to define monocytic differentiation.

4. Lymphoblasts express a nuclear enzyme, terminal deoxynucleotidyl transferase (TdT). TdT is involved in immunoglobulin and T-cell receptor gene rearrange-ments. It can be detected by immunoperoxidase stain or flow cytometry.

D. **Immunophenotyping (flow cytometry).** Flow cytometry can be used both to di-agnose and to classify acute leukemia.

1. Flow cytometric analysis of myeloblasts typically demonstrates expression of CD13, CD33, and CD117 on the cell surface. Other immunophenotypic

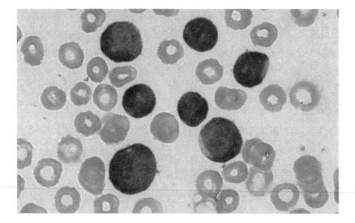

FIGURE 17–2. Lymphoblasts with inconspicuous nucleoli and scant cyto-plasm.

markers help to define subtypes of AML, including CD14 in M4–M5, glycophorin A expression in M6, and von Willebrand factor and CD41 (GPIIb-IIIa) in M7. CD34 is a stem cell marker that may be expressed on the surface of both myeloid and lymphoid blasts.

2. ALL is most commonly subclassified by immunophenotype.

   a. Some 70% of adult ALL is leukemia of precursor B cells. There is rearrangement of the immunoglobulin heavy chain genes in precursor B lymphoblasts. These blasts express CD10, CD19, cytoplasmic CD22, cytoplasmic μ-heavy chain, and TdT.

   b. One fourth of adult ALL has a T-cell phenotype, expressing a TdT and a subset of the antigens CD1a, CD2, CD3, CD4, CD5, CD7, and CD8. There is monoclonal T-cell receptor gene rearrangement in the malignant T lymphoblasts. Patients with T-cell ALL often present with a mediastinal mass.

   c. Some 5% of adult ALL patients have lymphoblasts with a mature B-cell immunophenotype. The B cells express surface immunoglobulin but lack expression of TdT. Lymphoblasts with a mature B-cell phenotype morphologically appear as L3 blasts.

E. **Cytogenetic and molecular genetic abnormalities.** Nonrandom chromosomal translocations, deletions, and additions are found in the leukemic blasts in most adults with acute leukemia. Identification of cytogenetic abnormalities in leukemic blasts is important for determination of prognosis and selection of postremission therapy.

1. A few cytogenetic changes are pathognomonic for various subtypes of acute leukemia and are helpful diagnostically.

   a. The translocation t(15;17)(q22;q21) is found only in APL and is due to a fusion of the *PML* gene on chromosome 15 with the retinoic acid receptor α (*RARα*) gene on chromosome 17.

   b. The translocations t(8;14), t(2;8), and t(8;22) are found only in mature B-cell ALL and Burkitt's lymphoma. These chromosomal rearrangements result in dysregulation and overexpression of the *c-myc* gene on chromosome 8 by juxtaposition of the enhancer elements of the immunoglobulin heavy or light chain gene loci.

2. However, some cytogenetic abnormalities can be found in either AML or ALL. For example, the Philadelphia chromosome, t(9;22)(q34;q11), which is characteristic of chronic myelocytic leukemia, can also be found in fewer than 5% of adult AML and 25%–30% of adult ALL blasts.

VI. INITIAL MANAGEMENT AND SUPPORTIVE CARE

A. **Transfusion support.** Curative therapy of acute leukemia depends on effective transfusion support.

1. The threshold for RBC transfusion depends on the patient's physiologic state; younger patients generally tolerate a lower hemoglobin level than elderly patients with cardiopulmonary disease.

2. Recent studies of patients with acute leukemia have established a platelet count of 10,000/μL as a reasonable threshold for prophylactic platelet transfusion, except for patients with fever, chemotherapy-induced mucositis, and DIC, in which case more than 20,000/μL is appropriate.

3. Patients with acute leukemia should receive leukocyte-depleted RBC and platelet transfusions to prevent transmission of cytomegalovirus, alloimmunization,

febrile transfusion reactions, and refractory response to platelet transfusion therapy.

4. Irradiated blood products are often prescribed to prevent transfusion-associated graft versus host disease, especially for patients undergoing allogeneic HSC transplantation. Graft versus host disease is a rare, fatal complication of transfusion characterized by skin rash, diarrhea, hepatic function abnormalities, and bone marrow aplasia.

B. **Management of leukostasis.** Leukostasis is a medical emergency. Patients with leukocytosis and circulating blasts should be referred for emergency evaluation by a hematologist, because the rate of increase in white blood cells (WBCs) or the development of leukostasis cannot be accurately predicted.

1. Intravenous hydration and leukapheresis are used for urgent reduction of the peripheral blood blast count. Hydroxyurea, a ribonucleotide reductase inhibitor, may be used for rapid cytoreduction before definitive diagnosis. If the blasts have lymphoid morphology, the addition of high-dose steroids may be helpful.

2. Alternatively, if the specific diagnosis has been confirmed, appropriate induction chemotherapy can be initiated.

3. Arbitrary RBC transfusion should be avoided in patients with extreme leukocytosis because it may acutely raise whole blood viscosity and precipitate leukostasis.

C. **Management of disseminated intravascular coagulation.** Replacement of plasma coagulation factors and platelets is the primary therapy for DIC. Therapy involves the use of fresh frozen plasma, cryoprecipitate (to elevate the fibrinogen), and platelet concentrates. In certain cases, there may be an adjuvant role for heparin or antifibrinolytic agents.

D. **Management of tumor lysis syndrome.** Despite the various methods used to manage tumor lysis syndrome, induction chemotherapy for acute leukemia may bring on acute renal failure, and temporary hemodialysis may be necessary.

1. Intravenous hydration should be prescribed to ensure brisk saline diuresis.

2. Allopurinol usually prevents the accumulation of uric acid.

3. Urine alkalinization increases the solubility of uric acid and helps prevent urate nephropathy, especially if the serum uric acid concentration is elevated at diagnosis.

E. **Other forms of management.** The following may be helpful in the management of patients with acute leukemia.

1. Placement of a subcutaneously tunneled central venous catheter (e.g., Hickman catheter) is advisable before beginning induction chemotherapy. Venous access is a prognostic factor for the treatment of acute leukemia.

2. Assessment of cardiac function (e.g., radionuclide ventriculogram) is typically performed in anticipation of administration of an anthracycline chemotherapy agent, especially in older patients with a history of cardiovascular disease.

3. Patients who may be eligible for subsequent allogeneic HSC transplantation should have tissue typing performed on a sample of peripheral blood.

VII. ACUTE MYELOCYTIC LEUKEMIA

A. **Prognostic factors in adult acute myelocytic leukemia.** The probability of achieving complete remission and long-term disease-free survival is influenced by a number of factors.

1. **Age.** Advanced age is an important negative prognostic factor. Only 45%–50% of AML patients over 60 years of age achieve complete remission, and

overall survival from diagnosis in this population is only 5%–10%. Conversely, in patients under 40 years of age, the complete remission rate is 75% and overall survival at 4 years is 35%–40%.

2. **Cytogenetic abnormalities in leukemic blasts.** The prognosis for adults with AML varies with specific cytogenetic changes found in the leukemic blasts at diagnosis.

   a. Two important translocations, each found in 5%–10% of adults with AML, affect the genes encoding subunits of the heterodimeric transcription factor core binding factor (CBF). CBF regulates expression of many genes involved in HSC differentiation. The translocation t(8;21)(q22;q22) results from fusion of the *AML1* gene on chromosome 21 (encoding a CBFα subunit) with the *ETO* gene on chromosome 8. The pericentric inversion of chromosome 16, inv(16)(p13;q22), results from fusion of the genes for CBFβ and the smooth muscle myosin heavy chain. The t(8;21) and inv(16) are usually found in FAB types M2 and M4eo AML, respectively. These two translocations have been associated with an excellent prognosis. AML patients with t(8;21) and inv(16), now referred to as CBF AML, have a 90% probability of entering complete remission with a single cycle of induction chemotherapy. Furthermore, 70%–80% of patients with CBF AML are alive and disease free at 5 years after high-dose cytarabine consolidation chemotherapy.

   b. Many other chromosomal translocations and deletions result in a worse outcome for adult AML patients. For example, deletion of the long arm of chromosome 5 or 7, monosomy 5 or 7, the Philadelphia chromosome t(9;22), most deletions or translocations involving chromosome band 11q23, inv(3)(q21;q26), and karyotypes with multiple chromosomal abnormalities have all been individually associated with lower complete remission rates and decreased probability of disease-free survival.

3. Patients with a history of a bone marrow disorder also do poorly.

   a. Elderly patients with AML are more likely to have an antecedent myelodysplastic syndrome. The risk of progression from myelodysplastic syndrome to AML is related to older age, number of cytopenias, the presence of specific cytogenetic abnormalities, such as monosomy 7, del(7)(q) or complex karyotypic changes, and percentage of bone marrow myeloblasts.

   b. Patients with myeloproliferative disorders may also develop AML. The risk is highest in patients with chronic myelocytic leukemia, but patients with polycythemia vera, myeloid metaplasia, and essential thrombocythemia have a 10% risk of developing AML.

   c. AML will also develop in 5%–10% of patients with aplastic anemia in remission after immunosuppressive therapy. These secondary leukemias tend to be more resistant to cytotoxic chemotherapy.

4. **Treatment-related acute myelocytic leukemia.** AML can be a devastating complication of curative chemotherapy for another malignancy. Two classes of cytotoxic agents have been associated with secondary AML.

   a. The alkylating agents (e.g., cyclophosphamide, chlorambucil, melphalan, nitrogen mustard, busulfan) can cause myelodysplastic syndrome or AML, usually within 5 years of treatment. Deletions of chromosomes 5/5q or 7/7q and multiple cytogenetic changes characterize alkylating agent–induced AML.

   b. Topoisomerase II inhibitors such as the epipodophyllotoxins (e.g., etoposide, teniposide) and doxorubicin can lead to AML with monocytic differentiation (M4, M5) without a preceding myelodysplastic syndrome.

5. **Multidrug resistance.** AML blasts often demonstrate multidrug resistance at presentation. The *MDR1* gene encodes P-glycoprotein, a 170-kd transmembrane protein that is an adenosine triphosphate–dependent drug efflux pump normally expressed in HSCs, the hepatocyte membrane of the bile canaliculus, capillary endothelial cells of the brain, and renal tubular cells. Expression of P-glycoprotein is more common in the AML blasts of elderly patients, in whom it has been associated with a lower rate of complete remission.

6. **Other prognostic factors.** Other factors that are predictive of AML relapse include failure to attain complete remission with a single cycle of induction chemotherapy, hyperleukocytosis at presentation (i.e., WBC > 100,000/μL), and expression of the HSC marker CD34.

B. **Treatment.** Curative therapy of AML can be divided into two phases: induction chemotherapy and postremission therapy.

1. **Induction chemotherapy.** The goal of induction chemotherapy is to obtain complete remission, which is specifically defined as fewer than 5% blasts in a bone marrow sample, no peripheral blood blasts, transfusion independence, normal hematopoiesis (i.e., absolute neutrophil count > 1500/μL, platelet count > 100,000/μL, and hemoglobin > 9 g/dL), and resolution of all extramedullary leukemic infiltrates.

   a. The **anthracycline drug daunorubicin** 45–60 mg/m^2 by intravenous push each day for 3 days **plus cytarabine** 100–200 mg/m^2 by continuous intravenous infusion each day for 7 days—that is, the 3 + 7 regimen—has remained the standard induction chemotherapy regimen since its introduction 30 years ago. Induction chemotherapy with daunorubicin and cytarabine results in complete remission in 50%–75% of adults with AML. However, 10%–25% of patients succumb to the toxicities of induction chemotherapy.

   b. **Toxicity of induction therapy.** Daunorubicin plus cytarabine in the 3 + 7 regimen results in temporary severe marrow hypoplasia. Therefore, patients require intensive supportive care during induction chemotherapy. Patients often complain of painful ulceration of the oral mucosa, dysphagia, dyspepsia, and diarrhea due to mucositis. Opioid analgesics and topical anesthetics are usually prescribed. Topical (nystatin) or systemic (fluconazole) antifungals help prevent oropharyngeal candidiasis. Patients who demonstrate evidence of previous exposure to herpes simplex virus should receive prophylactic acyclovir. Induction chemotherapy results in predictable severe myelosuppression lasting 21–28 days. Most patients develop febrile neutropenia. In the absence of a positive microbiologic culture, empiric antibiotics are needed to treat infection by enteric gram-negative bacteria (especially *Pseudomonas* species), cutaneous gram-positive cocci (*Staphylococcus* and *Streptococcus* species), and fungi (*Candida* and *Aspergillus* species). Neutropenic enterocolitis (i.e., typhlitis) is an especially severe complication of induction chemotherapy.

   c. Adult patients with AML fail to enter complete remission for two reasons: resistance of the leukemic blasts to induction chemotherapy and mortality during chemotherapy-induced marrow aplasia due to neutropenic infection or thrombocytopenic hemorrhage (less common). Several approaches have been investigated in an effort to increase the response rate to induction chemotherapy. Several randomized trials evaluated the addition of the myeloid colony-stimulating factors **granulocyte colony-stimulating factor (G-CSF) and granulocyte-macrophage colony-stimulating factor (GM-CSF)** versus placebo after completion of induction chemotherapy in patients with newly diagnosed AML.

(1) Both G-CSF and GM-CSF shortened by several days the chemotherapy-induced neutropenia.

(2) Randomized trials have also demonstrated a significant clinical benefit from G-CSF (i.e., filgrastim) in terms of length of hospitalization, parenteral antibiotic use, duration of fever, and need for antifungal therapy.

(3) Yeast-derived GM-CSF (i.e., sargramostim) treatment was associated with an improvement in overall survival.

(4) The addition of G-CSF or GM-CSF to standard induction chemotherapy did not improve the complete remission rate in any of these studies.

2. **Postremission therapy.** Induction chemotherapy results in only a thousand-fold reduction in the number of leukemic blasts. Because there are approximately 10^{12} blasts present at the time of diagnosis, a significant leukemic burden remains after successful remission induction. Therefore, postremission therapy is necessary to prevent relapse.

   a. Chemotherapy of similar intensity to induction therapy (i.e., **consolidation chemotherapy**) has been shown to be effective. Typically, patients receive two to four monthly cycles of an anthracycline for 2 days and standard-dose cytarabine by continuous intravenous infusion for 5 days. Only 10% of patients in their first complete remission achieve long-term disease-free survival with standard consolidation chemotherapy.

   b. Intensification of postremission therapy cures more patients with AML in first remission than standard consolidation or maintenance chemotherapy. There are three choices for intensive postremission therapy in AML patients, including high-dose cytarabine-based regimens, allogeneic bone marrow transplantation, and autologous bone marrow transplantation.

3. **Relapse.** Primary refractory disease and relapse after complete remission continue to be major problems in the care of adults with AML.

   a. If patients do not attain complete remission with induction chemotherapy, the prognosis is grim. Allogeneic HSC transplantation can salvage 10%–20% of patients with primary refractory AML and result in long-term disease-free survival.

   b. The single most important factor predictive of attaining a second complete remission is the length of the first remission; the longer the first remission, the greater the chance of attaining a second remission. If the first remission has been more than 2 years, it is reasonable to prescribe standard induction chemotherapy. Patients with duration of first remission of less than 1 year have a poor prognosis.

VIII. ACUTE PROGRANULOCYTIC LEUKEMIA

A. **Diagnosis.** Of all cases of adult AML, 5%–15% are APL. The therapeutic approach to adults with APL (i.e., M3 AML) is different from that to other AML patients. Therefore, APL must be recognized at presentation.

   1. The blasts are characterized by abundant primary cytoplasmic granules, at times obscuring the nucleus, and frequent Auer rods (Fig. 17–3).

   2. The nucleus is often bilobed or displays sliding plate morphology.

   3. The cytoplasm demonstrates intense cytochemical staining for myeloperoxidase. The nuclear features and myeloperoxidase content are diagnostically helpful for recognition of the microgranular variant of APL.

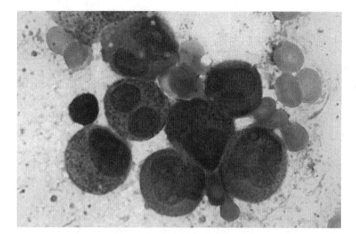

FIGURE 17-3. Acute progranulocytic leukemia. Note the large primary granules and bilobed immature nuclei (isthmus cells and sliding plates).

4. Patients with APL have a younger median age (30–40 years), often present with leukopenia, and have evidence of DIC or fibrinolysis at diagnosis.
5. The diagnosis of APL depends on either cytogenetic or molecular genetic detection of the *PML-RARα* fusion.

B. **Prognostic factors.** Advanced age, leukocytosis at presentation, and expression of the cell surface marker CD56 have all been associated with a worse outcome in APL, even with current therapy.

C. **Treatment of acute progranulocytic leukemia**
   1. **ALL-*trans*-retinoic acid (ATRA, tretinoin)** is a vitamin A analog that can bind to the *PML-RARα* fusion protein and interfere with its function. ATRA induces complete remission in more than 85% of newly diagnosed APL patients. The usual dose of ATRA is 45 mg/m^2/day in two divided oral doses with meals. ATRA does not cause blast lysis or marrow aplasia but instead induces the differentiation of the APL blasts. Resolution of DIC occurs rapidly.
      a. Mucocutaneous dryness, headache, pseudotumor cerebri, hypertriglyceridemia, and abnormal liver function tests are common adverse effects of high-dose vitamin A therapy.
      b. Patients with active APL treated with ATRA can develop a capillary leak syndrome characterized by weight gain, edema, fever, hypoxia, pulmonary infiltrates, and pleuropericarditis. This retinoic acid or APL differentiation syndrome occurs within a few days to 3 weeks of ATRA initiation and is often associated with a rapidly rising WBC count. Unless recognized early and treated with steroids, the APL differentiation syndrome can be rapidly fatal. Coadministration of ATRA with induction chemotherapy decreases the incidence of the APL differentiation syndrome from 25% to less than 5%.
   2. A new agent, **arsenic trioxide (ATO),** has recently been added to the armamentarium against APL. ATO induces apoptosis in APL cells. Patients are usually treated with ATO 0.15 mg/kg by intravenous infusion over 2 hours daily until remission. The rate of complete remission is 85%, with most patients attaining molecular remission (i.e., no evidence of the *PML-RARα* fusion by reverse transcriptase polymerase chain reaction amplification) after ATO consolidation therapy. The toxicities of ATO include nausea, emesis, diarrhea, rash, cardiac toxicity (i.e., prolongation of the QT interval, atrioventricular block, and torsade de pointes), neurotoxicity, and serum hepatic enzyme elevations. ATO has also been associated with hyperleukocytosis and the APL differentiation syndrome.

D. **General treatment approach**
   1. Patients receive induction therapy with ATRA and an anthracycline drug with or without cytarabine. The complete remission rate is ≥ 90%.
   2. Maintenance therapy with ATRA with or without oral antimetabolite chemotherapy has been shown to be important for prolonged disease-free survival. Approximately 70% of adult APL patients can be cured with this approach.
   3. Arsenic trioxide is used for the treatment of relapsed APL patients.

IX. ACUTE LYMPHOCYTIC LEUKEMIA

A. **Prognostic factors in acute lymphocytic leukemia**
   1. **Age.** In contrast to the excellent prognosis of children 2–9 years of age, the overall disease-free survival rate of adults with ALL is approximately 30%. Patients older than 60 years of age have less than a 10% chance of disease-free survival after complete remission. Infants also have a worse prognosis.
   2. **Cytogenetic abnormalities.** The presence of the Philadelphia chromosome and translocations involving chromosome band 11q23 are associated with a high risk of relapse with standard chemotherapy. The lymphoblasts from most infants younger than 1 year of age with ALL have translocations involving the *MLL* gene on chromosome 11q23, accounting for the poor prognosis in this age group. Conversely, the translocation t(12;21)(p12;q22) that is due to fusion of the *TEL* and *AML1* genes is found in 25% of childhood ALL cases and is associated with an excellent prognosis. This genetic event is not typically found in adults with ALL.
   3. **Immunophenotype.** Adults with T-cell ALL do better than those with the precursor B-cell type. Although coexpression of one or two myeloid antigens can be frequently detected in ALL blasts, recent studies have failed to demonstrate any effect on prognosis. Mature B-cell ALL (i.e., L3 ALL) has previously been associated with a poor prognosis; however, intensive chemotherapy regimens that include fractionated cyclophosphamide, high-dose methotrexate, and central nervous system prophylaxis have resulted in survival rates of 50%–70%.
   4. Other negative prognostic factors include hyperleukocytosis at presentation, failure to achieve complete remission within 4 weeks of beginning induction therapy, and elevated serum lactate dehydrogenase.

B. **Treatment**
   1. Most children with ALL are cured with standard chemotherapy. Unfortunately, the remarkable successes that have been realized in the treatment of ALL in children over the past 40 years have only partially been achieved in adults.
   2. Many drugs are active in ALL, including antimetabolites (thioguanine, mercaptopurine, methotrexate), anthracyclines (daunorubicin, doxorubicin), glucocorticosteroids, vincristine, cytarabine, cyclophosphamide, L-asparaginase, and epipodophyllotoxins (etoposide, teniposide).
   3. Standard therapy typically consists of a 2- to 3-year program.
      a. Remission induction chemotherapy with four or five drugs is the first phase of the program. The complete remission rate in ALL patients treated with anthracycline, glucocorticosteroid, and vincristine-based induction chemotherapy is 80%–90%.
      b. Intensive chemotherapy is administered immediately after attaining complete remission and 6 months later. The central nervous system, including the cerebrospinal fluid, provides a sanctuary site for leukemic blasts. Without

treatment that is specifically designed to reach lymphoblasts in this sanctuary site, 50%–75% of patients relapse in the central nervous system. Prophylaxis includes intrathecal administration of chemotherapy (i.e., methotrexate, cytarabine) with or without cranial irradiation.

c. Finally, prolonged maintenance chemotherapy has been shown to extend disease-free survival, especially in children with ALL. Unfortunately, despite this prolonged, intensive therapy, the relapse rate remains high in adult patients.

4. For patients at high risk for relapse (e.g., Philadelphia chromosome, *MLL* gene rearrangements, hyperleukocytosis at presentation, failure to attain complete remission within 4 weeks), allogeneic HSC transplantation in the first complete remission using a human leukocyte antigen–matched family member donor is preferable to 2–3 years of standard chemotherapy. However, for adults and children with standard-risk ALL, overall survival and disease-free survival are equivalent with standard chemotherapy for 2–3 years and HSC transplantation. Adults who relapse after complete remission should ultimately undergo allogeneic HSC transplantation once a second remission is attained.

X.   SUMMARY

In the past 3 decades we have seen remarkable advances in our knowledge of the molecular pathogenesis of leukemia. However, improvement in the clinical outcome of adult patients with acute leukemia has been more modest. Nonetheless, at the beginning of the 21st century, we have witnessed the successful clinical application of our understanding of the pathogenesis of two types of leukemia, APL and chronic myelogenous leukemia. Pharmacologic targeting of the novel fusion proteins in these two diseases (ATRA in APL and imatinib mesylate [Gleevec, an abl tyrosine kinase inhibitor] in chronic myelogenous leukemia) has resulted in complete remissions without the usual toxicities of cytotoxic chemotherapy. As we learn more about the molecular pathways that control cell proliferation and differentiation, new therapeutic approaches to acute leukemia are likely to evolve.

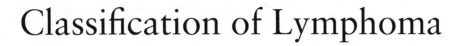
Classification of Lymphoma

- WILLIAM G. FINN

I. INTRODUCTION

Lymphoma (also called **malignant lymphoma**) is a neoplasm of cells derived from lymphocytes or lymphocyte precursors. The distinction between lymphoma and lymphoid leukemia is often confusing. As a general rule, a neoplasm of lymphocytes or lymphocyte precursors that manifests primarily as a tumor of **lymph nodes or related organs** (e.g., spleen, liver, other solid tissue) is considered lymphoma. A neoplasm of lymphocytes or lymphocyte precursors that manifests primarily as a proliferation of abnormal cells in the **blood and bone marrow** is considered **lymphoid leukemia.** However, leukemia may eventually spread to involve the lymph nodes or related organs, and lymphoma may eventually spread to involve the bone marrow and blood. The difference between leukemia and lymphoma in leukemic phase is confusing, but if one realizes that the difference is largely semantic (i.e., any hematopoietic malignancy can involve blood, bone marrow, lymph nodes, or related organs), the nomenclature becomes a matter of convention and hopefully less confusing.

II. PRINCIPLES OF THE CLASSIFICATION OF LYMPHOMA

Malignant lymphoma can be divided into two main categories: non-Hodgkin lymphoma and Hodgkin disease (also called Hodgkin lymphoma).

A. **Non-Hodgkin lymphoma** is a broad category that includes a number of types of lymphomas that all originate from lymphocytes or lymphocyte precursors.

   1. **Overview**

      a. Generally, the classification of non-Hodgkin lymphoma is based on the degree to which the cells in a particular type of non-Hodgkin lymphoma mimic normal lymphocytes in different compartments of the lymph node (Fig. 18–1), in bone marrow, in the thymus, in the spleen, or in other lymphoid organs. For example, lymphoma composed of cells that look and act like cells of the normal germinal center of the lymphoid follicle is called **follicular lymphoma.** Lymphoma composed of cells that look and act like cells of the normal mantle zone of the lymphoid follicle is called **mantle cell lymphoma.** Lymphoma composed of cells that look and act like cells of the normal marginal (parafollicular) zone is called **marginal zone lymphoma.**

      b. Although lymph node follicles are populated by B lymphocytes, some lymphomas display T-cell phenotypes. In the Western Hemisphere, B-cell lymphomas far outnumber T-cell lymphomas; therefore, this chapter focuses on the principles of classification of B-cell lymphomas.

      c. Mastering the classification and diagnosis of lymphoma is something that

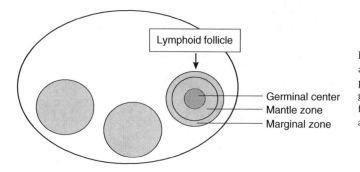

FIGURE 18–1. Normal lymph node architecture. The elements of the lymphoid follicle are highlighted. Marginal zones are more evident in splenic follicles than lymph node follicles but are included here for illustration.

few physicians do in an entire career. Therefore, what follows is a basic, overview of some of the subtypes of non-Hodgkin lymphoma and how these subtypes fit into the concept of normal lymph node anatomy and physiology. For a more comprehensive overview of lymphoma subtypes, see the list of suggested reading at the end of this chapter.

2. Non-Hodgkin lymphoma arising from naïve (prefollicular) B lymphocytes
   a. The terms **small lymphocytic lymphoma** (SLL) and **chronic lymphocytic leukemia** (CLL) are essentially synonymous, because they represent the same disease process manifesting in different ways.
      (1) If the disease involves lymph nodes or other solid organs but not blood, it is called SLL.
      (2) If the disease involves blood with or without lymph nodes, it is called CLL.
   b. B-cell CLL is the most common lymphoid malignancy in the Western Hemisphere. It is characterized by an increase in fairly normal appearing lymphocytes in the peripheral blood or by an infiltration of these lymphocytes in the lymph nodes, spleen, or other solid organs (Fig. 18–2).
   c. In the past, immunophenotyping studies (i.e., studies analyzing the pattern of surface protein expression on malignant lymphoid cells) revealed that the cells of CLL and SLL resembled naïve B cells. In other words, they mimic the profile seen in B cells before antigen-driven differentiation within the germinal center of the lymphoid follicle. Practically speaking, this means the cells express immunoglobulin (Ig) of the IgM or IgD class (as opposed to IgG or IgA), exhibit very low-density surface Ig expression, contain intracytoplasmic Ig, and express the marker CD5, which is usually restricted to T lymphocytes. Thus, the presence of CD5 antigen on a **B-cell** population can help in the diagnosis of CLL and SLL. More recently, the resemblance of CLL cells to naïve B cells has been questioned (see II.A.2.e.).
   d. Both CLL and SLL are slowly progressing diseases. They are generally considered incurable by standard therapy, but many people lead fairly normal lives despite the disease. Therapy (if necessary) is generally aimed toward relief of symptoms and improvement of quality of life.
   e. **Important caveat.** For the sake of illustration, CLL and SLL are listed here as neoplasms of naïve prefollicular B cells. This model is based on the surface marker expression pattern and homing patterns of the lymphocytes of CLL and SLL. However, recent genotypic data reveal that many (or most) typical examples of CLL and SLL are composed of cells with gene rearrangement patterns more similar to postfollicular (memory) B cells. This

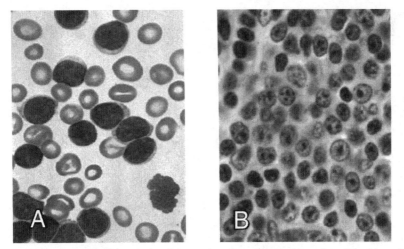

FIGURE 18–2. High-power photomicrographs of chronic lymphocytic leukemia and small lymphocytic lymphoma. **A.** High-power photomicrograph of a peripheral blood smear showing CLL marked by a proliferation of mature, fairly unremarkable-appearing lymphocytes. **B.** High-power photomicrograph of a lymph node biopsy showing infiltration of the lymph node by CLL and SLL. In histologic sections the small lymphocytes are admixed with occasional larger cells with prominent nucleoli. These larger cells coalesce to form proliferation centers, a hallmark of CLL and SLL in lymph node sections.

has resulted in a reappraisal of our basic understanding of the biology of CLL and SLL and is the topic of ongoing research.

3. **Non-Hodgkin lymphoma arising from the germinal center of the lymphoid follicle**
    a. **Follicular lymphoma** is also a common B-cell lymphoma in the Western Hemisphere.
        (1) Histologically, follicular lymphoma cells closely mimic the cells of the normal germinal center of the lymphoid follicle, even to the point that the tumor actually forms follicles.
        (2) Microscopic evaluation reveals a pattern that can be confused with reactive follicular hyperplasia. However, the follicles of follicular lymphoma generally do not respect the normal anatomic architecture of the lymph node, and follicles appear to proliferate throughout the lymph node (Fig. 18–3*A*). At closer look, the follicles of follicular lymphoma usually contain a fairly monotonous population of lymphoma cells (Fig. 18–3*B*). Unlike other cancers, follicular lymphoma generally displays **fewer** mitotic figures and **less** cell turnover than its benign counterpart, follicular hyperplasia.
        (3) In most follicular lymphoma cases, the malignant cells harbor a translocation between chromosomes 14 and 18, abbreviated t(14;18). This chromosomal abnormality juxtaposes the *bcl*-2 gene to the Ig heavy-chain gene. Because *bcl*-2 is involved in triggering programmed cell death (apoptosis), t(14;18) appears to play a role in the development of follicular lymphoma by preventing normal programmed cell death within the follicular B lymphocytes.
        (4) As with CLL and SLL, follicular lymphoma is an indolent, usually incurable disorder.
    b. **Large cell lymphomas** consist of cells that look like the largest cells that occupy normal follicles.

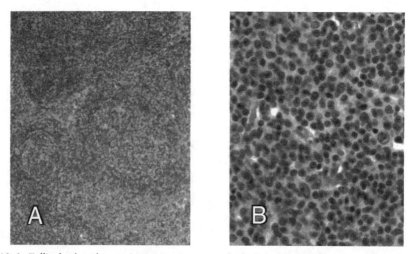

FIGURE 18–3. Follicular lymphoma. **A.** Low-power view of a lymph node biopsy showing follicular lymphoma. Note the haphazard proliferation of lymphoid follicles. **B.** High-power view of follicular lymphoma showing predominance of small cleaved follicle center cells.

(1) Sometimes large cell lymphomas display a follicular pattern. However, large cell lymphoma usually lacks follicular architecture.

(2) Lymphomas that do not form lymphoid follicles are called **diffuse** lymphomas. Therefore, most large cell lymphomas are called **diffuse large cell lymphomas** (Fig. 18–4). When the lymphoma cells can be identified as B cells, the term **diffuse large B-cell lymphoma** is used.

(3) Diffuse large B-cell lymphoma is an aggressive disease if untreated, unlike follicular lymphoma. Ironically, its aggressiveness makes it quite responsive to chemotherapy, and a significant fraction (perhaps up to half) of patients with diffuse large B-cell lymphoma may be cured by therapeutic intervention.

c. **Burkitt lymphoma** does not form follicles and is generally not considered a variant of follicular lymphoma. It is mentioned here because some have hypothesized that the cell type of Burkitt lymphoma originates in the germinal center.

(1) In the United States, Burkitt lymphoma most commonly arises in the lymphoid tissue of the distal small intestine. In Africa, Burkitt lymphoma most commonly arises in the lymph nodes of the head and neck region.

(2) Burkitt lymphoma has been linked to infection with Epstein-Barr virus, which is thought to play a causative role, particularly in the African type.

(3) Burkitt lymphoma is also linked to an alteration of the c-*myc* oncogene, and the cells of Burkitt lymphoma generally harbor a translocation between chromosomes 8 and 14, abbreviated t(8;14), that involves the c-*myc* oncogene on chromosome 8.

(4) Burkitt lymphoma is highly aggressive. The cells of Burkitt lymphoma proliferate at a higher rate than virtually any other human neoplasm (Fig. 18–5). However, this makes the disease amenable to aggressive chemotherapeutic intervention. Relapse after therapy is fairly common, but a fraction of these patients may be cured.

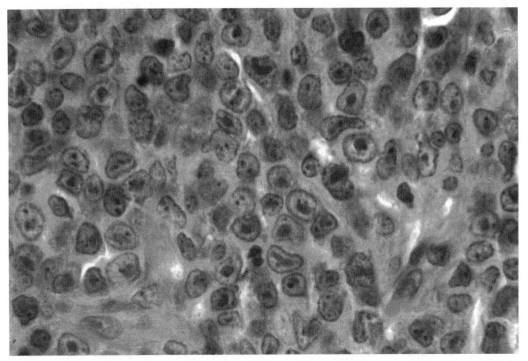

FIGURE 18–4. Diffuse large B-cell lymphoma. Note the sheets of large cells with prominent nucleoli on this high-power view.

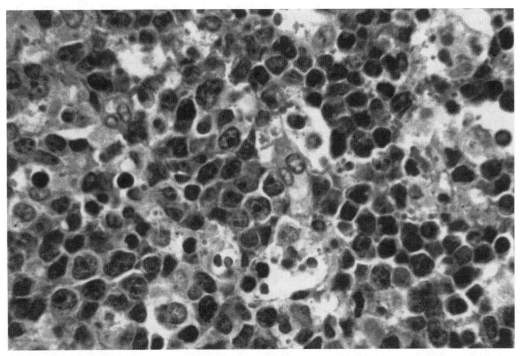

FIGURE 18–5. High-power view of Burkitt lymphoma. This lymphoma is marked by a very high rate of cell proliferation, generally manifested by numerous mitotic figures and scattered individual benign phagocytic histiocytes, imparting a starry sky pattern.

4. **Non-Hodgkin lymphoma arising from the mantle zone of the lymphoid follicle: mantle cell lymphoma**

   a. Although initially recognized more than 25 years ago, mantle cell lymphoma has only recently been appreciated as a distinct type of lymphoma.

   b. Mantle cell lymphoma consists of cells that seem to represent the neoplastic counterpart of mantle zone lymphocytes of the normal lymphoid follicle (i.e., the cuff surrounding the germinal center).

   c. Mantle cell lymphoma is distinct histologically, immunophenotypically, genetically, and clinically.

      (1) Histologically, mantle cell lymphoma is usually diffuse (Fig. 18–6A). In a minority of cases, however, the involved lymph nodes show a pattern of expansion of neoplastic mantle zones surrounding benign germinal centers (Fig. 18–6B).

      (2) Mantle cell lymphoma shares some immunophenotypic features with CLL and SLL (see II.A.2.). Specifically, it usually expresses Ig of the IgM or IgD class, and importantly, it also expresses the CD5 antigen. (CD5 is expressed on normal T cells, so its presence on a B-cell lymphoma is important to the diagnosis.)

      (3) Mantle cell lymphoma is associated with a chromosomal translocation between chromosomes 11 and 14, abbreviated t(11;14). This translocation juxtaposes the gene for cyclin D1 (also called *bcl*-1) on chromosome 11 to the Ig heavy-chain gene on chromosome 14. Cyclin D1 plays a key role in entry of a cell into the cell cycle (i.e., the process that leads to cell division) and is thought to play a role in the development of mantle cell lymphoma.

      (4) Although mantle cell lymphoma shares some common features with CLL and SLL, the distinction between these lymphoma types is important. CLL and SLL are incurable but usually follow a long, slowly progressive clinical course. Mantle cell lymphoma is also incurable by standard therapy but is clinically more aggressive, with median survival of 3–5 years after diagnosis.

5. **Non-Hodgkin lymphoma arising from the marginal (parafollicular) zone of the lymphoid follicle.** This includes B-cell monocytoid lymphoma, low-grade mucosa-associated lymphoid tissue (MALT) lymphoma, and splenic marginal zone lymphoma.

   a. **Marginal zone lymphomas** are a group of recently recognized low-grade lymphomas described in the 1980s and 1990s.

   b. The cells that constitute these lymphomas resemble the small lymphocytes normally seen in the parafollicular (marginal) zone of normal splenic lymphoid follicles (Fig. 18–7). Specifically, these cells have slightly bent or bean-shaped nuclei and abundant cytoplasm that imparts distinct spacing between the nuclei of each cell in a histologic section.

   c. Recently, much attention has been focused on a type of marginal zone lymphoma known as extranodal marginal zone B-cell lymphoma of mucosa-associated lymphoid tissue, or simply MALT lymphoma (Fig. 18–8).

      (1) Lymphoid tissue is present throughout the gastrointestinal tract (e.g., Peyer patches in the small intestine) and is known as MALT. Therefore, MALT lymphomas are thought to represent the neoplastic counterpart to normal MALT.

      (2) MALT lymphomas can arise in any mucosal site but are most common in the stomach, salivary glands, and lacrimal glands.

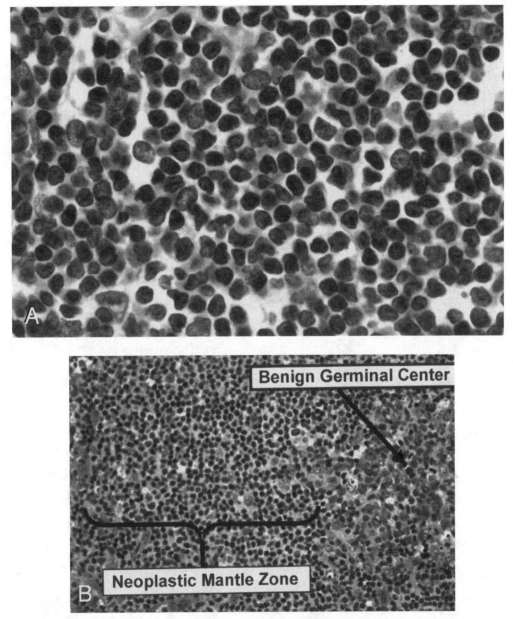

FIGURE 18–6. Mantle Cell Lymphoma. **A.** High-power view of mantle cell lymphoma showing a diffuse pattern of growth. **B.** Mantle cell lymphoma occasionally appears as expanded neoplastic mantle zones surrounding benign germinal centers, mimicking the distribution of the normal mantle zone.

(3) In the stomach and duodenum, MALT lymphomas have been linked to infection with *Helicobacter pylori*, better known as a cause of peptic ulcer disease. Antibiotic therapy aimed at eradicating *H. pylori* can be a highly effective therapy for early-stage MALT lymphoma of the stomach.

6. **Non-Hodgkin lymphoma arising from T cells**
   a. T-cell lymphomas are uncommon in the Western Hemisphere, although they are quite prevalent in the East (e.g., Japan).

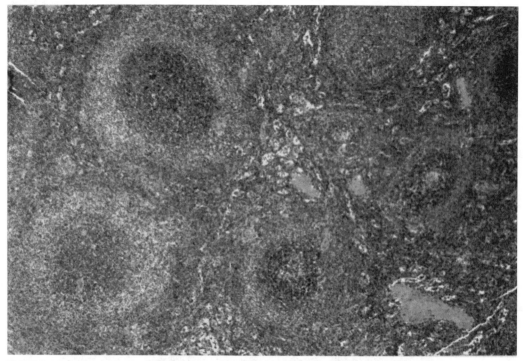

FIGURE 18–7. Low-power view of splenic marginal zone lymphoma. Note the markedly expanded pale marginal zones surrounding the normal follicles of the splenic white pulp.

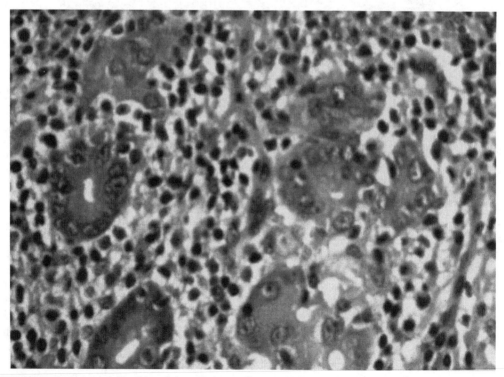

FIGURE 18–8. Low-grade B-cell lymphoma of mucosa-associated lymphoid tissue involving the stomach. Note the destruction of gastric glands by the infiltrate of small lymphocytes.

    b. Clinically and histologically, T-cell lymphomas are diverse and not easily categorized. For this reason, most T-cell lymphomas are officially categorized as T-cell lymphoma, unspecified. Nonetheless, several distinct (albeit rare) forms of T-cell lymphoma exist.

    c. T-cell lymphoma is not a focus of this chapter. See the list of additional reading at the end of this chapter.

B. Hodgkin disease (Hodgkin lymphoma)

    1. Overview

        a. Hodgkin disease is a distinct type of lymphoma. Clinically, it is marked by a tendency to spread in contiguous fashion, from lymph node group to lymph node group. This pattern of spread is in contrast to non-Hodgkin lymphoma, which may spread in a less predictable fashion, most likely via seeding of the bloodstream by lymphoma cells, in addition to the more predictable lymphatic spread.

        b. Hodgkin disease is also distinct histologically. The infiltrate seen under the microscope in a lymph node affected by Hodgkin disease consists largely of an inflammatory (i.e., nonneoplastic) reaction to the neoplastic cells. The neoplastic cells themselves are a small minority of cells in the infiltrate and appear cytologically distinct.

        c. The actual neoplastic cell type of Hodgkin disease is known as the Reed-Sternberg cell (or Hodgkin cell).

        (1) Classic Reed-Sternberg cells are large, with bilobed nuclei. Each nuclear lobe contains a large nucleolus imparting an owl's-eye appearance (Fig. 18–9).

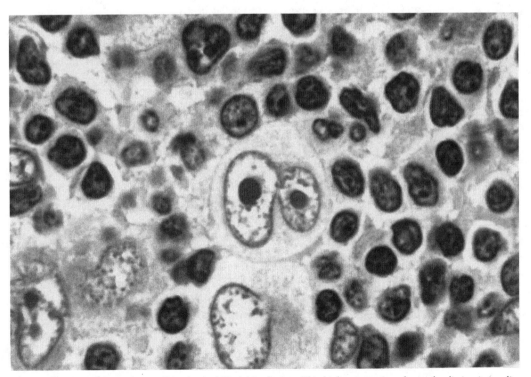

FIGURE 18–9. Reed-Sternberg cell in classical Hodgkin disease. This high-power view shows the distinctive owl's-eye appearance.

       (2) For decades, no one knew exactly what the Reed-Sternberg cell represented. Indeed, no one was sure it was a lymphoid cell; hence the term *Hodgkin disease* as opposed to the more recent *Hodgkin lymphoma*.

       (3) Recently, molecular genetic analysis has revealed strong evidence that Reed-Sternberg cells are derived from B cells of the germinal center.

       (4) Nonetheless, Hodgkin lymphoma still warrants its own category because its clinical presentation, histology, and response to specific types of therapy are distinct.

  2. **Subclassification of Hodgkin disease**

    a. Hodgkin disease is typically divided into four histologic subtypes.

      (1) **Nodular sclerosis** (named for prominent sclerosis of involved nodes, yielding sclerotic nodules)

      (2) **Mixed cellularity** (named for the prominence of the mixed inflammatory infiltrate and lack of sclerosis)

      (3) **Lymphocyte depleted** (named for the presence of sheets of Reed-Sternberg cells, with little inflammatory background)

      (4) **Lymphocyte predominant** (a distinct and separate disease)

    b. The **lymphocyte predominant** type of Hodgkin disease behaves much like a low-grade B-cell non-Hodgkin lymphoma. The term **classical Hodgkin disease** has emerged to signify all types of Hodgkin disease other than the lymphocyte predominant type. Therefore, a more useful conceptualization of Hodgkin disease is as follows:

      (1) **Classical Hodgkin disease**

        (a) **Nodular sclerosis (most common)**

        (b) **Mixed cellularity**

        (c) **Lymphocyte depleted (extremely rare)**

      (2) **Lymphocyte predominant Hodgkin disease**

    c. The **lymphocyte depleted** type of Hodgkin disease is extremely rare. Most cases that used to be called lymphocyte depleted Hodgkin disease are now categorized as either variants of nodular sclerosis Hodgkin disease or as variants of large-cell non-Hodgkin lymphoma.

    d. Generally, most cases of classical Hodgkin disease are of the nodular sclerosis type.

III. GROUPING LYMPHOMAS BY CLINICAL BEHAVIOR

The beginning of the chapter discusses classifying lymphomas according to the theoretical origins of the neoplastic cell in each lymphoma subtype. It is sometimes more helpful to conceptualize lymphomas by how clinically aggressive they are or how well they respond to certain types of therapy.

  A. **Lymphomas that are indolent (slow growing) but usually incurable**

    1. CLL and SLL

    2. Follicular lymphoma except the large-cell type

    3. Some marginal zone lymphomas; gastric MALT lymphoma is often curable in the early stages

  B. **Lymphomas that are fairly aggressive if untreated but may be cured with appropriate therapy**

    1. Hodgkin disease

    2. Follicular lymphoma, large-cell type

    3. Diffuse large B-cell lymphoma

  C. **Lymphomas that are fairly aggressive and incurable:** mantle cell lymphoma

D. **Lymphomas that are extremely aggressive if untreated but potentially curable with therapy**
1. Burkitt lymphoma
2. Lymphoblastic lymphoma

IV. SUMMARY

Lymphoma is a neoplasm of cells derived from lymphocytes or lymphocyte precursors. Lymphoma is broadly categorized as either Hodgkin disease (also called Hodgkin lymphoma) and non-Hodgkin lymphoma.

A. Non-Hodgkin lymphomas are usually classified according to the degree to which the cells of a particular lymphoma mimic cells in normal lymph nodes and other lymphoid organs. For example, lymphomas consisting of cells mimicking those found in the germinal center of the lymphoid follicle are called follicular lymphomas. Non-Hodgkin lymphomas vary widely in their clinical behavior and response to treatment; therefore, accurate classification of these disorders is important.

B. Hodgkin disease is a distinct form of lymphoma characterized histologically by a prominent reactive (inflammatory) infiltrate surrounding individual large cells known as Reed-Sternberg cells. Clinically, Hodgkin disease initially presents in the mediastinum and tends to spread contiguously from one lymph node group to the next. Therapy is usually quite effective, and a majority of patients with Hodgkin disease can be cured with standard treatments.

SUGGESTED READING

Aster J, Kumar V. White cells, lymph nodes, spleen, and thymus. In: Cotran RS, Kumar VK, Collins T, eds. *Robbins Pathologic Basis of Disease*. 6th ed. Philadelphia: Saunders, 1999:645–674.

Finn WG, Kroft SH. New classifications for non-Hodgkin's lymphoma. In: Tallman MS, Gordon LI, eds. *Diagnostic and Therapeutic Advances in Hematologic Malignancies*. Boston: Kluwer Academic, 1999:1–26.

Harris NL et al. A revised European–American classification of lymphoid neoplasms: A proposal from the International Lymphoma Study Group. *Blood* 1994; 84:1361–1392.

Jaffe ES, Harris NL, Stein H, Vardiman JW, eds. *World Health Organization Classification of Tumours: Pathology and Genetics of Tumours of the Haematopoietic and Lymphoid Tissues*. Lyon: IARC, 2001.

Clinical Evaluation and Management of Lymphoma

• MARK S. KAMINSKI

I. INTRODUCTION

Hodgkin disease, also known as Hodgkin lymphoma, and non-Hodgkin lymphoma are two malignant disorders arising from cells that populate the lymph nodes.

II. DIAGNOSIS OF LYMPHOMA

A. Establishing the histopathologic diagnosis of either Hodgkin disease or non-Hodgkin lymphoma is crucial because the prognosis and treatment regimen for each disease is different.

B. Differential diagnosis of **palpable lymphadenopathy** includes careful history and physical examination as well as consideration of all possible causes.
   1. The **history and physical examination** should focus on:
      a. Age of the patient (e.g., pediatric, adult)
      b. Local or systemic symptoms (e.g., infection, trauma)
      c. Size, location, history of nodes (e.g., rapid, slow, or indolent growth) (Table 19–1)
   2. **Causes of lymphadenopathy** include:
      a. Infections, such as common cold, local acute or chronic infection, infectious mononucleosis, tuberculosis, syphilis, toxoplasmosis, cytomegalovirus, HIV, cat-scratch fever
      b. Drugs (e.g., phenytoin)
      c. Connective tissue disorders (e.g., systemic lupus erythematosus, dermatomyositis, scleroderma)
      d. Metastatic cancer
      e. Primary lymphoid malignancies (e.g., Hodgkin disease, non-Hodgkin lymphoma)

III. DISTINCTIONS BETWEEN HODGKIN DISEASE AND NON-HODGKIN LYMPHOMA

A. **Epidemiologic factors**
   1. Hodgkin disease is about one-third as common as non-Hodgkin lymphoma. In the United States, there were about 60,000 new cases of non-Hodgkin

TABLE 19–1 • Distinctions Between Palpable Lymph Nodes

Normal	Reactive	Malignant
Small (0.5–1.0 cm)	Moderately large (< 2 cm)	Large (> 1 cm, especially > 2 cm)
Soft, flat, ellipsoid, fixed	Firm, spherical, movable	Firm, spherical, especially matted
Nontender	Tender or nontender	Usually nontender
Usually multiple	Single to multiple (depends on disease)	Single or multiple (depends on type of cancer)
Usually high neck, submandibular, submental areas; occasionally inguinal	Usually cervical	Any anatomic nodal area
Usually stable	Should resolve 1–2 mo after acute process stops	Progressive growth

lymphoma in 2000, and non-Hodgkin lymphoma is associated with an estimated 25,000 deaths per year and a prevalence of approximately 250,000.

2. The incidence of non-Hodgkin lymphoma is rising rapidly, while the incidence of Hodgkin disease is not rising. Non-Hodgkin lymphoma now ranks fifth among cancers in incidence and cause of death from cancer.

3. Hodgkin disease has a bimodal age distribution; it peaks at 20–29 years of age and again at 60 years of age and older. The incidence of non-Hodgkin lymphoma increases with age.

4. Both Hodgkin disease and non-Hodgkin lymphoma have a moderate male predominance.

B. **Clinical presentation**

1. Differences in clinical presentation arise in part from distinct differences in the pattern of spread of disease. Hodgkin disease generally spreads in a contiguous fashion from one anatomic lymph node group to another. Non-Hodgkin lymphoma is less predictable in its spreading pattern. It can have characteristics of blood dissemination and lymphatic contiguity.

2. Hodgkin disease rarely involves the mesenteric nodes, central nervous system (CNS), skin, gastrointestinal tract, or Waldeyer ring. These sites are much more likely to be affected by non-Hodgkin lymphoma.

3. Gross splenomegaly is rare in Hodgkin disease; it is more common in non-Hodgkin lymphoma.

4. Fever, night sweats, and weight loss (i.e., B symptoms) can accompany both disorders. However, pruritus and pain soon after drinking alcohol (i.e., non-B symptoms) are much more likely to be associated with Hodgkin disease.

C. **Staging**

1. The prognosis and treatment of Hodgkin disease and non-Hodgkin lymphoma are greatly influenced by the stage (degree of known spread) of the disease. Staging is especially important in Hodgkin disease because it is used to decide whether radiation therapy is appropriate as the sole treatment or should be given after chemotherapy and to what field.

2. The **Ann Arbor staging system** (Table 19–2) is used for both Hodgkin disease and non-Hodgkin lymphoma.

3. The tools used to stage Hodgkin disease and non-Hodgkin lymphoma are similar. These tools are used to determine the overall stage and identify prognostic factors that may influence the outcome within stages of the disease.

TABLE 19–2 • The Ann Arbor Staging Classification

Stage[a]	Description
I	Involvement of a single lymph node region (I) or a single extralymphatic organ or site (IE)
II	Involvement of two or more lymph node regions on same side of diaphragm (II) or local involvement of an extralymphatic organ or site and one or more lymph node regions on same side of diaphragm (IIE)
III	Involvement of lymph node regions on both sides of diaphragm (III), which may also be accompanied by involvement of the spleen (III$_s$) or by local involvement of an extralymphatic organ or site (IIIE) or both (III$_s$E).
IV	Diffuse or disseminated involvement of one or more extralymphatic organs or tissues, with or without lymph node involvement

[a]Letters following the roman numerals are used to subclassify the stage. Fever, night sweats, or unexplained loss of 10% or more of body weight in the 6 mo preceding diagnosis is denoted by B. A indicates absence of these symptoms. E indicates involvement of an extralymphatic site; S indicates splenic involvement.
Adapted from Hoffman R et al. Hematology: Basic Principles and Practice. New York: Churchill-Livingstone, 1991.

  a. History
     (1) Unexplained fever
     (2) Weight loss
     (3) Night sweats
     (4) Pruritus
     (5) Alcohol intolerance
     (6) Fatigue
     (7) Pain
     (8) Overall performance status
     (9) Overall tempo of the disease
  b. Physical examination
     (1) Areas of palpable lymphadenopathy
     (2) Size of liver and spleen
     (3) Bony tenderness
     (4) Neurologic abnormalities
  c. Laboratory studies
     (1) Complete blood count, differential and platelet count, erythrocyte sedimentation rate (especially for Hodgkin disease)
     (2) Serum alkaline phosphatase, lactic dehydrogenase, albumin, uric acid
     (3) Renal function (creatinine, blood urea nitrogen [BUN])
     (4) Liver function tests
  d. Radiologic studies
     (1) Chest radiograph
     (2) Computed tomography scan of the chest, abdomen, and pelvis
     (3) Bone scan or bone radiograph if symptoms of bone involvement are present
     (4) Gallium or positron emission tomography (PET) scan, especially when other radiologic studies are equivocal
  e. Biopsies
     (1) Diagnostic biopsy of affected lymph node (reviewed by experienced hematopathologist)
     (2) Bone marrow biopsy, especially when treatment may be modified

(3) Biopsy of suspicious disseminated extranodal sites (e.g., pulmonary or liver lesions) if clinically indicated

4. Staging laparotomy (e.g., splenectomy, liver biopsy, lymph node sampling) was a tool widely used before the advent of computed tomography scans and sensitive nuclear medicine scans. It has now been abandoned as a staging tool.

IV. TREATMENT OF HODGKIN DISEASE

A. **Early stages: IA, IB, IIA**

1. **Radiation therapy alone.** Until recently, the mainstay of treatment for early-stage Hodgkin disease was radiation therapy. Because of the contiguity of spread of Hodgkin disease to adjacent lymph node groups, radiation was given to the clinically involved areas and the next contiguous clinically uninvolved nodal groups. This approach resulted in the development of standard radiation fields (i.e., mantle, paraaortic, pelvic) to fit the individual situation.

2. **Chemotherapy followed by radiation.** With the recognition that within the clinical stages of disease certain prognostic factors can influence outcome (Table 19–3) and that large-field radiation is associated with the development of second malignancies, heart disease, and lung disease, chemotherapy has been increasingly incorporated into the treatment plan. The use of chemotherapy before radiation is designed to eradicate disease in the next contiguous clinically uninvolved nodal groups. Beginning with chemotherapy treatment allows the fields of radiation to be limited to clinically involved areas, thereby lessening the exposure of the patient to radiation. A standard approach is administration of an abbreviated course of chemotherapy (usually four cycles) followed by involved-field radiation. The most widely accepted chemotherapy regimen is doxorubicin (Adriamycin), bleomycin, vinblastine, and dacarbazine (ABVD).

3. **Chemotherapy alone.** The complete elimination of radiation from the treatment regimen is controversial and is still the subject of research.

4. **Overall results.** Regardless of the approach used, a 5-year freedom from relapse rate of at least 80% is expected for patients with early-stage disease with no unfavorable factors. However, the longer patients are followed, the more treatment-related mortality increases; thus, death from Hodgkin disease is becoming less of a concern than the late consequences of treatment (see IV.D.).

B. **Later stages: IIB, IIIA, IIIB, IVA, IVB**

1. **Chemotherapy alone.** Chemotherapy is the primary form of treatment in advanced cases of Hodgkin disease. The role of radiation therapy as consolida-

---

TABLE 19–3 • Unfavorable Factors in Hodgkin Disease

Early-Stage Disease	Advanced Disease
Bulky disease[a]	Albumin < 4.0 g/dL
Any mass > 10 cm	Hemoglobin < 10.5 g/dL
Erythrocyte sedimentation rate > 50 mm/hr	Leukocytosis ($> 15,000/\mu$L)
More than three sites of disease	Lymphopenia ($600/\mu$L or $< 8\%$ of total WBC)
	Male
	Older than 45 years of age
	Stage IV disease

[a]Ratio of maximum mediastinal mass width to maximum intrathoracic diameter $> 1:3$

tion after chemotherapy is controversial. ABVD is the most commonly used regimen, although other regimens are continually being tested.

2. **Overall results.** As with early-stage disease, a number of adverse prognostic factors affect the outcome of late-stage disease (Table 19–3). The prognosis according to the number of unfavorable factors is shown in Table 19–4.

C. **Salvaging treatment failures**

1. Chemotherapy, usually ABVD, is used at the time of relapse for patients treated with radiation therapy alone. The success rate of inducing a second remission is approximately 60%.

2. For patients who relapse after receiving chemotherapy as part of the initial treatment, salvage with standard-dose chemotherapy is far less successful.

3. High-dose chemotherapy with autologous stem cell transplantation is generally preferred for patients relapsing after standard-dose chemotherapy. Long-term success with this treatment is up to 40% in some series. However, salvage after transplant is dismal, and there are no known curative options.

D. **Complications of treatment**

1. Despite the high rate of success in the treatment of Hodgkin disease, long-term follow-up indicates a continuous pattern of mortality related to the agents used in therapy. Death from complications of treatment now approximates, if not exceeds, death from Hodgkin disease in certain stages.

2. Secondary leukemias were the first major concern to emerge. Previously, the risk of developing leukemia was approximately 5% at 5–7 years after exposure to chemotherapy. This risk appears to have decreased with the broad use of ABVD rather than the previously used alkylating agent–containing regimen nitrogen mustard, vincristine (Oncovin), procarbazine, and prednisone (MOPP).

3. Solid tumors (e.g., breast, lung, sarcoma) have now emerged as the principal problem. There appears to be no plateau to the incidence over time.

4. Lung fibrosis and early coronary artery disease are among late problems.

5. It is hoped that reducing the fields of radiation and the radiation dose will curb the incidence of these late events. Alterations in chemotherapeutic regimens may also help.

E. **Lymphocyte predominant Hodgkin lymphoma.** This disease is often categorized with the other histologic types of Hodgkin disease. However, there is considerable doubt that this entity should be classified as Hodgkin disease. Its clinical behavior and immunophenotype are more akin to low-grade or follicular B-cell

TABLE 19–4 • Prognosis for Advanced Hodgkin Disease According to the Number of Unfavorable Factors

Number of Factors	Proportion of Population (%)	Freedom From Progression at 5 Years (%)
0	7	84
1	22	77
2	29	67
3	23	60
4	12	51
5+	7	40

(Abstracted from Hasenclever DH, Diehl V, et al. A prognostic score for advanced Hodgkin's disease. *N Engl J Med* 1998;339:1506–14)

non-Hodgkin lymphoma. The therapeutic recommendations for this disease are in flux.

V.   TREATMENT OF NON-HODGKIN LYMPHOMA

A. **Overview.** Treatment recommendations are highly dependent on the histologic type of disease. Therefore, it is imperative that a thorough and expert review of pathologic specimens be performed before initiation of treatment and in some cases before staging.

1. Although imperfect and dated, the Working Formulation for Clinical Usage is still a useful guide. It is based on the morphologic appearance of the lymphoma along with its known usual clinical behavior and response to treatment. In general, it divides the non-Hodgkin lymphomas into three major categories: **low-, intermediate-,** and **high-grade non-Hodgkin lymphoma.**

2. Over time, our knowledge of the biology of the various non-Hodgkin lymphomas has expanded and allowed us to classify them in a more sophisticated way. The Revised European-American Lymphoma (REAL) classification scheme, which is undergoing continual revision, has also enabled the inclusion of disease entities that previously either were not recognized or did not fit well into the Working Formulation.

B. **Indolent, usually incurable non-Hodgkin lymphomas.** These lymphomas account for approximately 30%–40% of lymphomas. The median age of presentation is 50–60 years. The most common types are the follicular lymphomas, followed by the small lymphocytic lymphomas. Chronic lymphocytic leukemia (CLL) (see V.C.) can be regarded as a type of small lymphocytic lymphoma when circulating lymphoma cells are detected in the blood. More than 80% of these lymphomas are diagnosed in an advanced stage. Despite the advanced stage of the disease, most patients are not symptomatic, and the disease often behaves in an indolent manner (i.e., stays stable in size for long periods, slowly increases in size, or decreases in size). The natural history of the disease is typically long, with median survivals of 7–10 years.

1. **Initial observation.** Given that treatment may lessen the quality of life and that the disease appears incurable, can be slow growing, may not produce symptoms for some time, and may spontaneously regress, some patients can be observed without treatment until intervention is clinically necessary (i.e., when symptoms emerge, the pace of the disease increases, blood counts are compromised, or a vital organ is at risk).

   a. Approximately 20% of patients have spontaneous regression without receiving treatment. Although regression can be complete and last for months or years, it is temporary.

   b. Studies have indicated that there is no difference in the survival of patients who receive immediate treatment compared to those who are just observed (Figure 19–1).

   c. The median time from diagnosis to treatment using this observational approach is approximately 2–3 years.

2. **Chemotherapy.** Paradoxically, these are among the most responsive neoplasms to initial treatment with chemotherapy. However, relapse of disease is inevitable (median of 2–3 years after initial treatment), regardless of the intensity of treatment.

   a. There is a range of choices for initial chemotherapy, from single agents to multiagent combinations.

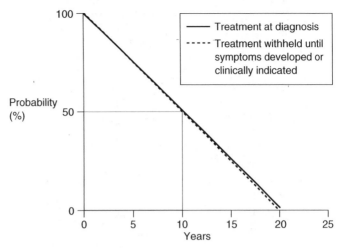

FIGURE 19–1. Survival of patients with indolent lymphoma with or without initial treatment.

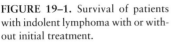

(1) Commonly used single-agent regimens include chlorambucil (pill form), fludarabine (a purine analog), or cyclophosphamide.

(2) Multiagent combinations include cyclophosphamide, vincristine, and prednisone (CVP); cyclophosphamide, hydroxydaunomycin (doxorubicin), vincristine (Oncovin), and prednisone (CHOP); and fludarabine, mitoxantrone (Novantrone), and dexamethasone (FND).

   b. Upon relapse, treatment with the same or a different, more intense chemotherapy regimen is often successful. However, with each relapse the remission becomes shorter until the disease resists treatment. Eventually, the patient dies of either the disease or complications of treatment.

3. **Radiation therapy.** At times, only one site of disease may cause symptoms. In these instances, local radiation may be appropriate to palliate symptoms. Long-term local control of disease is frequently possible with this approach, with patients enjoying long disease-free intervals (median of close to 10 years) and long overall survival (median of approximately 17 years). However, in most instances the disease is widespread, and there is no curative treatment. In these cases, survival curves continue on a downward slope without clear evidence of a plateau (Figure 19–2). In addition, the indolent lymphoma may transform to an aggressive form of disease, which portends a poorer prognosis.

4. **Stem cell transplantation.** This approach is rarely used as an initial treatment because toxicity can be severe and early mortality from complications can occur, especially with allotransplants. Stem cell transplantation is generally reserved for patients with a poor prognosis (e.g., short remission, transformation to an aggressive lymphoma).

5. **Monoclonal antibodies.** Rituximab is a chimeric monoclonal antibody (human–mouse hybrid) directed against the CD20 antigen expressed by nearly all lymphomas of B-cell origin (approximately 85% of lymphomas). When it is given by intravenous infusion weekly for 4 weeks, the response rate in patients with indolent lymphomas that have relapsed after chemotherapy is approximately 50% (mostly partial remissions). The median response duration is approximately 9–12 months. Recently, this antibody has been used in combination with chemotherapy; it is believed to sensitize tumor cells to chemotherapy.

6. **Radiolabeled monoclonal antibodies.** Anti–CD20 antibodies tagged with radionuclides, such as iodine-131 (Bexxar) and yttrium-90 (Zevalin), have been

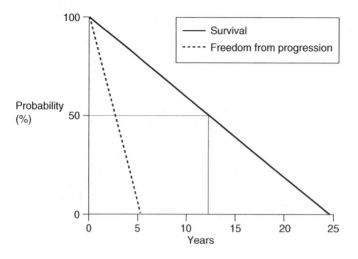

FIGURE 19–2. Survival and freedom from progression in indolent lymphoma.

shown to produce higher overall response rates (60%–80%) and higher complete response rates (20%– 40%) in patients with chemotherapy-relapsed or refractory indolent lymphomas than their unlabeled counterparts. For example, iodine-131 used as initial therapy for follicular lymphoma has demonstrated a 95% response rate and a 74% complete response rate. The main side effect of radiolabeled monoclonal antibodies is reversible bone marrow suppression.

7. **Interferon.** This biologic has activity in indolent lymphoma and has generally been used in combination with chemotherapy or as a single agent after chemotherapy in an effort to maintain remission. Data from various studies are conflicting as to whether overall survival is improved by the addition of interferon to chemotherapy.

8. **Vaccines.** Studies are under way to determine whether vaccines directed against the surface immunoglobulin idiotype displayed on malignant B cells can prolong remission after initial treatment with chemotherapy.

9. **Antibiotics.** Mucosa-associated lymphoid tissue (MALT) lymphoma of the stomach is the only indolent lymphoma that may be curable with antibiotics. If MALT lymphoma is associated with a *Helicobacter pylori* infection of the stomach, antibiotic eradication of the infection results in frequent and complete remissions.

10. **T-cell lymphomas.** Although almost all lymphomas are of B-cell lineage, a form of T-cell lymphoma involving the skin (i.e., mycosis fungoides) can also be included in the indolent lymphoma category. T-cell lymphomas typically present with plaque-like lesions and can be treated with **ultraviolet light, radiation therapy,** and **various topicals** (e.g., nitrogen mustard, retinoids). In some cases, the disease can progress to invade lymph nodes or to produce tumors on the skin, in which case the prognosis becomes poorer. Treatment in these stages can include **chemotherapy, interferon,** and **interleukin-2 conjugated to diptheria toxin (Ontak).**

C. **Chronic lymphocytic leukemia.** CLL can be considered part of the spectrum of small lymphocytic lymphomas. It is the most common leukemia in the Western Hemisphere, affecting 20 in 100,000 persons older than 60 years of age. The diagnosis is often incidental on routine blood screening, and patients frequently have no symptoms. There is a monoclonal lymphocytosis in the blood (i.e., absolute lymphocyte count of at least $10,000/\mu L$). More than 95% of cases of CLL are derived from B-cell lineage. The prognosis depends on the stage of disease (Table 19–5). Median survival ranges from 12 or more years for stage 0 to 1.5 years for stage 4.

1. As with the other indolent lymphomas, some patients with CLL can be observed without initial treatment.
2. The most effective drug for the treatment of CLL is **fludarabine** (a purine analog), which is increasingly being used as initial therapy. However, oral chlorambucil with or without prednisone can also be used with reasonable success. The choice of treatment depends on the anticipated tolerance of either treatment and the desired rapidity of response. The prognosis for patients who are resistant to fludarabine is dim. However, an antibody to CD52 (Campath-1H) has recently been shown to be effective in patients who are resistant to fludarabine and do not have bulky lymphadenopathy. Rituximab in high doses has also shown efficacy. It is now being combined with fludarabine or fludarabine plus cyclophosphamide in studies of initial treatment.
3. In selected cases, autologous or allogeneic stem cell transplants, including subablative transplants, have shown promise.

D. **Aggressive, potentially curable non-Hodgkin lymphomas.** These are the most common lymphomas. By far the most common type is diffuse large B-cell lymphoma. Other recognized entities include anaplastic large cell lymphoma; peripheral T-cell lymphoma, unspecified; and peripheral T-cell lymphoma, natural killer cell lymphoma. It is more common to diagnose these lymphomas in a lower stage than indolent lymphomas. Because of their rapid growth and propensity to invade vital organs, staging and treatment of these lymphomas should be initiated soon after diagnosis. Certain sites of involvement (i.e., bone marrow, sinuses, testes) pose a higher risk of CNS involvement. The International Prognostic Index identifies risk factors for prognosis, including age, stage, lactate dehydrogenase, number of extralymphatic sites, and performance status. Table 19–6 identifies the prognosis based on the number of risk factors.

1. Chemotherapy, the primary treatment for aggressive non-Hodgkin lymphomas, can be curative. Unfortunately, despite numerous combinations of drugs tried over the years, no treatment regimen has been found to be superior to CHOP.
   a. Patients with low-stage disease and no other adverse factors have a good prognosis. The usual recommended treatment for patients with localized disease is CHOP for 3–4 cycles followed by local radiation therapy.

TABLE 19–5 • RAI Clinical Staging System

Stage	Description
0	Lymphocytosis only (in blood and marrow)
1	Lymphocytosis plus enlarged nodes
2	Lymphocytosis plus enlarged spleen and/or liver with or without enlargement of nodes
3	Lymphocytosis plus anemia (hemoglobin < 110 g/dL), with or without enlarged nodes, spleen, or liver
4	Lymphocytosis plus thrombocytopenia (platelets $< 100 \times 10^9/\mu L$, with or without anemia and/or enlarged spleen, or liver

Adapted with permission from Rai KR et al. Clinical staging of chronic lymphocytic leukemia. *Blood* 1975;46:219.

TABLE 19–6 • International Prognostic Index for Aggressive Non-Hodgkin Lymphoma

IPI	Expected Complete Remission Rate	Predicted 2-Year Survival Rate	Predicted 5-Year Survival Rate
0–1	87%	84%	73%
2	67	66	51
3	55	54	43
4–5	44	34	26

IPI, International Prognostic Index. Each risk factor [age > 60, stage III or IV, LDH elevation, ≥ 2 extralymphatic sites, and performance status ≥2 (on a scale from 0–4)] is assigned a value of one. The number of IPI values (0–5) is indirectly correlated with prognosis.

    b. The outcome for patients who are considered intermediate high risk or high risk is suboptimal. The standard treatment is CHOP alone, but studies are under way to determine whether adding anti–CD20 antibodies to the regimen or consolidating CHOP with autologous stem cell transplantation can improve prognosis.

    c. Elderly patients have a poorer prognosis overall, partially because they are less likely to tolerate intensive treatments.

    d. Probably fewer than 20% of patients who do not achieve a complete remission with initial therapy can be cured.

  2. The most successful salvage approach is with stem cell transplantation (usually autologous). Unfortunately, many patients are too old to withstand the toxicity of such an approach. In addition, success of the transplant depends on whether the patient's disease is still sensitive to chemotherapy, which may be less than 50% of the time. Thus, new approaches to treatment are clearly needed.

E. Moderately aggressive incurable non-Hodgkin lymphomas. A prime example of such a lymphoma is mantle cell lymphoma. This B-cell lymphoma has a clear male predominance and a median survival of 3–4 years. It usually presents in an advanced stage, often with splenomegaly, circulating lymphoma cells, or intestinal involvement.

  1. Although it usually initially responds to chemotherapy, such as CHOP, remissions are short.

  2. Resistance to salvage regimens, including transplantation, is frequent.

F. Highly aggressive, potentially curable non-Hodgkin lymphomas. These include Burkitt lymphoma and lymphoblastic lymphoma.

  1. Despite their tendency for rapid proliferation, these lymphomas are often responsive to chemotherapy.

  2. Special attention must be paid to possible CNS involvement. If none is found, CNS prophylaxis with intrathecal chemotherapy with or without cranial radiation is indicated.

  3. Lymphoblastic lymphoma is treated for the most part like acute lymphocytic leukemia (see Chapter 17, IX.B.).

VII.   SUMMARY

The curability of Hodgkin disease is one of the great success stories of 20th century medicine. Most patients can now expected to be cured with chemotherapy with or without radiation therapy. However, this success has its price in that second malignancies and organ toxicity from treatment have emerged as serious problems developing several years after treatment. The emphasis of current research is the search for ways to decrease the late consequences of treatment while maintaining the high level of cure.

The non-Hodgkin lymphomas are a diverse collection of lymphoid malignancies ranging in clinical behavior from indolent to rapidly progressive and in prognosis from curable to incurable. New treatment modalities besides those of traditional chemotherapy and radiation therapy (e.g. monoclonal antibodies, radiolabeled antibodies, vaccines) are likely to make a significant impact in the near future on the natural history of these diseases.

SUGGESTED READING

Hoffman R, ed. *Hematology: Basic Principles and Practice*. 2nd ed. New York: Churchill Livingston, 1995.

Cheson BD, ed. *New Frontiers in Cancer Therapy: Monoclonal Antibody Therapy of Hematologic Malignancies*. Abingdon, UK: Darwin Scientific, 2001.

CHAPTER 20

Plasma Cell Disorders

- ANDRZEJ J. JAKUBOWIAK

I. INTRODUCTION

Plasma cell disorders constitute a spectrum of benign and malignant neoplasms. The most common malignant plasma cell disorder is multiple myeloma. It constitutes slightly more than 10% of hematologic malignancies. While progress has been made in prolonging the life of patients with multiple myeloma, only rarely are patients cured.

II. OVERVIEW OF PLASMA CELL DISORDERS

A. **Key concepts**
   1. All plasma cell disorders are characterized by the accumulation and proliferation of neoplastic plasma cells.
   2. The cause of plasma cell disorders is unknown.
   3. The hallmark of all plasma cell disorders is excessive production of monoclonal immunoglobulins (Ig) by a malignant clone of plasma cells, which appears as an M spike (or monoclonal band) in serum protein electrophoresis (SPEP).
   4. The diagnosis of a specific plasma cell disorder is critical for the selection of therapy.
B. **Plasma cells and their function**
   1. Plasma cells are formed as a result of terminal differentiation of B lymphocytes.
   2. Plasma cells are present in various lymphoid tissues and are most abundant in bone marrow.
   3. Plasma cells are two to three times the size of peripheral lymphocytes. They contain eccentric nuclei and highly differentiated cytoplasm that is rich in rough-surfaced endoplasmic reticulum.
   4. The main function of plasma cells is production of antibodies as part of the humoral immune response.
   5. Antibodies secreted by plasma cells in response to antigen stimulation constitute a group of serum proteins, Ig.
   6. The Ig produced by plasma cells are composed of four polypeptide chains: two identical heavy chains and two identical light chains (Fig. 20–1). The structure of the heavy chain determines the class of Ig.
   7. There are five major classes of Ig: IgG, IgM, IgA, IgD, and IgE. The heavy chain portion of an Ig is identical within a class and its c-terminus is called a crystallizable fragment (Fc); it is the complement-binding region. The opposite portion of the Ig, the antibody-binding fragment (Fab), is involved in

Antigen-binding sites

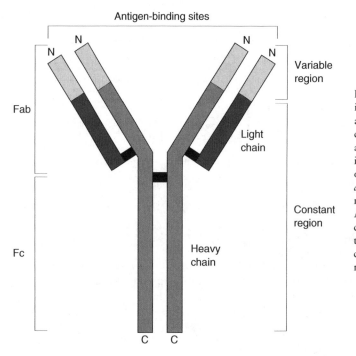

FIGURE 20–1. Structure of Ig. Two identical heavy chains (*darker bars*) are connected with two identical light chains (*lighter bars*) via linkers. Variable regions involved in antigen binding are at the N terminus portion (*N*) of the heavy and light chains (*shaded area*). Constant regions at the C terminus (C) determine the class of Ig. Antibody-binding fragments (Fab) and crystallizable fragments (Fc) are obtained after enzymatic digestion and correspond to variable and constant regions, respectively.

the recognition of a variety of specific antigens and has a specific, variable protein sequence referred to as idiotype.

8. Malignant plasma cells appear similar to their normal counterparts and retain many of their functions, including production of Ig. They also have features characteristic of malignant cells, such as more diffuse chromatin and the presence of one or several nucleoli (Fig. 20–2).

C. **Pathogenesis of plasma cell disorders**

1. A neoplastic clone of plasma cells is produced as a result of malignant transformation of the B-cell precursor of plasma cells.

2. The transformation process is associated with multiple chromosomal translocations in all clonal cells of all patients.

3. Chromosome translocations at the Ig gene locus on chromosome 14 appear to be an early event preceding clonal expansion.

4. The development of a full malignant phenotype may require additional genetic events, including various losses and gains of whole or fragmented chromosomes.

5. Deletion of 13q is present in approximately 50% of patients and is associated with a poor outcome.

6. Defining the role of the variety of chromosomal translocations in plasma cell disorders is critical for understanding the pathogenesis of the disease, providing prognostic information, and designing molecularly targeted therapies.

D. **Diagnosis of plasma cell disorders: analysis of monoclonal proteins**

1. **Serum protein electrophoresis (SPEP)** is an older technique used to separate plasma proteins into several major groups. Negatively charged serum proteins migrate in an electric field in agarose gel toward the anode. Their mobility is inversely proportional to their size.

   a. Separated serum proteins form distinct peaks based on their charge and the amount of the protein in plasma. Closest to the anode are prealbumins, fol-

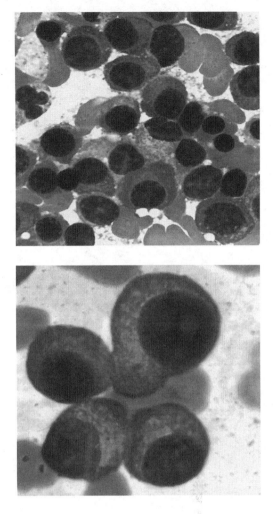

FIGURE 20–2. Malignant plasma cells from bone marrow biopsy aspirate. **A.** Low-power view with plasma cell sheet. **B.** High-power view with atypical plasma cells. Note the dispersed chromatin and nucleoli.

lowed by albumins, α_1-globulins, α_2-globulins, β-globulins, and γ-globulins (Fig. 20–3).

   b. Most Ig travel in the γ region, but they are also present in the α_2-globulin and β-globulin regions.

   c. A broad peak in the γ-region indicates normal distribution of polyclonal Ig. An increase in the γ-globulin region may be diffuse and broad, indicating a polyclonal inflammatory response (e.g., hepatitis), or sharp, as seen in plasma cell dyscrasias with monoclonal Ig (Fig. 20–4).

  2. Immunofixation (Fig. 20–5), which determines the type of Ig, and **quantitative measurement of Ig** are used to evaluate abnormal SPEP and when a plasma cell disorder is suspected. These techniques determine the following:

   a. Monoclonal versus polyclonal elevation of γ-globulins

   b. The class of monoclonal protein and identification of the light chain

   c. Accurate quantitation of monoclonal Ig

   d. Other causes of M bands on SPEP (e.g., hyperfibrinogenemia)

   e. Small peaks of monoclonal gammopathies concealed in the normal β- or γ-peaks

 E. Classification of plasma cell disorders (Fig. 20–6)

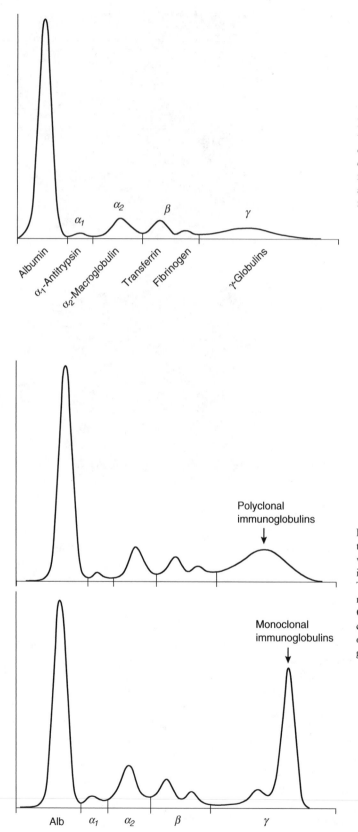

FIGURE 20–3. Normal serum protein electrophoresis. Different peaks contain a variety of serum proteins, including the examples indicated in the figure. γ-Globulins are present generally in the γ region, but small amounts may be present in the β- and α_2-peaks.

FIGURE 20–4. Abnormal serum protein electrophoresis. **A.** Polyclonal elevation of globulins as seen in chronic inflammatory states. **B.** Monoclonal Ig. The elevation of other than monoclonal proteins in this region, such as C-reactive protein, may mimic monoclonal gammopathy. *Alb*, albumin; α_1, α_1 antitrypsin; $\alpha_2 = \alpha_2$ globulin; $\beta = \beta_2$ globulin; $\gamma = \gamma$ globulin.

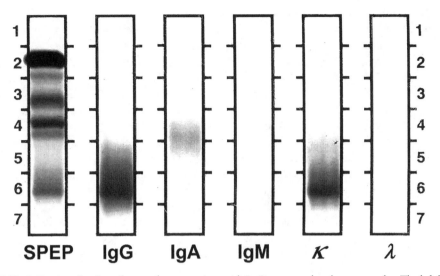

FIGURE 20-5. Immunofixation of serum from a patient with Ig G κ- monoclonal gammopathy. The left lane represents regular serum protein electrophoresis (SPEP) with a monoclonal band in the γ-globulin region (level 6). Lanes to the right contain antibodies against heavy and light chains, as indicated, allowing determination of a specific gammopathy for this patient.

III.   MULTIPLE MYELOMA AND PLASMACYTOMA

A. Epidemiology of multiple myeloma

1. Multiple myeloma affects predominantly older patients, and the incidence increases with age. The median age is 68 years for women and 70 years for men. It is rare (i.e., < 2%) in people younger than 40 years of age.
2. Multiple myeloma is the most common hematologic malignancy (2.1% of all malignancies) in African Americans and is the second most common (1.1%) in whites.
3. Multiple myeloma is more common in men than women. The average age-adjusted incidence is 4.3–9.6 in 100,000 men and 3–6.7 in 100,000 women.
4. The incidence of multiple myeloma has been increasing over the past several decades.

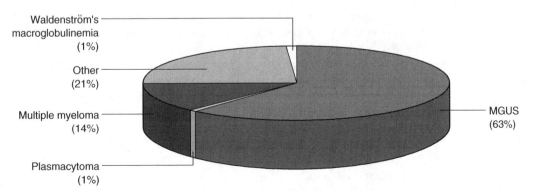

FIGURE 20-6. Representation of diseases with monoclonal gammopathies. The category of other diseases with monoclonal γ-globulins may include lymphoproliferative disorders, connective tissue diseases, and heavy chain disease. *MGUS,* monoclonal gammopathy of unknown significance.

B. **Clinical presentation of multiple myeloma and plasmacytoma**
  1. Multiple myeloma may develop unnoticed for years. The first signs and symptoms may be present when it is already in an advanced stage.
  2. Typically, patients complain of fatigue, weakness, back pain, or recurrent infections.
  3. A small subset of patients may be diagnosed with solitary plasmacytoma. Signs and symptoms are limited to local infiltration of bone or soft tissue.
  4. Signs and symptoms are generally related to infiltration of the bone marrow or other tissues by malignant clones of plasma cells or increased amounts of monoclonal protein in the serum and tissues.
      a. Presentations related to infiltration of tissues by plasma cells:
         (1) **Anemia and cytopenias** due to infiltration of the bone marrow and inhibition of normal hematopoiesis
         (2) **Bone pain** as the result of accumulation of plasma cells in local areas of the bone marrow
             (a) Patients typically present with back pain due to growth in vertebral bodies.
             (b) Other frequent sites include the ribs, clavicles, and femurs.
         (3) **Cord compression** due to the extension of plasma cell tumors from vertebral bodies compromising the spinal canal
             (a) Cord compression is a frequent first presentation.
             (b) It is considered a **medical emergency.**
         (4) **Pathologic fractures** due to local osteolytic destruction of bones
         (5) **Infections** due to defects in both humoral and cell-mediated immunity. (The function of nonmalignant plasma cells and lymphocytes is inhibited by the proliferating malignant clone.)
         (6) **Hypercalcemia** due to destruction of bones and malignancy
         (7) **Plasma cell leukemia** if plasma cells are detected in circulation with other normal blood elements (rare)
         (8) **Impairment of functions of visceral organs** (e.g., kidney, liver, brain, spleen) because of infiltration with plasma cells (rare)
      b. Presentations due to circulating monoclonal proteins include:
         (1) **Renal failure** (myeloma in the kidney), mostly due to the deposition of light chains (frequently the κ-chain); **amyloidosis** (see VI); and **hypercalcemia**
         (2) Headaches, impaired vision, mental status changes, and congestive heart failure
             (a) These presentations are due to **hyperviscosity syndrome** associated with large amounts of circulating monoclonal Ig.
             (b) A high percentage of IgM patients have hyperviscosity syndrome.
         (3) **Bleeding** due to interference by monoclonal proteins with proteins of the hemostatic system
         (4) **Neuropathies** due to amyloid or light chain deposition in perineural and perivascular tissues
C. **Laboratory evaluation of multiple myeloma and plasmacytoma**
  1. If multiple myeloma or plasmacytoma is suspected, **SPEP** should be ordered. Indications for SPEP include:
      a. **Laboratory test results**
         (1) Anemia and cytopenia
         (2) Rouleaux formation on peripheral blood smear
         (3) Elevation of total serum protein or an increased albumin–globulin gap

 (4) Hypercalcemia
 (5) Renal insufficiency or proteinuria
 (6) Ig deficiency
 b. **Radiologic test results**
 (1) Osteoporosis
 (2) Osteolytic lesions
 (3) Pathologic fractures
 c. **Syndromes**
 (1) Unexplained congestive heart failure
 (2) Peripheral neuropathy
 (3) Carpal tunnel syndrome
2. Identification of monoclonal protein on SPEP should prompt an additional diagnostic workup.
 a. **Immunofixation and quantitative measurement of Ig.** These tests are performed to determine the type of monoclonal protein and its quantity (see II.D.2). Most cases have elevation on IgG (60%), IgA (20%), and light chains (20%) only. Rarely, IgM, IgD, IgE, multiple M proteins, or heavy chains are detected.
 b. **A 24-hour urine protein secretion and electrophoresis of concentrated urine proteins.** Typical for multiple myeloma is the excretion of light chains (i.e., Bence Jones proteins). If detected, these light chains should be measured. Intact monoclonal proteins are rarely detected in significant amounts in urine. Heavy chains are found in urine in cases of heavy chain disease.
 c. **Complete skeletal survey.** All bones, including the skull and long bones, should be radiographed to look for lytic lesions (i.e., punch-out lesions in bones where local accumulation of plasma cells results in bone resorption) (Fig. 20–7).
 d. **Unilateral bone marrow aspiration and biopsy.** Positive samples are analyzed for cytogenetic abnormalities. Special stains with Congo red are performed to rule out amyloidosis.

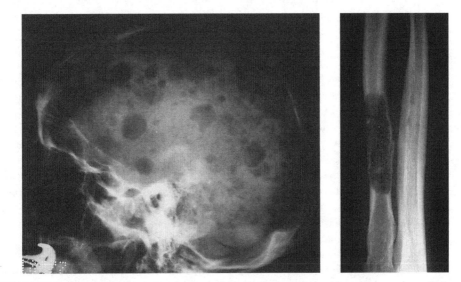

FIGURE 20–7. Radiograph of lytic lesions in the skull. **A.** Skull of a patient with multiple myeloma. **B.** Long bone.

    e. Additional tests may include:

      (1) Magnetic resonance imaging of the spine if the skeletal survey or symptoms suggest cord or nerve root compromise

      (2) Computed tomography when local accumulation of plasma cells in soft tissues or bones is suspected

      (3) Tissue biopsy of suspected plasmacytoma

      (4) Serum viscosity when symptoms or high levels of serum paraprotein (especially IgM) suggest hyperviscosity syndrome

      (5) Serum β_2-microglobulin and plasma cell labeling index for prognostic risk assessment

D. Diagnostic criteria and staging of multiple myeloma

  1. Diagnosis of multiple myeloma is made when one major and one minor criterion or three minor criteria are present.

    a. **Major criteria:**

      (1) Plasmacytoma on tissue biopsy

      (2) Marrow plasmacytosis ($>$ 30% plasma cells)

      (3) Monoclonal protein spike greater than 3.5 g/dL for IgG, greater than 2 g/dL for IgA, and greater than 1 g/24 hr of λ- or κ-light chain in urine

    b. **Minor criteria:**

      (1) Marrow plasmacytosis (10%–30% plasma cells)

      (2) Monoclonal protein spike smaller than for the major criteria ($<$ 3.5 g/dL for IgG, $<$ 2.0 g/dL for IgA, and $<$ 1g/24 hr of λ- or κ-light chain in urine)

      (3) Lytic bone lesions

      (4) Suppressed levels (below normal range) of uninvolved Ig

  2. Patients diagnosed with multiple myeloma are staged for treatment recommendations. Usually, the Durie-Salmon staging system is used (Table 20–1).

E. Treatment of multiple myeloma

  1. Stage I and smoldering myeloma are followed by observation. They usually have an indolent course. Treatment may not be needed for years if at all.

  2. Treatment is indicated for patients with stages II and III of multiple myeloma. Although patients usually respond to therapy, rarely is the malignant clone eradicated. The disease is typically characterized by relapses and progression.

    a. Initial management includes **chemotherapy.** The most commonly used combinations are melphalan and prednisone (MP) and vincristine, doxorubicin (Adriamycin), and dexamethasone (VAD). Many other combinations and agents (e.g., thalidomide) are being used and discovered.

    b. **Autologous bone marrow transplantation** is recommended after initial therapy for responding and eligible patients. It has been shown to prolong overall survival and disease-free survival but is not considered curative (Fig. 20–8).

    c. **Allogeneic bone marrow transplantation** and minitransplant are potentially curative, but at the price of high toxicity. These procedures are usually not recommended outside of a clinical trial.

    d. For patients with lytic lesions, **pamidronate or other bisphosphonates** are used to prevent skeletal fractures and to slow progression of the disease in the bones.

    e. **Radiation therapy** is used for painful lesions and when lesions compromise vital organs (e.g., spinal cord).

  3. Certain medical problems (e.g., hypercalcemia, pathologic fractures, renal failure) require specific medical management in addition to myeloma-directed therapy.

TABLE 20–1 • Durie-Salmon Staging System for Multiple Myeloma

Stage	Criteria	Myeloma Cell Mass ($\times 10^{12}$ cells/m^2)
I	All of the following: Hemoglobin > 10 g/dL Serum calcium level ≤ 12 mg/dL (normal) Normal bone or solitary plasmacytoma on x-ray Low M-component production rate: IgG < 5 g/dL IgA < 3 g/dL Bence Jones protein < 4 g/24 h	< 0.6 (low)
II	Not fitting stage I or III	0.6–1.2 (intermediate)
III	Any one or more of the following: Hemoglobin < 8.5 g/dL Serum calcium level > 12 mg/dL Multiple lytic bone lesions on x-ray High M-component production rate: IgG > 7 g/dL IgA > 5 g/dL Bence Jones protein > 12 g/24 h	> 1.2 (high)

Subclassification	Criteria
A	Normal renal function (serum creatinine level < 2.0 mg/dL)
B	Abnormal renal function (serum creatinine level ≥ 2.0 mg/dL)

Reprinted with permission from the National Comprehensive Cancer Network. NCCN *Practice Guidelines in Oncology*. V.1.2001 "Multiple Myeloma," Table 1.

F. **Treatment of plasmacytoma**
1. Patients with **solitary osseous plasmacytoma** need a similar diagnostic workup as patients with multiple myeloma (see III.C.). If systemic myeloma is excluded, treatment is limited to local radiation therapy. After the completion of radiation therapy, patients are followed regularly for life to rule out progression to multiple myeloma, which may not take place for years.
2. Similar to osseous plasmacytoma, **solitary extraosseous plasmacytoma** is treated with radiation therapy. This form of plasmacytoma occurs in a broader age group, including children and young adults. It is less likely to progress to multiple myeloma, so close observation is needed only for a limited time.

IV. MONOCLONAL GAMMOPATHY OF UNKNOWN SIGNIFICANCE

A. **Epidemiology**
1. Monoclonal gammopathy of unknown significance (MGUS) is the most frequent monoclonal gammopathy.
2. Similar to multiple myeloma, the incidence of MGUS is highest in the older population.
B. **Clinical presentation**
1. The diagnosis of MGUS is a diagnosis of exclusion. When monoclonal

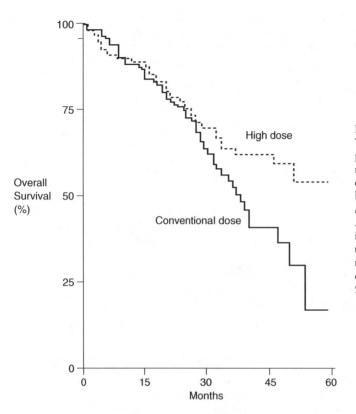

FIGURE 20–8. Kaplan-Meier curves. These curves depict overall survival of patients treated with conventional chemotherapy (*solid line*) and high-dose chemotherapy followed by autologous bone marrow transplantation (*dotted line*). (Adapted with permission from Attal M et al. A prospective, randomized trial of autologous bone marrow transplantation and chemotherapy in multiple myeloma. Intergroupe Français du Myelome. *N Engl J Med*, 1996;335: 91–97.)

gammopathy is found and there is no evidence of multiple myeloma, Waldenström macroglobulinemia (WM), primary amyloidosis, or other defined conditions with monoclonal gammopathies (i.e., the patient is asymptomatic without cytopenias or lytic lesions), then MGUS is diagnosed.

2. Some patients develop multiple myeloma or related disorders, although it is impossible to predict which patients will progress. The median interval from diagnosis of MGUS to progression to multiple myeloma is approximately 10 years.

C. **Laboratory evaluation**

1. Detection of monoclonal gammopathy should prompt diagnostic evaluations similar to that for multiple myeloma (see III.C.).

2. M bands should not exceed 3.5 g/dL for IgG, 2 g/dL for IgA, and 1 g/24 hr for Bence Jones proteins.

3. Bone marrow plasma cells should not exceed 10%.

D. **Treatment**

1. In general, MGUS is a benign condition. Up to 75% of patients have either stable disease or only a slow increase in M protein and never require treatment. Therefore, MGUS requires only observation.

2. Follow-up surveillance should include M-protein quantitation every 3 months, skeletal survey every year, and 24-hour urine for Bence Jones proteins every year.

V. WALDENSTRÖM MACROGLOBULINEMIA

A. **Clinical presentation**

1. WM is essentially a low-grade lymphoma characterized by clonal expansion of lymphoplasmacytoid cells secreting IgM monoclonal protein.

2. Clinical presentation is related to:
   a. **Bone marrow infiltration** (e.g., fatigue and weakness due to anemia, infections due to a low white blood cell count, and suppression of cells involved in immune surveillance)
   b. **Visceral organ infiltration** (e.g., lymphadenopathy, liver and spleen enlargement, cutaneous lesions)
3. Because IgM is a large pentamer molecule, high amounts of circulating monoclonal protein may result in the development of hyperviscosity syndrome [see III.B.4.b.(2)], bleeding due to coagulopathy, and peripheral neuropathy more frequently than in multiple myeloma.
4. Cryoglobulinemia and cold agglutinin hemolytic anemia are infrequently but specifically associated with WM.
5. Bone diseases and renal failure, two hallmarks of multiple myeloma, are infrequent in WM.

B. **Laboratory evaluation**
1. The workup includes SPEP with immunofixation, quantitative Ig, and bone marrow biopsy and aspirate, similar to the workup for multiple myeloma (see III C).
2. Serum viscosity should always be obtained.
3. Biopsy of enlarged lymph nodes or masses and computed tomography of the chest, abdomen, and pelvis are almost always required, similar to the workup of low-grade lymphoma.
4. Skeletal surveys and 24-urine collections are usually not needed.
5. Cryoglobulins and cold agglutinins in patients with suggestive symptoms of cryoglobulinemia or cold agglutinin syndrome.

C. **Diagnostic criteria and staging**
1. Diagnosis of WM is established by the presence of characteristic lymphoplasmacytoid cells on biopsy specimens in combination with IgM monoclonal gammopathy and clinical syndrome. However, bone marrow biopsy may be sufficient to establish a pathologic diagnosis.
2. WM should be differentiated from MGUS, multiple myeloma, and chronic lymphocytic leukemia.
3. Staging is according to the Ann Arbor system (see Table 19–2).

D. **Treatment**
1. Similar to multiple myeloma and low-grade lymphoma, WM is considered incurable. Treatment is indicated when patients develop complications or symptoms related to paraprotein or organ infiltrations. Typical indications for treatment include:
   a. Fatigue, symptomatic anemia, infections, and symptomatic splenomegaly
   b. Hyperviscosity syndrome
   c. Cryoglobulinemia, hemorrhages, cold agglutinin disease, and peripheral neuropathy
2. Treatment modalities include plasmapheresis, chemotherapy, and immunotherapy.
   a. **Plasmapheresis** is frequently required urgently for rapid removal of excess circulating IgM (i.e., in hyperviscosity syndrome, peripheral neuropathy, and cryoglobulinemia).
   b. **Chemotherapy** regimens are similar to those used for low-grade lymphoma and chronic lymphocytic leukemia—typically fludarabine or CVP (cyclophosphamide, vincristine, prednisone)—and for multiple myeloma (VAD).
   c. **Immunotherapy** includes anti–CD20 antibodies (e.g., rituximab).

3. Responses are frequently achieved, but the disease inevitably recurs and follows a progressive course.
4. Bone marrow transplant is not considered to be a part of WM therapy.

VI.   AMYLOIDOSIS

A. Overview
1. Amyloidosis is a rare disorder in which the patient's organs are infiltrated by fibrillar deposits of amyloid.
2. Classification of amyloidosis is based on the structure of the 80-angstrom subunit fibril protein:
   a. AL amyloidosis: Ig light chain (primary or myeloma) Amyloid
   b. AH amyloidosis: Ig heavy chain (primary or myeloma) Amyloid
   c. AA amyloidosis: Apolipoprotein (Apo) serum AA (secondary amyloidosis) Amyloid
   d. $A\beta_2M$ amyloidosis: β_2-microglobulin (hemodialysis) Amyloid
   e. $A\beta$ amyloidosis: $A\beta$ protein precursor ($A\beta$PP, Alzheimer disease) Amyloid
   f. ATTR amyloidosis: transthyretin (familial and senile) Amyloid
3. Only AL amyloidosis, and extremely rarely AH amyloidosis, are associated with monoclonal plasma cell disorders. This chapter covers only AL amyloidosis.
4. AL amyloidosis is produced by monoclonal plasma cells and is homogenous and homologous to the Fab region of λ- or, more frequently, κ-light chains.

B. Clinical presentation
1. AL amyloidosis has the affinity to form deposits in visceral organs such as the kidneys, heart, liver, spleen, nerve sheets, tongue, gastrointestinal tract, and skin, with related end-organ dysfunction.
2. Most patients with amyloidosis have no coexistent multiple myeloma, but amyloidosis is also present in 15% of multiple myeloma patients.
3. Presenting symptoms include:
   a. Fatigue, dyspnea, and ankle edema (as a result of congestive heart failure or nephrotic syndrome)
   b. Macroglossia
   c. Periorbital purpura (raccoon eyes)
   d. Paresthesias (peripheral neuropathy)
   e. Bleeding (gastrointestinal tract involvement)
   f. Splenomegaly
   g. Carpal tunnel syndrome (deposition of amyloid in carpal ligaments)
   h. Weight loss (common)

C. Laboratory evaluation
1. Diagnosis of amyloidosis is frequently challenging. No blood test, radiograph, or scan is diagnostic for this disease. Therefore, amyloidosis should be suspected with any unexplained presenting symptoms noted above.
2. When AL amyloidosis is suspected, a gingival or rectal biopsy specimen should be obtained and stained with Congo red. Other possible biopsy sites include the subcutaneous fat, bone marrow, and kidney. Congo red staining produces apple-green birefringence under polarized light.
3. The remaining workup is similar to the workup for multiple myeloma (see III.C.).

D. Treatment of AL amyloidosis
1. With an established diagnosis, observation is not an option and treatment is indicated.

2. Treatment is similar to the treatment of multiple myeloma: chemotherapy with MP, a high dose of dexamethasone, or VAD. Chemotherapy may slow or rarely stop amyloid deposition; however, in contrast to multiple myeloma, responses to chemotherapy are infrequent.

3. Autologous bone marrow transplantation should be considered early for eligible patients, as it provides the best chance for the most durable responses.

4. Patients with isolated cardiac amyloidosis may be candidates for cardiac transplantation.

5. Most patients die of the disease within 1–2 years of diagnosis.

VII. SUMMARY

Multiple myeloma and related disorders are a therapeutic challenge to hematologists. Although much is known about the diagnosis and pathogenesis of these disorders, effective therapies are still being sought.

SUGGESTED READING

Anderson KC et al. Recent advances in the biology and treatment of multiple myeloma. *Hematology American Society of Hematology Education Program Book*. 2000:63–88.

Anderson KC. Multiple myeloma. Advances in disease biology: therapeutic implications. *Semin Hematol* 2001;38:6–10.

Kyle RA. Multiple myeloma: diagnostic challenges and standard therapy. *Semin Hematol* 2001;38:11–14.

Ludwig H, Meran J, Zojer N. Multiple myeloma: an update on biology and treatment. *Ann Oncol* 1999; 10:S31–S43.

Munshi NC, Tricot G, Barlogie B. Plasma cell neoplasms. In: DeVita VT, Hellman S, Rosenberg SA, eds. *Cancer Principles & Practice of Oncology*, 6th ed. Philadelphia: Lippincott Williams & Wilkins, 2001: 2465–2499.

CHAPTER 21

Pediatric Hematology

- GREGORY YANIK

I. INTRODUCTION

Modern hematology is indebted to the work of pediatric hematologists over the past century. The origin and development of blood cells and the basic understanding of hemoglobinopathies, granulocyte, and platelet function were pioneered in pediatric hematology.

II. EMBRYONIC HEMATOPOIESIS

A. Development of the human hematopoietic system begins early in embryonic life, in conjunction with the rapid embryonic growth seen after fertilization. Because oxygen delivery is required to sustain this growth, the development of an embryonic hematopoietic system is essential during this period. Differences between fetal and adult hematopoiesis are related to the nature of embryonic development within the fetus, interactions between the fetus and the mother, and changes necessary for the fetus to adapt to extrauterine life.

B. Embryonic and fetal hematopoiesis follows a stepwise process from the **yolk sac** to the **liver** to the **bone marrow.** The yolk sac is the major site of hematopoiesis during the first trimester; hepatic hematopoiesis predominates during the second trimester; and bone marrow hematopoiesis predominates thereafter.

1. The earliest hematopoietic cells are derived from vessels in the yolk sac and appear 15–20 days after gestation. Identifiable stem cells and primitive erythroblasts, leukocytes, and megakaryocytes are all present at this time. Hematopoiesis in the yolk sac declines and typically ceases by 10–12 weeks' gestation.

2. Hepatic hematopoiesis arises from pluripotent stem cells during the second month of gestation. Between 9 and 24 weeks' gestation, the liver becomes the primary site for hematopoiesis. During this period, hematopoietic precursors are also seen in the spleen, thymus, lymph nodes, and kidneys. Lymphocyte growth and activity begins in the thymus after 10 weeks' gestation and in the lymph nodes after 12 weeks' gestation.

3. Medullary hematopoiesis begins at approximately 4 months of gestational age, occurring in the cartilaginous spaces in long bones. By 20 weeks' gestation, the marrow space is fully cellular, with full representation of all cell lines. As marrow production increases during this period, hepatic hematopoiesis declines. At term, only a few nucleated red blood cells (RBCs) remain in the liver, with the marrow space remaining the predominant site for blood cell production.

C. During times of hematologic stress, adults have the ability to increase marrow output up to eight times normal. Fatty marrow is converted to active red marrow for this purpose. In a fetus, however, the same ability to increase marrow production is not present. The marrow space of a fetus is fully cellular; therefore, fetal hematopoietic activity can be increased only by stimulating extramedullary hematopoiesis (i.e., liver, spleen). The hepatosplenomegaly seen in infants with severe erythroblastosis fetalis (see X) results from the increased extramedullary hematopoiesis required to compensate for the active *in utero* hemolysis.

III.   EMBRYONIC AND FETAL HEMOGLOBIN SYNTHESIS

A. In contrast to adulthood, the major form of hemoglobin (Hb) during the embryonic period is not Hb A_1 ($\alpha_2\beta_2$) (see Fig. 2–5).
   1. Within 2 weeks of gestation, primitive erythroblasts in the yolk sac are already synthesizing the most primitive Hb, Gower 1 ($\zeta_2\varepsilon_2$).
   2. Synthesis of the α- and γ-chains begins in the yolk sac by 4–8 weeks' gestation. Synthesis of the ζ- and ε-chains decreases as that of the α- and γ-chains increases.
   3. By 6 weeks' gestation, Hb F ($\alpha_2\gamma_2$) has become the major Hb of fetal life. Hb F constitutes more than 95% of the total Hb in a fetus until 34–36 weeks' gestation, after which synthesis of Hb A ($\alpha_2\beta_2$) increases dramatically.
   4. At birth, term infants typically have 50%–95% Hb F and the remainder Hb A.
   5. By 6 months of postnatal age, Hb F values decline to 1%–3% and then persist at those levels throughout life.
B. The switch from fetal to adult Hb is delayed in infants who are small for gestational age, have chronic intrauterine anoxia, or have been born to diabetic mothers.

IV.   RED BLOOD CELLS DURING INFANCY AND CHILDHOOD

A. **Overview**
   RBC, Hb, and hematocrit measurements increase markedly during weeks 30–40 of gestation in the developing fetus. After birth, these values decline rapidly. Infants develop physiologic anemia by 2 months of age, with a mean Hb value of 11 g/dL. In premature infants, this fall in Hb is more pronounced, often declining to 9–10 g/dL by 4–6 weeks of age. Gradually a rise in Hb ensues. At 14 years of age, Hb levels reach 16 g/dL in boys and 14 g/dL in girls.

   The RBCs of a newborn are markedly **macrocytic** at birth, having a mean corpuscular volume (MCV) typically greater than 100 fL; the MCV does not decline to adult levels until 1 year of age. The average life span of an infant's RBC is 60–80 days, whereas the life span in an adult is 120 days. This shortened RBC survival in infants is secondary to the unique membrane composition, hemoglobin, and metabolic features of the infant RBC. RBC values for infants and children are shown in Table 21–1.
B. **Neonatal red blood cell membrane.** In general, the RBCs of neonates have decreased membrane deformability (i.e., increased rigidity); decreased membrane permeability to water, bicarbonate, and chloride; and decreased permeability to potassium influx through the membrane.
C. **Hemoglobin in neonatal red blood cells.** The Hb of neonatal RBCs has increased oxygen affinity, as characterized by a left shift of the oxyhemoglobin dissociation curve. A progressive decline in oxygen affinity with a resultant right shift of the oxyhemoglobin dissociation curve occurs after birth. Neonatal RBCs are more

TABLE 21–1 • Normal Red Blood Cell Values for Infants and Children

Age	Hb (g/dL)	Hct (%)	RBC (× 10⁶/μL)	MCV (fL)	MCH (pg)	MCHC (g/dL)	Retics (%)
28-week fetus	14.5	45	4.0	120	40	31	5–10
Newborn	17–18[a]	55	5.0–5.5	108	35	32	3–7
2 weeks	16–17	50	4.5	112	30	33	0.8
2 months	11.3	33	4.0	88	27	34	0.7
12 months to 6 years	12.0	37	4–4.5	80	27	34	1.0
7–12 years	13.0	38	4.5	80–82	27	34	1.0
> 12 years	14–16	42–47	4.5	87	29	34	1.0

Hb, hemoglobin; Hct, hematocrit; MCH, mean corpuscular hemoglobin; MCHC, mean corpuscular hemoglobin concentration; MCV, mean corpuscular volume; RBC, red blood cell; retics, reticulocyte count.
[a]Hemoglobin values in cord blood of newborns range from 13.7 to 20.1 g/dL (mean 16.8 g/dL).

fragile than those of adults, with an increased susceptibility to oxidation and denaturation. Neonatal RBCs have decreased levels of methemoglobin reductase, leading to increased levels of methemoglobin in RBCs. Methemoglobinemia is more common during infancy than any other time. Methemoglobin reductase levels typically normalize within the first 6–12 months after birth.

D. **Erythropoietin levels in neonatal red blood cells.** Erythropoietin production rises with gestational age and reaches significant levels after 34 weeks' gestation. A fall in erythropoietin occurs in the first 5–8 weeks of life and correlates with the period of physiologic anemia; during this time erythropoiesis virtually ceases. Erythropoietin production increases dramatically in infants with congenital cyanotic heart diseases or congenital hemolytic anemias.

V. WHITE BLOOD CELLS DURING INFANCY AND CHILDHOOD

A. At birth, **leukocytosis** is present, with mean white blood cell (WBC) values of 19 × 10³/μL and 60% neutrophils. By the second month of life, WBCs total 12 × 10³/μL, with 35% neutrophils and 60% lymphocytes. This relative **lymphocytosis** persists until 4–6 years of age, at which time the WBC count declines to a mean value of 8 × 10³/μL, with 65% neutrophils and 30% lymphocytes. These values persist into adulthood.

B. African American children and children of certain Jewish sects have been shown to have lower WBC values than other racial groups. WBC values in infancy are summarized in Table 21–2.

VI. PLATELETS IN INFANCY AND CHILDHOOD

A. Though platelet counts may show great variability (100–300 × 10³/μL) at birth, platelet counts less than 100 × 10³/μL are uncommon at any gestational age.

B. Platelet counts in healthy preterm and full-term infants correspond to those of adults.

VII. COAGULATION FACTORS IN INFANCY AND CHILDHOOD

A. The coagulation system is not static in infants; marked changes occur from the prenatal period to roughly 6 months of age. These changes are caused by decreased rates of hepatic synthesis of coagulation factors, increased rates of clearance,

TABLE 21–2 • Normal White Blood Cell Values in Infancy and Childhood

Age	WBC ($10^3/\mu L$)	PMN ($10^3/\mu L$)	Lymphocytes ($10^3/\mu L$)	Monocytes ($10^3/\mu L$)	Eosinophils ($10^3/\mu L$)	Basophils ($10^3/\mu L$)
Birth	18.0	11.0	5.5	1.0	0.4	0.1
7 days	12.0	5.5	5.0	1.5	< 0.1	< 0.1
14 days	11.4	4.7	5.7	1.0	< 0.1	< 0.1
1 month	10.8	3.8	6.0	0.7	0.3	< 0.1
6 months	11.9	3.8	7.2	0.6	0.3	< 0.1
1 year	11.4	3.5	7.0	0.6	0.3	< 0.1
4 years	9.1	3.8	4.4	0.6	0.3	< 0.1
8 years	8.3	4.4	3.3	0.4	0.2	< 0.1
16 years	7.8	4.4	2.8	0.4	0.2	< 0.1

PMN, polymorphonuclear cells; WBC, white blood cells.

and the synthesis of fetal forms of many factors. Marked differences are noted between the fibrinolytic and anticoagulant systems of infants and adults. In fact, thromboembolic complications related to deficiencies in anticoagulant factors are fairly common during the neonatal period (Table 21–3).

B. Values for vitamin K–dependent factors, prekallikrein, factor XII, high-molecular-weight kininogen, and fibrinolytic and anticoagulant factors typically normalize by 6 months of age.

1. Because newborns have a physiologic deficiency of vitamin K–dependent factors at birth, the prothrombin time and activated partial thromboplastin time are increased during this period; therefore, these measurements may be difficult to interpret in newborns. However, the thrombin time should be normal in newborns and can be used to assess clotting activity.

2. Preterm infants exhibit even lower levels of vitamin K–dependent factors than term infants and thus are particularly at risk for spontaneous hemorrhage or thromboembolic complications. For example, protein C (a vitamin K–dependent anticoagulant) may be low in preterm infants, leading to an increased incidence of thrombotic complications (e.g., catheter-related thrombosis).

VIII. FACTORS INFLUENCING BLOOD COUNTS AT BIRTH

A. Prenatal factors
1. Premature birth
2. Congenital bone marrow abnormalities (e.g., Blackfan-Diamond syndrome)
3. ABO or Rh incompatibility between maternal and infant RBCs

TABLE 21–3 • Plasma Coagulation Protein Levels at Birth

Normal at Birth	Decreased at Birth
Fibrinogen	Factors II, VII, IX, X (vitamin K–dependent factors)
Factors V, VIII, XIII	Factors XI and XII, PK, HK
vWF	Antithrombin, protein C, protein S, plasminogen

HK, high-molecular-weight kininogen; PK, prekallikrein; vWF, von Willebrand factor.

4. Maternal infections, such as **TORCH** syndrome (**TO**xoplasmosis, **R**ubella, **C**ytomegalovirus infection, **H**erpes simplex). Maternal TORCH infections are commonly associated with neonatal thrombocytopenia or hemolytic anemias.

5. Maternal drug use

6. Maternal illness (e.g., diabetes mellitus, autoimmune disorders, malignancy). The transplacental passage of antiplatelet immunoglobulin G antibodies in mothers affected with systemic lupus erythematosus or maternal immune thrombocytopenic purpura may be associated with thrombocytopenia in affected infants.

B. **Perinatal factors**

Perinatal factors influencing neonatal blood counts may include fetomaternal transfusion (measured by the Kleihauer-Betke test), obstetric hemorrhage (e.g., placenta abruptio, early or delayed cord clamping), maternal infection (e.g., herpes simplex virus, HIV, hepatitis B), perinatal hypoxia or anoxia, and neonatal anomalies (e.g., hemangiomas, tumors).

In addition to the blood count, the blood volume may be affected by perinatal factors. The blood volume at the time of birth ranges from 80–89 mL/kg in term infants to 105 mL/kg in preterm infants. Blood volumes may be increased by as much as 60% with prolonged delays in umbilical cord clamping at the time of delivery. On the other hand, holding an infant above the level of the placenta at delivery may contribute to anemia in a newborn.

C. **Postnatal factors.** Acquired neonatal infections, congenital heart defects, congenital hemolytic disorders (i.e., disorders of RBC membrane, Hb, or RBC enzymes) are a few of the common conditions that may affect RBC counts shortly after birth. Congenital RBC membrane and enzyme disorders are commonly associated with hemolysis, unconjugated hyperbilirubinemia, and clinical jaundice during the perinatal period.

IX.   ROLE OF IRON IN CHILDHOOD

A. The most important determinants of iron content at birth are birthweight and initial Hb level.

1. Placental iron transport is negligible in the first two trimesters and rises progressively in the third trimester. For example, whereas a 1-kg preterm infant may have less than 50 mg of body iron, term infants may have more than 300 mg of available iron. Thus, preterm infants are extremely susceptible to the development of iron deficiency unless iron supplementation is begun soon after birth.

2. Unless maternal iron stores are severely depleted, maternal iron status usually has little effect on a newborn's iron status. Hb values in infants born to mothers with iron deficiency are usually normal. Maternal iron supplements do not alter the iron supply to the fetus.

B. At the moment of delivery, only 65% of fetal blood is within the infant; the remainder is in the placental circulation. Uterine contractions in the next 3 minutes increase this proportion to 85%. Immediate clamping of the umbilical cord after delivery may decrease body iron content by 15%–30%.

C. For most term infants, ferritin levels are high (100–200 ng/mL) at birth, increase rapidly during the first 2 months of life (during the period of physiologic anemia), and decline markedly as infant erythropoiesis resumes. Ferritin levels typically range from 20–60 ng/mL throughout the remainder of childhood. A serum ferritin level less than 10 ng/mL at any age indicates low reserves.

D. In early teen years, a corresponding acceleration of iron absorption is required to accommodate the rapid expansion of blood volume and muscle mass. Adults typically require absorption of 0.5–1 mg of iron daily, whereas this increases to 1.6 mg/day in teenage males and 1.4 mg/day in menstruating females.

X.   ERYTHROBLASTOSIS FETALIS

A. **Overview.** Erythroblastosis fetalis is defined as **hemolytic disease** of the fetus or newborn caused by a maternal–fetal **blood group incompatibility.** The research devoted to the description and prevention of this disorder has greatly influenced modern clinical medicine, with the development of the Rh blood group system, the direct antiglobulin test by Coombs, intrauterine transfusions, exchange transfusion therapy, and clinical use of Rh immune globulin. Before the implementation of RBC sensitization therapy, more than 10,000 deaths annually in the United States were attributed to this condition. In approximately 97% of cases, erythroblastosis fetalis is caused by anti–Rh(D) antibody, with the remaining 3% of cases caused by a variety of other antibodies to less common RBC groups.

B. **Pathophysiology.** Passage of fetal Rh(D) positive RBCs across the placental barrier to an Rh-negative mother is the primary method of maternal alloimmunization. Approximately 10%–15% of Rh-negative women who bear children of Rh-positive men become sensitized. Though the fetal blood occasionally leaks into maternal circulation during pregnancy, the major cause of sensitization is fetomaternal bleeding at the time of delivery.

1. The amount of blood transferred across the placental barrier correlates with the risk of sensitization. The transfer of 0.1 mL of ABO-compatible blood can lead to sensitization in 3% of susceptible mothers, versus a 60% sensitization rate if more than 5 mL of blood is transferred.

2. Obstetric complications (e.g., preeclampsia, abruptio placentae, spontaneous abortion) and obstetric procedures (e.g., amniocentesis, cesarean section, therapeutic abortion) are factors that may induce maternal Rh sensitization.

3. In general, the maternal response to Rh sensitization is the development of an anti–Rh antibody that is initially immunoglobulin M but is soon replaced by an immunoglobulin G antibody. In subsequent pregnancies, the immunoglobulin G can cross the placenta and attach to fetal Rh-positive cells. Fetal RBCs with anti–Rh antibodies (immunoglobulin G form) attached to them are removed from fetal circulation by the mononuclear phagocyte system of the developing fetus. The effects of the anti–Rh antibody on the fetal circulation are those associated with any immune hemolytic anemia.

   a. The antibody coats the RBCs, leading to their destruction in tissues of the mononuclear phagocyte system, particularly the spleen.

   b. The fetus compensates by increasing RBC production in the bone marrow, liver, and spleen, with resulting hepatomegaly and splenomegaly.

   c. Anemia develops and leads to cardiac dilatation, hypertrophy, and subsequent high-output failure.

   d. Hypoalbuminemia develops as normal liver functions are affected.

   e. Hepatic dysfunction subsequently leads to development of hydrops in the infant. A generalized edema (hydrops fetalis) develops and eventually leads to intrauterine death. The development of hydrops typically occurs between 20 and 40 weeks' gestation.

4. If the fetus can compensate sufficiently (**compensated hemolysis**), it will be born alive with some degree of erythroblastosis fetalis.

5. The concomitant presence of ABO incompatibility (e.g., mother group O, father group A or B) reduces the frequency of sensitization to Rh(D) by 50%–75%. The mother's anti–A or anti–B antibodies destroy fetal group A or group B RBCs, preventing them from entering the mother's circulation before the Rh antigen on the infant's RBCs can elicit a primary immune response.

C. **Clinical presentation.** Physical and laboratory findings both contribute to the diagnosis of erythroblastosis fetalis.

1. Most infants are not jaundiced at birth because the placenta effectively clears the bilirubin. However, **jaundice** develops soon after delivery.

2. Approximately 30% of affected infants are born with only mild signs; **pallor** caused by anemia is usually the principal finding on examination. In addition to pallor, varying degrees of **hepatomegaly, splenomegaly,** and **edema** are common.

3. Laboratory findings may include anemia with an increased reticulocyte count, a positive Coombs test, nucleated RBCs in circulation, polychromatophilia, increased bilirubin, and decreased platelets. Hypoglycemia is often noted in severe cases.

4. The increased bilirubin and clinical jaundice seen in erythroblastosis fetalis result from increased hemolysis of RBCs, producing increased amounts of degraded Hb pigments. Unconjugated (indirect) fat-soluble bilirubin can enter neurons in the basal ganglia, resulting in neurologic damage (i.e., **kernicterus**). The newborn infant lacks adequate levels of glucuronyl transferase to conjugate bilirubin. Kernicterus refers to the yellow coloring induced by bilirubin in the cerebellum and basal ganglia. If not treated with exchange transfusion, kernicterus may lead to a severe encephalopathy, which may present as lethargy, high-pitched crying, increased spasticity, or hypotonia. Infants who survive the initial encephalopathy typically develop severe neurologic sequelae.

D. **Routine prenatal care.** Careful prenatal monitoring is required when erythroblastosis fetalis or Rh hemolytic disease is suspected.

1. Prenatal care should include the determination of the mother's ABO and Rh status and an antibody screen. Rh-negative women with a history or laboratory evidence of Rh sensitization should have their anti–Rh antibody titers determined and followed during pregnancy to determine the degree of sensitization. Antibody titers of 1:16 or 1:32 may be associated with hydrops. The father's blood should also be tested for ABO, Rh, and Rh zygosity.

2. Amniocentesis is considered if there is a history of erythroblastotic stillbirth or a severely affected child or if the maternal anti–Rh antibody titer is elevated.

3. Spectrophotometric measurements are performed on the amniotic fluid to calculate the level of bilirubin as an index of fetal hemolysis. The result can be compared to previously established predictors of the fetal condition and used to determine the most suitable time for delivery or whether intrauterine fetal transfusion is required.

4. Fetal transfusions are done with transabdominal punctures into the fetal peritoneal cavity cells or by ultrasound-guided direct intravascular transfusion into an umbilical vein using compatible Rh-negative RBCs.

5. Delivery is usually timed for 2, 3, or 4 weeks before term, depending on the anticipated severity of the disease. At delivery, the cord blood is examined with the Coombs test and for bilirubin and Hb levels. Exchange transfusions remove excessive bilirubin (limiting the risk of kernicterus) and are indicated if the unconjugated bilirubin level is above 20 mg/dL. The technique involves removing 10- to 20-mL aliquots of blood and replacing with group O (or ABO

compatible) Rh-negative blood. The procedure is repeated until approximately twice the infant's blood volume has been exchanged. This removes about 85% of the infant's RBCs, 50% of the anti–Rh antibody, and 50% of the bilirubin. Exchange transfusions are repeated as many times as necessary to keep the bilirubin level below 20 mg/dL.

E. **Prevention.** Prevention of Rh sensitization is much more efficient and desirable than treatment. **Rh immunoglobulin** (concentrated fraction of γ-globulin that contains anti–Rh antibody) can prevent Rh sensitization when injected intramuscularly into unsensitized Rh-negative mothers within 72 hours after delivery of an Rh-positive child.

1. The mother must be Rh negative and not sensitized to Rh (i.e., must not have circulating anti–Rh antibodies); the infant must be Rh positive with RBCs not coated with anti–Rh antibodies.

2. Use of Rh immunoglobulin has reduced the incidence of Rh sensitization to less than 0.1% of first pregnancies and 1.3% of second pregnancies compared to 7% and 13%, respectively, in untreated control subjects.

3. Rh immunoglobulin should be considered when there is an increased risk of blood crossing the placental barrier (e.g., post amniocentesis, post therapeutic or spontaneous abortion, other obstetric procedures).

4. The routine administration of 300 μg of Rh immunoglobulin to all unsensitized Rh-negative women is recommended at 28 weeks' gestation.

F. **ABO incompatibility.** Hemolytic disease of the newborn is not restricted to Rh incompatibility but may also involve ABO incompatibility between the mother and infant. Compared to Rh-associated erythroblastosis, ABO hemolytic disease has a milder clinical presentation. The disorder is almost exclusively limited to group O mothers giving birth to group A or B infants. In this instance, maternal immunoglobulin G class antibodies (anti–A or anti–B antibodies) cross the placenta, coat fetal RBCs, and cause an A–O or B–O erythroblastosis. From a clinical standpoint, the condition is usually mild and does not usually require repeated tests during pregnancy or early delivery. At delivery, a direct antibody test is performed on cord blood in addition to Hb and bilirubin levels. The infant's bilirubin levels are followed. Exchange transfusion is performed only if high bilirubin levels are encountered; however, this is rarely the case.

XI. SUMMARY

Hematopoiesis is an ever-changing process in a neonate. A complete set of interactions between the fetal and the maternal hematopoietic system takes place during fetal development. These interactions may persist through birth, as manifested by conditions such as erythroblastosis fetalis. Knowledge of these complex interactions will lead to a much greater understanding of hematologic disorders that may develop in adult years.

SUGGESTED READING

Andrew M, Paes B, Johnston M. Development of the hemastatic system in the neonate and young infant. *Am J Pediatric Hematol Oncol* 1990;12:95–104.

Miller DR, Baehner RL. *Blood Diseases of Infancy and Childhood.* 6th ed. St. Louis: Mosby, 1990.

Christensen RD. *Hematologic Problems of the Neonate.* Philadelphia: Saunders, 2000.

Blood Banking

- ROBERTSON D. DAVENPORT

I. INTRODUCTION

Blood transfusion is the oldest and most frequently performed type of human tissue transplantation. Although there were experiments with both animal and human blood transfusion before the 19th century, it was only relatively recently that transfusion became a standard form of therapy. The first human blood group, ABO, was described in 1900. Anticoagulation of blood with citrate, first described in 1914, permitted storage of blood and so-called indirect transfusion. The first hospital blood bank in the United States was established in 1936.

II. BLOOD DONATION

A. Blood donations may be allogeneic (for another person), autologous (for later transfusion to the donor), or directed (designated for a particular recipient).

B. The Food and Drug Administration establishes criteria for acceptability of blood donors. These include measures to protect the donor's health (e.g., minimum hematocrit, minimum time between donations) and measures to protect the recipient (e.g., history or risk factors for infectious diseases). Donors undergo a focused medical history, limited physical examination, and hematocrit screening.

   1. For allogeneic and directed donations, the hematocrit must exceed 38%, and donations may be no more frequent than every 8 weeks or 5 times per year.
   2. The criteria for autologous donations are less stringent because the blood is used for transfusion to the donor. Autologous blood may be donated every 4 days, up to 4 days before surgery. The patient's hematocrit must exceed 34% before donation.

C. A single blood donation is 450 mL ($\pm$ 45 mL) of whole blood. This is usually processed into components of red blood cells (RBCs), plasma, and platelets (Table 22–1). Apheresis (the process of removing whole blood, separating a portion, and returning the rest to the donor) may be used for blood component donation. Apheresis has less effect on blood volume, so a greater amount of the intended component can be collected from one donor. RBCs, platelets, and plasma can be collected by apheresis as well as by whole blood donation. Leukocyte components that include granulocytes, mononuclear cells, and hematopoietic progenitor cells are collected only by apheresis because a whole blood donation does not contain sufficient numbers of these cells to be therapeutically effective.

TABLE 22–1 • Blood Components for Transfusion

Whole blood
Red blood cells
Plasma
Cryoprecipitated antihemophilic factor
Platelets
Granulocytes
Mononuclear cells
Hematopoietic progenitor cells

III.   DONOR TESTING

A. Blood donations are tested for markers of infectious diseases that may be transmitted by transfusion (Table 22–2). Donations are tested for antibodies to pathogens (indicates previous exposure), viral antigens, and most recently, viral genetic material. The testing requirements and methods for blood donors are evolving. Progress in infectious disease testing has outpaced clinical studies, so the risks of infectious disease transmission are not known with certainty.

B. The transfusion-transmitted diseases tested for in donor blood are HIV, hepatitis B, hepatitis C, syphilis, and human T-cell lymphoma/leukemia virus types I and II.

C. Infectious disease testing is not necessarily the most important factor in reducing transfusion-transmitted diseases. The greatest progress in reducing the rate of serious transfusion-transmitted disease has come from the exclusion of donors with risk factors in their medical histories.

IV.   CHARACTERISTICS OF DONATED BLOOD

Blood components stored in the liquid state undergo **changes that affect post-transfusion efficacy** (Table 22–3).

A. Stored **RBCs** lose 2,3-diphosphoglycerate and leak potassium. They also age.

1. Although potassium concentrations in the supernatant of stored RBCs may reach 35 mEq/dL, the total amount of extracellular potassium in a unit is less than the daily requirement of an adult. This usually poses no problem except for transfusion of newborns. The metabolic changes in stored RBCs are reversible after transfusion.

TABLE 22–2 • Current Infectious Disease Testing

Hepatitis B surface antigen (HB_sAg)
Hepatitis B core antibody (anti-HB_c)
Hepatitis C virus antibody (anti-HCV)
HIV-1 and HIV-2 antibody (anti–HIV-1 and anti–HIV-2)
HIV p24 antigen
HTLV-I and HTLV-II antibody (anti–HTLV-I and anti–HTLV-II)
Serologic test for syphilis
HIV and HCV genome (NAT)

HTLV, human T-cell lymphoma/leukemia virus; NAT, nucleic acid test.

TABLE 22–3 • Changes in Blood Components During Storage

Red blood cells
    Hemolysis
    Leakage of potassium
    Decreased 2,3-diphosphoglycerate
    Senescence
Plasma (liquid)
    Decreased factor V
    Decreased factor VIII
Platelets
    Activation
    Granule release
Leukocytes (in cellular components)
    Activation
    Cytokine generation
    Apoptosis

2. An irreversible change in RBCs is an aging process similar to senescence *in vivo.* By the end of the storage period (35 or 42 days, depending on the preservative solution) as many as 25% of transfused RBCs will be cleared from circulation within 24 hours.

B. The labile **coagulation factors V and VIII** are gradually lost from liquid plasma. After 7 days of storage at 4°C, the factor V and VIII activity of plasma is about 50% of the initial value. Other coagulation factors are not affected by storage temperature.

C. **Platelets** must be stored at room temperature with constant gentle agitation to maintain hemostatic activity. During storage, platelets undergo a variety of changes, including expression of activation markers, degranulation, and apoptosis-like events. These events result in lower posttransfusion survival of stored platelets and the release of mediators that may cause transfusion reactions.

D. **Leukocytes** in stored RBCs and platelets also undergo activation during storage, which results in the release of cytokines and other biologic response modifiers. These activation products can cause transfusion reactions and changes in the immune status of the recipient. However, methods of blood component preparation that significantly reduce the number of leukocytes can abrogate many of these reactions.

   1. Pyrogenic cytokines, such as interleukin-1 and tumor necrosis factor, may cause febrile reactions.

   2. Chemokines, such as interleukin-8, may affect the function of circulating leukocyte populations and may cause impaired immune and inflammatory responses.

   3. Lipid mediators similar to platelet-activating factor may prime neutrophils to respond briskly to secondary inflammatory stimuli.

V. BLOOD GROUP SEROLOGY AND PRETRANSFUSION TESTING

A. **Formation of antibodies**

   1. Blood transfusion would be relatively simple if it were not for **immune responses** in transfusion recipients that cause antibodies to form against cellular

antigens with rejection of the transfused cells. Such antibodies may be **naturally occurring** or may be made in **response to previous exposure.**

   a. Antibodies in the ABO system are naturally occurring. They usually form in the first months of life as a result of exposure to environmental bacterial antigens. Typically, anti-A and anti-B are immunoglobulin (Ig) M and IgG, fix complement, and cause rapid intravascular hemolysis.

   b. In contrast, antibodies to most other blood groups (e.g., Rh system) are not naturally occurring. Previous transfusion or pregnancy is required before a patient will make such antibodies. Typically these antibodies are IgG, do not fix complement, and cause extravascular hemolysis, although there are exceptions. Blood groups outside of the ABO system vary considerably in immunogenicity. Many patients do not make RBC antibodies despite repeated transfusion.

  2. **Autoantibodies,** antibodies to the patient's own RBCs, also occur and may cause hemolysis, such as autoimmune hemolytic anemia (AIHA). Autoantibodies may be secondary to certain diseases, such as systemic lupus erythematosus or chronic lymphocytic leukemia. In some cases, RBC autoantibodies may be benign and not cause cell destruction. Autoantibodies usually react with epitopes common to virtually all blood donors.

B. **Detection of antibodies**

  1. It is necessary to detect RBC antibodies before transfusion to provide **compatible blood.** Such tests are based on **agglutination,** the clumping of RBCs caused by cross-linking of cells by antibodies. Antibodies in the ABO system and some other IgM antibodies can directly agglutinate RBCs. Most IgG antibodies require a second antibody, anti-IgG (also called antihuman globulin or Coombs serum), for detection by agglutination.

   a. RBCs coated with IgG in circulation, as in AIHA or during a hemolytic transfusion reaction, are detected by the direct antiglobulin test (DAT). The DAT is also known as the Coombs test, after the individual who described it.

   b. Circulating antibodies in the plasma may be detected by the indirect Coombs test. Test RBCs are incubated with serum, excess unbound IgG is washed away, and the RBCs are tested for bound antibody with antiglobulin serum.

   c. Serologic reactions are temperature dependent. Anti-A and anti-B are readily detected at room temperature, but detection of most IgG RBC antibodies requires testing at 37°C.

   d. Not all RBC antibodies are clinically significant in terms of causing accelerated RBC destruction.

  2. Testing for RBC antibodies is also useful in the **diagnosis of some anemias.**

   a. The DAT is used to detect IgG on the surface of RBCs in warm AIHA.

   b. A DAT performed with anticomplement serum can detect complement activation products (e.g., C3b) on the RBC surface; this test is typically positive in cold hemagglutinin disease.

   c. Some drug-induced hemolytic anemias also have a positive DAT.

   d. RBC autoantibodies may be found in autoimmune diseases such as systemic lupus erythematous.

C. **Pretransfusion testing**

  1. **Routine pretransfusion testing** consists of **ABO typing** (testing for A and B antigens and the corresponding anti-A or anti-B in the serum); **Rh typing,** that is, testing for the Rh(D) antigen; and **screening for other RBC antibodies.**

   a. This screening is an indirect Coombs test using RBCs for two or three group O selected donors of known phenotype that are positive for the most common clinically significant RBC antigens.

b. If there are problems with concluding the ABO type or if the antibody screen is positive, further testing is required before compatible blood can be provided.

c. RBC antibodies are identified using panels of typed donor cells. When an antibody is identified, donor units are typed to find ones that are negative for that specificity.

2. **The final check of RBC compatibility is the cross-match.** Serologic cross-matching involves incubating the donor's RBCs with the recipient's serum, checking for agglutination, and performing an antiglobulin test. The most important purpose of cross-matching is to detect ABO incompatibility. If the patient has a negative antibody screen, it is also possible to perform an electronic cross-match using a computer to verify ABO compatibility.

3. In **emergencies,** when there is no time to perform full pretransfusion testing, **group O RBCs can usually be given safely.**

a. Group O Rh-negative RBCs are often selected to avoid sensitization to Rh(D). However, group O Rh-negative individuals constitute only 15% of blood donors, so this resource is limited.

b. Group O Rh-positive RBCs may be used, particularly if there is no risk of later hemolytic disease of the newborn.

c. In addition, the patient may have antibodies to other RBC antigens. Good communication between the treating physician and the blood bank is essential in emergencies.

VI. SUMMARY

Criteria for the acceptability of blood donors are established to protect the health of the donor and the recipient. Donors are screened for risk factors for transfusion-transmitted disease. Donations are also tested for hepatitis B, hepatitis C, HIV, and other pathogens. Blood donations are typically processed into RBCs, platelet concentrates, and plasma. Stored blood components undergo changes that can influence the effectiveness of transfusion. RBCs lose 2,3-diphosphoglycerate and become senescent. Platelets activate and degranulate during storage. Labile coagulation factors are gradually lost from plasma in the liquid state. Serologic testing is performed before transfusion to ensure compatibility. The patient may have RBC antibodies that are naturally occurring, the result of previous exposure through transfusion or pregnancy, or as a manifestation of disease. Alloantibodies are directed against foreign RBCs, while autoantibodies react with the patient's own cells. Routine pretransfusion testing includes determination of ABO and Rh type and screening for RBC antibodies. If unexpected RBC antibodies are found, the antigen specificity is determined and antigen-negative RBCs are provided. RBC serology is also used for diagnosis of anemias, autoimmune diseases, and some drug reactions.

SUGGESTED READING

Mintz PD, ed. *Transfusion Therapy: Clinical Principles and Practice.* Bethesda, MD: American Association of Blood Banks, 1999.

Triulzi DJ, ed. *Blood Transfusion Therapy: A Physi-*

cian's Handbook. Bethesda, MD: American Association of Blood Banks, 1999.

Vengelen TV, ed. *Technical Manual.* 13th ed. Bethesda, MD: American Association of Blood Banks, 1999.

CHAPTER 23

Transfusion Therapy

- ROBERTSON D. DAVENPORT

I. INTRODUCTION

There are no absolute indications and few absolute contraindications to blood transfusion. Therefore, all decisions about blood transfusion must be driven by clinical considerations, such as the cause of bleeding or red cell loss, amount and rate of blood loss, underlying diseases (e.g., cardiac, respiratory), risks of future bleeding, and extent of physiologic compensations.

II. COMPONENTS OF BLOOD

A. **Red blood cells**
   1. Red blood cells (RBCs) (previously called packed RBCs) are the product of a single whole-blood donation from which most of the plasma and usually the platelets have been removed.
   2. RBC transfusion provides oxygen-carrying capacity. The critical level of hemoglobin is difficult to determine. There is no single hemoglobin or hematocrit trigger at which a patient needs to be transfused. In a normovolemic 70-kg adult, one unit of RBCs usually increases the hemoglobin by 1.5 g/dL or the hematocrit by 2%–3%.
   3. General indications for RBC transfusion are given in Table 23–1.
   4. RBC transfusions should be given on a unit-by-unit basis with assessment of the clinical response after each transfusion.
   5. Pretransfusion testing (see Chapter 22) is necessary to ensure compatibility of RBC transfusions.
B. **Platelet concentrates**
   1. Platelet concentrates are made from either a single whole-blood donation (random-donor platelets) or by apheresis (single-donor platelets).
   2. Platelet transfusions contain about 300 mL of plasma with ABO antibodies and coagulation factors.
   3. There is no single criterion for determining the need for a platelet transfusion, although there are some guidelines.
      a. Platelet counts less than 10,000/μL are associated with mucosal bleeding and may present a risk of intracerebral hemorrhage.
      b. The minimum platelet count necessary for surgical hemostasis is controversial, although many patients can tolerate surgery with a platelet count of 50,000/μL.
      c. Administration of $3–7 \times 10^{11}$ platelets (the amount in a pool of five random-donor platelet concentrates or one apheresis platelet concentrate) ideally

TABLE 23–1 · Indications for Red Blood Cell Transfusion

Indications	Transfusion Guidelines
Symptomatic anemia (e.g., tachycardia, tachypnea, cyanosis)	Clear indication
Blood loss > 15% total blood volume	May be indication for RBC transfusion, particularly with expectation of continued bleeding
Chronic hypoproliferative anemia (e.g., myelodysplastic transfusion syndrome)	May require periodic RBC
Sickle cell disease	May require transfusion during sickle cell crisis or to prevent sickle cell crisis

should raise the platelet count of a 70-kg patient by 30,000/μL; however, this is often not achieved.

4. Platelet transfusions are used to treat or prevent bleeding caused by thrombocytopenia or platelet dysfunction. For example, hypoproliferative thrombocytopenia with a risk of hemorrhage (e.g., platelet count < 10,000/μL) is an indication for platelet transfusion. However, there are also several contraindications to platelet transfusion.
   a. Patients with immune thrombocytopenic purpura rapidly clear transfused platelets as they do their own platelets. Therefore, platelet transfusion is rarely indicated.
   b. Some consumptive states, such as heparin-induced thrombocytopenia and thrombosis syndrome and thrombotic thrombocytopenic purpura, can be exacerbated by platelet transfusion. Platelet transfusion should be undertaken with great caution in such situations.
5. When performing a platelet transfusion, the expected posttransfusion platelet increment may not occur.
   a. Nonimmune factors are the most frequent causes of refractory response to platelet transfusion. They include splenomegaly, sepsis, disseminated intravascular coagulation (DIC), bleeding, and drug effects.
   b. Immune factors may also cause refractoriness to platelet transfusion.
      (1) Autoantibodies or alloantibodies to platelet antigens can cause rapid clearance of transfused platelets.
      (2) Platelets express class I human leukocyte antigens (HLA) and platelet-specific antigens. Immunization to HLA antigens is common in multiply transfused and previously pregnant patients. Production of platelet-specific antibodies is uncommon but may cause refractory response to platelet transfusions.
   c. Patients who are refractory to platelet transfusion may benefit from HLA-matched or platelet cross-match–negative platelet concentrates. Using leukocyte-reduced RBC and platelet components can largely prevent refractoriness to platelet transfusions. Full pretransfusion testing as for RBCs is not required for platelet transfusions.
C. Plasma
   1. Plasma is prepared from either a single whole-blood donation (fresh frozen plasma) or by apheresis and promptly frozen to maintain activity of labile proteins.

2. Indications for plasma transfusion are listed in Table 23–2.
   a. Plasma is usually transfused for coagulation factor replacement. For congenital deficiency of factor VII, VIII, or IX, von Willebrand factor (vWF), antithrombin III, C1 inhibitor, and protein C, high-quality purified factor concentrates are available and are preferred over plasma.
   b. Plasma may be indicated in multiple-factor deficiency states, such as liver disease and the dilutional coagulopathy that can accompany massive transfusion. However, the role of plasma transfusion in chronic liver disease is limited. Cirrhotic patients have multiple defects of hemostasis that plasma transfusion cannot correct.
   c. Plasma transfusion can rapidly reverse the anticoagulant effect of warfarin.
   d. Plasma transfusion and plasma exchange are both effective in thrombotic thrombocytopenic purpura and hemolytic uremic syndrome.
   e. The role of plasma transfusion in DIC is controversial. However, plasma does supply coagulation inhibitors that may be depleted in severe intravascular coagulation associated with acral cyanosis and digital ischemia.
3. Several types of plasma can be used for transfusion.
   a. Solvent/detergent treated (S/D) plasma is manufactured from pools of plasma units by a process that inactivates lipid-enveloped viruses, particularly HIV, hepatitis B, and hepatitis C, and carries little risk of transmitting these viruses. The coagulation factor content of S/D plasma is more uniform than that of fresh frozen plasma. Some plasma proteins, such as protein S and antiplasmin, are reduced in S/D plasma.
   b. Cryoprecipitated antihemophilic factor (cryoprecipitate) is manufactured from frozen plasma that is thawed at 4°C. The resultant precipitate contains factor VIII, vWF, factor XIII, and fibrinogen.
      (1) Cryoprecipitate was a major advance in the treatment of hemophilia A and von Willebrand disease. Today, however, the use of factor VIII–vWF concentrate has largely replaced cryoprecipitate in the treatment of von Willebrand disease.
      (2) Cryoprecipitate may be effective in controlling bleeding in uremia, although this indication has not been rigorously tested.
      (3) Because of the high fibrinogen content of cryoprecipitate, it is useful for making fibrin glue when mixed with thrombin. This preparation can be used to achieve surgical hemostasis. Presently, cryoprecipitate is used to replace fibrinogen in DIC, liver disease, and congenital deficiency states.

TABLE 23–2 • Indications for Plasma Transfusion

Coagulation factor deficiency[a]
Disseminated intravascular coagulation
Reversal of warfarin anticoagulation
Dilutional coagulopathy (as seen in massive transfusion)
Hemorrhage in liver disease
Thrombotic thrombocytopenic purpura

---

[a]Consider using factor concentrates in place of plasma.

III.   COMPLICATIONS OF TRANSFUSION

A. **Transfusion reactions** are a diverse group of adverse consequences of transfusion that usually occur during or shortly after transfusion (Table 23–3).

1. **Acute hemolytic transfusion reactions** occur within 24 hours of transfusion and are usually characterized by intravascular hemolysis with hemoglobinemia and hemoglobinuria.

   a. Acute hemolytic transfusion reactions result when preformed antibody binds to transfused RBCs and activates complement. ABO incompatibility is the most common cause of an immediate hemolytic transfusion reaction.

   b. Most hemolytic transfusion reactions occur because of a human error in obtaining and labeling the pretransfusion specimen, in laboratory processing, or in transfusing the wrong patient. **The importance of proper labeling of the pretransfusion blood specimen and identification of the recipient cannot be overemphasized.**

   c. The initial clinical presentation is usually fever and chills. Pain, nausea, vomiting, hypotension, and dyspnea may occur. Later sequelae of acute hemolytic transfusion reactions include renal failure, DIC, and death.

2. **Delayed hemolytic transfusion reactions** occur 1 day to several weeks after transfusion. These usually result in extravascular hemolysis with a falling hematocrit and a rise in unconjugated hyperbilirubin.

   a. Delayed hemolytic reactions are usually caused by immunoglobulin (Ig) G RBC antibodies that do not activate complement and are not detected by routine pretransfusion testing. Such antibodies may be a brisk primary immune response or an amnestic secondary response.

   b. These reactions may be clinically silent or may cause fever and leukocytosis. In patients with sickle cell anemia, a hemolytic transfusion reaction may precipitate a sickle cell crisis.

3. **Febrile nonhemolytic reactions** are common in multiply transfused patients and usually resolve in a few hours.

   a. Febrile reactions are caused by cytokines that accumulate in blood components during storage or by recipient antibodies to donor leukocytes.

   b. Febrile reactions cause fever and chills and must be differentiated from hemolytic reactions.

   c. Antipyretics (e.g., acetaminophen) may be useful in preventing or treating febrile reactions. Removal of leukocytes from stored blood components may also prevent many of these reactions.

4. **Allergic reactions** are also common in multiply transfused patients.

TABLE 23–3 • Transfusion Reactions

Acute (intravascular) hemolytic reaction
Delayed (extravascular) hemolytic reaction
Febrile nonhemolytic reaction
Allergic (urticarial) reaction
Bacterial contamination
Transfusion-related acute lung injury
Posttransfusion purpura
Nonimmune hemolysis
Hypotensive reaction
Graft versus host disease

---

    a. Allergic reactions are associated with transfusion of plasma and the plasma residual in cellular blood components. Although the exact mechanism of allergic reactions is unclear, they may be caused by recipient antibodies to plasma proteins.

    b. Most allergic reactions are mild and consist of urticaria, flushing, or itching. Occasionally, more severe allergic reactions include nausea, vomiting, or dyspnea.

    c. Rarely, severe allergic reactions result in anaphylaxis. Patients with IgA deficiency may make anti-IgA as the result of previous transfusion and are at risk for anaphylactic reactions. If anti-IgA is identified as a cause, RBCs and platelets can be washed free of plasma proteins before transfusion. IgA-deficient plasma is available from rare donor registries.

5. **Bacterial contamination** of blood components is rare but very serious when it occurs.

    a. Bacteria can enter donated blood from contaminated equipment, donor skin, or asymptomatic bacteremia in the donor.

    b. A few bacteria in the initial blood collection can grow to very high levels during storage. The organisms involved depend on the component type.

        (1) *Yersinia* and *Pseudomonas* can grow in refrigerated RBCs.

        (2) Gram-negative and gram-positive organisms can grow in platelet concentrates at room temperature.

    c. Transfusion of a contaminated unit usually results in septic shock. The mortality rate is high. Unfortunately, these reactions are unpredictable and little can be done to prevent them.

6. **Transfusion-related acute lung injury** occurs during or shortly after transfusion, resolves within 48–72 hours, and does not progress to acute respiratory distress syndrome.

    a. These reactions are caused by neutrophil-activating substances that accumulate during storage or by the transfusion of antileukocyte antibodies that react with recipient white blood cells. Both mechanisms cause leakage of pulmonary capillaries.

    b. Transfusion-related acute lung injury presents as noncardiogenic pulmonary edema. The mortality rate is about 10%, depending on the patient's underlying status at the time of the reaction.

    c. Prestorage leukocyte depletion of blood components may prevent some of these reactions.

7. **Posttransfusion purpura** presents as profound thrombocytopenia 1–3 weeks after transfusion.

    a. The inciting transfusion can be RBCs, platelets, or plasma. The thrombocytopenia is immune mediated. It occurs as the patient has a primary immune response to a platelet-specific antigen. Initially, the antibody response cross-reacts with common epitopes on both autologous and allogeneic platelets. As the immune response matures, the antibody specificity narrows and cross-reaction ceases. At this time (usually 2–3 weeks after the onset of thrombocytopenia) the platelet count returns to normal.

    b. Treatment of posttransfusion purpura is dictated by clinical circumstances.

        (1) A stable patient may simply need to restrict activities and wait.

        (2) If bleeding occurs or there is a risk of intracranial hemorrhage, high-dose intravenous Ig is the most effective treatment.

        (3) Platelet transfusion is futile because the patient will clear transfused platelets as rapidly as autologous platelets.

8. **Nonimmune hemolysis** occurs when RBCs are exposed to nonphysiologic conditions (e.g., cold, heat, hypotonic solutions) or forced through small-bore needles.

   a. Nonimmune hemolysis presents as hemoglobinemia and hemoglobinuria and must be differentiated from a hemolytic transfusion reaction.

   b. Transfusion of hemolyzed blood may be well tolerated by some patients, but hyperkalemia and renal failure can occur. Nonimmune hemolysis must be recognized promptly to prevent additional hemolyzed blood from being transfused.

9. **Hypotensive reactions** must be differentiated from hemolytic reactions, bacterial contamination, and anaphylaxis.

   a. Hypotensive reactions occur because of bradykinin generation in the blood component during the transfusion process.

   b. Hypotensive reactions present as hypotension and tachycardia shortly after the beginning of a transfusion. If the transfusion is stopped promptly, blood pressure rapidly returns to normal. The transfusion can usually be resumed at a slow rate once the blood pressure stabilizes.

   c. Patients on angiotensin-converting enzyme inhibitors are at risk for hypotensive reactions from elevating bradykinin levels. In addition, rapid infusion of platelet concentrates often causes hypotension.

10. **Transfusion-associated graft versus host disease (GVHD)** occurs when viable transfused T lymphocytes engraft in the recipient and recognize the recipient as foreign.

   a. GVHD causes pancytopenia, fever, rash, diarrhea, and liver dysfunction several weeks after transfusion.

   b. Patients with cellular immune deficiencies (e.g., bone marrow transplant recipients, low-birth-weight infants, congenital immunodeficiency states) are at risk for GVHD. In addition, a blood transfusion from a first-degree relative can cause GVHD because of close similarity in HLA types.

   c. Transfusion-associated GVHD has a high mortality rate, with death caused by infection or bleeding. It can be prevented by γ-irradiation of blood components to prevent lymphocyte proliferation.

B. **Transfusion-transmitted infectious diseases.** Progress in donor screening and infectious disease testing in the past two decades has greatly reduced the incidence of transfusion-transmitted disease (Table 23–4).

1. **Viral hepatitis** is the most important transfusion-transmitted disease today.

   a. Posttransfusion **hepatitis B virus (HBV)** infection usually causes jaundice about 2 months after transfusion. A chronic carrier state develops in 5%–10% of cases. Approximately 25% of carriers have active hepatitis, often progressing to cirrhosis. The per unit risk of HBV transmission by blood transfusion is about 1:66,000 to 1:200,000.

   b. Acute **hepatitis C virus (HCV)** infection is relatively mild and often not icteric. However, chronic hepatitis develops in about 80% of cases; of these, 10%–40% progress to cirrhosis or hepatocellular carcinoma. Chronic hepatitis usually manifests after 10 years, cirrhosis after 20 years, and liver cancer after 30 years. Among the first-time blood donor population, the prevalence of HCV antibodies is about 1%. In the United States, transfusion accounts for a small percentage of all HCV cases. Worldwide, approximately one-quarter of HCV-infected individuals give a history of blood transfusion. The risk of HCV transmission from a unit of blood is about 1:500,000.

TABLE 23–4 • Transfusion-Transmitted Diseases

Viral hepatitis (B, C, and G)
HIV, AIDS
Cytomegalovirus
Human T-cell lymphoma/leukemia virus
Parvovirus
Chagas disease
Malaria
Babesiosis

---

    c. **Hepatitis G virus (HGV)** is a recently described RNA virus that is homologous to HCV. The transmission of HGV through blood transfusion has been clearly established. Many HGV-positive patients have HBV or HCV coinfection, presumably because of shared risk factors of infection. Screening for other hepatitis viruses has therefore reduced HGV transmission. About half of HGV-infected patients without other infections develop elevated transaminase levels but are usually not icteric. Chronic hepatitis occurs in less fewer 20% of HGV infections.

2. Transfusion transmission of **HIV** peaked in early 1985. Deferral of high-risk donors, HIV antibody testing, p24 antigen testing, and HIV genome testing have markedly reduced the risk of HIV transmission by transfusion. The natural history of transfusion-acquired HIV is similar to that of other routes of viral transmission. The current per unit risk of HIV transmission is about 1:1 million.

3. **Human T-cell lymphoma/leukemia virus types I and II (HTLV-I, HTLV-II)** are retroviruses not related to HIV. These viruses may cause T-cell lymphoma or a demyelinating peripheral neuropathy in about 5% of infected individuals. The incubation time from infection to clinical disease is typically about 20 years. Acute demyelinating neuropathy after transfusion-acquired HTLV-I can occur in immunosuppressed patients.

4. **Cytomegalovirus (CMV)** belongs to the herpesvirus group and can be transmitted by blood transfusion. In immunocompetent recipients, CMV causes mild mononucleosis-like symptoms, if any. CMV infection can be very serious in immunocompromised patients or if acquired *in utero*. Many blood donors have CMV antibody. The virus is latent in leukocytes of most blood donors with antibody. CMV transmission may be prevented by selecting blood components from seronegative donors or by removing leukocytes from blood components.

5. **Parvovirus B19** causes fifth disease in children and is associated with arthritis in adults. In persons with accelerated hematopoiesis, parvovirus can cause bone marrow failure (e.g., aplastic crisis of sickle cell disease). It can cause nonimmune fetal hydrops and death if acquired during gestation. Parvovirus is common in the general population and tends to occur in periodic outbreaks. Most transfusion recipients are not at risk for significant disease from parvovirus infection. The risk of transmission by transfusion depends on the prevalence in the population and ranges from about 1:1000 to 1:10,000.

6. A number of other blood-borne infections are rarely transmitted by blood transfusion.

    a. A few cases of transfusion-transmitted **malaria** are reported annually in the

United States. The implicated donors have lived in or traveled to endemic areas and are asymptomatic.

    b. **Babesiosis** is an intraerythrocytic parasitic infection carried by North American mammals and transmitted by tick bite. Transfusion-transmitted babesiosis can be severe in splenectomized patients.

    c. *Trypanosoma cruzi* causes **Chagas disease** and is endemic in parts of Central and South America. Chronic Chagas disease can result in dilated cardiomyopathy, though carriers are often asymptomatic. Several cases of transfusion-transmitted Chagas disease have occurred in North America. The implicated donors have been immigrants from endemic areas.

C. Hemolytic disease in the newborn and neonatal alloimmune thrombocytopenia

    1. **Overview.** Antibodies against blood cells can cause significant problems in the fetus during pregnancy or in the newborn period. Maternal antibodies to fetal RBC antigens can cause hemolytic disease of the newborn (HDN) (Fig. 23–1). This is described in detail in Chapter 21. Maternal antibodies to platelet antigens can cause neonatal alloimmune thrombocytopenia, and maternal antibodies to white cells can cause transient neutropenia in the newborn.

    2. **Etiology.** Similar to HDN, neonatal alloimmune thrombocytopenia is caused by maternal antibodies to fetal platelet antigens. The HPA-1a (Pl^{A1}) antigen is most commonly involved, but other platelet-specific antigens have been implicated. Occasionally, HLA antibodies may cause neonatal alloimmune thrombocytopenia.

    3. **Clinical presentation.** Neonatal alloimmune thrombocytopenia presents as severe thrombocytopenia with petechiae and bleeding at birth. Intracranial hemorrhage is the most serious consequence. Unlike HDN, neonatal alloimmune thrombocytopenia may occur with the first pregnancy. The affected fetus is at little risk for hemorrhage *in utero* but may be at significant risk at delivery. Thrombocytopenia continues until maternal antibody is cleared (usually within 1 week).

    4. **Treatment.** Neonatal alloimmune thrombocytopenia is treated with transfusion of antigen-negative platelets. The most readily available donor is usually the mother because she lacks the antigen to which she has made antibodies. The father is not a suitable platelet donor because he must carry the involved antigen. Transfusion of antigen-negative platelets usually results in a dramatic increase in the platelet count. If antigen-negative platelets are not available, transfusion of an unselected platelet concentrate will transiently increase the platelet count, but repeat transfusion is often required.

    5. **Prophylaxis.** Unlike HDN, there is no effective prophylaxis for neonatal alloimmune thrombocytopenia. If a pregnant woman already has had an affected

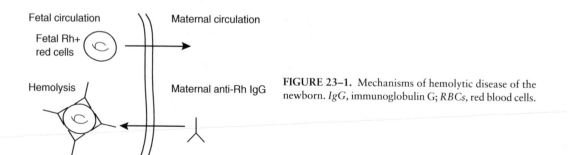

FIGURE 23–1. Mechanisms of hemolytic disease of the newborn. *IgG*, immunoglobulin G; *RBCs*, red blood cells.

child, prenatal diagnosis can be made by genotyping amniotic or chorionic villus cells. Percutaneous umbilical blood sampling is usually not indicated because of the low risk of bleeding *in utero* and the possibility of hemorrhage at the needle insertion site.

IV.   SUMMARY

Transfusion is generally safe but can result in adverse outcomes. Common transfusion reactions that usually have mild clinical effects include febrile and allergic reactions. More serious reactions, which are uncommon, include hemolysis, bacterial contamination, anaphylaxis, and transfusion-related acute lung injury. Some reactions can be prevented by judicious selection of appropriate components for transfusion. Proper patient identification and routine pretransfusion testing can prevent most hemolytic reactions. Serious transfusion-transmitted diseases are now rare due to progress in donor screening and testing. However, hepatitis and HIV transmission are still possible. Transmission of CMV, parvovirus B19, and blood-borne parasites can be a problem for selected patients. New infectious agents may emerge as threats to the safety of the blood supply, so continued vigilance is necessary to prevent transfusion-transmitted diseases.

SUGGESTED READING

Popovsky MA, ed. *Transfusion Reactions*, 2nd ed. Bethesda, MD: American Association of Blood Banks Press, 2001.

Stramer SL, ed. *Blood Safety in the New Millennium.* Bethesda, MD: American Association of Blood Banks Press, 2001.

CHAPTER 24

Bone Marrow Transplantation

• JOSEPH UBERTI, SAMUEL M. SILVER, AND JAMES L. M. FERRARA

I. INTRODUCTION

A. Hematopoietic stem cell (HSC) transplantation. The treatment and possible cure of certain malignant diseases depends on doses of chemotherapy or chemotherapy plus radiation therapy that exceed the tolerance of bone marrow. Without stem cell support, these patients undergo irreversible marrow toxicity leading to marrow aplasia (no production) and death. In HSC transplantation (frequently called bone marrow transplantation or stem cell transplantation), high-dose chemotherapy or chemoradiotherapy is administered in the hopes of eliminating the malignant disease. However, this high-dose therapy also eliminates or nearly eliminates (ablates) the patient's marrow. Therefore, high-dose therapy is followed by the infusion of HSCs, which allows full lymphohematopoietic reconstitution.

B. Definitions

1. **Autologous** ("from self "). The patient's own marrow or stem cells are removed, cryopreserved, and reinfused after high-dose chemotherapy.

2. **Allogeneic** ("different genes"). Marrow or stem cells are obtained from another individual, such as a human leukocyte antigen (HLA) matched sibling donor, HLA-mismatched family donor, or HLA-matched unrelated donor (see III.C.2.).

3. **Syngeneic** ("same genes"). Marrow or stem cells are obtained from an identical twin.

II. AUTOLOGOUS STEM CELL TRANSPLANTATION

A. Overview

1. In preclinical tumor models, a number of malignant cell lines have been shown to have a log-linear cell kill with radiation or anticancer drugs. This steep dose–response curve allows a small increment in the dose of the drug to increase the number of cancer cells killed by many logs. This principle has been shown to be effective in a number of tumor types. However, as the dose of chemoradiotherapy is increased, toxicities also develop. The dose of the drug and radiation is often limited by marrow toxicity. Marrow or peripheral stem cells can be obtained from these patients before the high-dose therapy, frozen alive (cryopreserved), and then reinfused after the high-dose therapy to reconstitute marrow function.

2. In autologous stem cell transplantation, the mechanism of cure is the high-dose chemotherapy. The "transplanted" HSCs are essentially a sophisticated support device that allows the high-dose therapy to be safely administered. Without this stem cell support, the patient would succumb to the consequences of marrow aplasia, including infection, bleeding, and profound anemia.

3. Autologous stem cell transplants are also used in some severe autoimmune diseases because treatment can be very immunosuppressive. Table 24–1 lists diseases treated with autologous stem cell transplantation.

B. **Phases of autologous stem cell transplantation**

1. **Harvesting.** During harvesting, bone marrow and/or peripheral HSCs are collected. The stem cell is a multilineage progenitor cell that gives rise to the entire lymphohematopoietic system. Approximately 1 in 2000 nucleated marrow cells is a stem cell and has the unique property of self-renewal; the daughter cells produced during cell division give rise to a stem cell and to more differentiated progenitor cells. These progenitor cells begin the pathway toward further differentiation and production of the mature circulating cells. Theoretically, all that is required for a stem cell transplant is the stem cell. However, with current technology, these cells are collected along with other more differentiated HSCs. The stem cell is identified as CD34$^+$ by immunophenotyping; it was previously identified by culture of bone marrow in a colony-forming unit, granulocyte macrophage (CFU-GM) assay. Early progenitor cells are also CD34$^+$.

   a. **Bone marrow harvesting** is the traditional method of collecting stem cells. Marrow is removed from the posterior superior iliac crest with the patient under general anesthesia. In the typical harvest, 1000 mL of marrow is aspirated, which requires entering the marrow space about 100 times.

   b. **Peripheral stem cell harvesting** is clearly an easier way to collect stem cells than traditional harvests in the operating room. More than 90% of autologous HSC transplants use peripheral stem cells.

      (1) Stem cells are normally found in low levels in the peripheral blood. Chemotherapy injures the marrow and alters the normal equilibrium of stem cells between the marrow and the blood. Administration of hematopoietic growth factors such as granulocyte colony-stimulating factor (G-CSF) also results in the release of stem cells from the marrow

TABLE 24–1 • Diseases Treated With Autologous Stem Cell Transplant

Malignancies	Severe Autoimmune Diseases
Breast cancer[a]	Scleroderma
	Lupus
Hodgkin disease	
Non-Hodgkin lymphoma	
Acute myeloid leukemia	
Germ cell tumors	
Neuroblastoma	
Multiple myeloma	
Ovarian cancer	

[a]Metastatic and high-risk local disease.

into the peripheral blood. The administration of G-CSF when patients are recovering from chemotherapy enhances the efflux of the stem cells into the blood.

    (2) The stem cells can be harvested from the peripheral blood via an apheresis machine that removes the stem cells by a centrifugation density gradient and returns to the patient the plasma and other formed elements.

2. **Cryopreservation of cells.** The collected bone marrow or peripheral blood stem cells are suspended in dimethyl sulfoxide and cryopreserved in liquid nitrogen. The dimethyl sulfoxide helps prevent ice crystallization in the cell. The cells can remain viable at liquid nitrogen temperatures for at least 5 years.

3. **Conditioning (the preparative regimen).** In the autologous transplant setting, the preparative regimen, which consists of high-dose chemotherapy and/or total-body irradiation (TBI), is administered before the transplant in an attempt to ablate the malignant disease. In contrast to allogeneic transplantation (see III), for autologous transplantation immunosuppression is not required to prevent graft versus host disease (GVHD) (see III.C.4.). The dose-limiting toxicity of the chemotherapy drugs selected should primarily affect the marrow. If the dose-limiting toxicity of the chemotherapy drugs affects other organ systems (e.g., vincristine causes damage to the peripheral nervous system), stem cell infusion will not prevent toxicity. Conditioning lasts several days and has both hematologic and other consequences (Table 24–2).

4. **Stem cell transplant.** Of all of the steps of the transplant process, this is the most anticlimactic (in contrast to solid organ transplants). It involves intravenous infusion of collected bone marrow or peripheral stem cells. The cryopreserved stem cells are thawed in the patient's room and then infused intravenously, as with a blood transfusion. These stem cells home from the peripheral circulation to the now empty marrow space.

5. **Recovery.** This time is a period of intensive supportive care. The patient is anemic, neutropenic (white blood cells [WBCs] < 500/μl), and thrombocytopenic (i.e., pancytopenic). The high-dose chemotherapy has additionally caused breakdown of the normal mucosal barriers in the mouth and gut. This mucosal breakdown increases susceptibility to infections. The mucosal damage to the

TABLE 24–2 • Consequences of Conditioning in Autologous Stem Cell Transplantation

Hematologic Consequences	Other Consequences
Marrow aplasia	Mucositis
Immunosuppression	Alopecia
	Pulmonary toxicity
	Nausea and vomiting
	Venoocclusive disease of the liver
	Rashes
	Dysesthesia
	Hyponatremia
	Hemorrhagic cystitis
	Cerebellar ataxia
	Cardiomyopathy
	Renal failure

mouth causes painful ulcerations and limits the ability to eat. Many patients require continuous infusions of opioids. Recovery lasts approximately 2 weeks.

  a. **Supportive care during recovery**

   (1) **Transfusions.** All blood products are irradiated to prevent engraftment of lymphocytes from the transfused unit that may cause transfusion-associated GVHD. Red blood cell (RBC) transfusions are used to keep the hematocrit over 25%. Platelet transfusions are used to keep platelets above 10,000/μL to minimize bleeding.

   (2) **Cytokine support.** Use of G-CSF hastens marrow recovery, particularly WBCs.

  b. **Possible complications during recovery**

   (1) **Infections.** When the neutrophil count goes below 500/μL, there is a marked susceptibility to bacterial and fungal infections. The disturbance of the mucosal barrier and intravascular access devices add to the patient's risk of infection. The longer a patient has no WBCs, the higher the risk. The patient is at greatest risk for infection during the neutropenic phase of the transplant, which occurs from the first day post transplant through the tenth day. The use of prophylactic antibiotics and antifungals, cytokines, and peripheral stem cells has dramatically decreased the incidence of severe infections.

    (a) The major infections encountered in autologous HSC transplants are gram-negative and gram-positive bacterial infections and fungal infections, particularly *Candida* and *Aspergillus*.

    (b) Herpes simplex virus (HSV) infections of the perioral area were previously a common cause of morbidity, but the use of prophylactic acyclovir has dramatically decreased this infectious process.

   (2) **Venoocclusive disease of the liver.** This small-vessel liver disease is related to the intensity of the preparative regimen. It usually presents with tender hepatomegaly, jaundice, and fluid retention. The patient is at the highest risk for this complication during the first week after the transplant. It is reversible in most cases; however, extreme fluid imbalances may cause respiratory failure.

   (3) **Interstitial pneumonia.** This complication may occur within the first 2 weeks after the transplant; however, it may not appear until 1–2 months post transplant. It may take many months to resolve. Possible causes include lung toxicity from chemotherapy or irradiation and viral infections.

  6. **Engraftment.** Engraftment is the period when production of WBCs, RBCs, and platelets occurs. The time to a neutrophil count recovery (the usual engraftment standard) has decreased with the use of cytokines (e.g., G-CSF) and peripheral blood stem cells instead of marrow. The time to a neutrophil count of 500/μL is 10–12 days as compared to 18 days or more when bone marrow was used without cytokine support. The time to platelet transfusion and RBC transfusion independence is 12 days.

C. **Outcomes of autologous stem cell transplantation.** Outcomes depend on the underlying disease and the status of the disease at the time of transplant.

  1. In terms of **survival rates,** when autologous and allogeneic transplants are compared for similar diseases, the following appear to be true:

   a. Treatment-related mortality is less with autologous transplants (typically < 3% during the first 100 days post transplant).

   b. Relapse rate is higher with autologous transplants (up to 70%).

2. The major cause of death in autologous transplants is relapse of disease.

3. A long-term complication in autologous transplants, rarely seen in allogeneic transplants, is secondary leukemia from chemotherapy or radiation therapy.

D. **Advantages and disadvantages of autologous stem cell transplantation**

1. **Advantages:**

  a. A ready source of stem cells (the patient is the donor)

  b. Low treatment-related mortality

   (1) Ten years ago, the mortality rate 100 days after the transplant was as high as 20%. At present the mortality rate is approximately 0.5%.

   (2) This is a much lower mortality rate than for allogeneic transplants, which can be as high as 40% in some groups.

  c. Low toxicity

   (1) Unlike allogeneic transplants, with autologous transplants no immunologic barriers must be crossed.

   (2) There is no GVHD; therefore, immunosuppressive medications such as cyclosporine and tacrolimus are unnecessary and infectious complications are fewer.

   (3) Graft failure (rejection) is rare.

2. **Disadvantages:**

  a. Tumor contamination

   (1) The cryopreserved stem cells may contain viable tumor cells.

   (2) When infused into the patient, these tumor cells may be a cause of post-transplant relapse.

  b. Lack of antitumor effect

   (1) There is no graft versus tumor effect, which occurs with allogeneic transplants.

   (2) The lack of antitumor effect may also be a cause of posttransplant relapse.

III. ALLOGENEIC STEM CELL TRANSPLANTATION

A. **Overview.** Allogeneic HSC transplantation is the administration of high-dose chemotherapy and/or radiation therapy for elimination of malignant disease and bone marrow followed by the infusion of normal donor HSCs. The donor HSCs are derived from an HLA-matched or HLA-mismatched family member (usually a sibling) or an unrelated donor.

B. **Indications for allogeneic transplantation**

1. **Malignancy**

  a. The most common use of allogeneic transplants is for hematologic malignancies, such as chronic myelocytic leukemia (CML), acute myelocytic leukemia, acute lymphocytic leukemia, myelodysplastic syndrome, multiple myeloma, and non-Hodgkin lymphoma.

  b. The curative potential of allogeneic transplants relies on three concepts:

   (1) Higher doses of chemotherapy may overcome the resistance to standard chemotherapy of some aggressive tumor cells. This higher dose of chemotherapy completely ablates the bone marrow. In this situation, the reinfusion of stem cells after high-dose chemotherapy or radiation therapy functions as a biologic marrow rescue.

   (2) Reinfusion of normal donor marrow or stem cells after high-dose chemotherapy reestablishes normal hematopoiesis.

   (3) Perhaps most important, the donor marrow eliminates the patient's

tumor through immunologic mechanisms. This is known as the graft versus tumor effect: the newly infused marrow and immunologic system from the donor can eliminate any tumor cells that may be present in the patient after the high-dose chemotherapy is administered.

   c. The decision as to when to proceed with transplant varies by disease.

     (1) In CML, allogeneic transplant is the only curative therapy and is therefore recommended for all patients under age 55 with CML.

     (2) In acute lymphocytic leukemia, many patients (especially children) are cured with conventional chemotherapy. Therefore, transplantation is recommended only for patients who relapse after standard therapy or patients who have high-risk features that indicate they are at a high risk for relapse.

   d. The cure rate of allogeneic HSC transplant after relapse is lower than during remission, and not all patients can achieve another remission after relapse.

2. Bone marrow failure. Allogeneic transplant remains the treatment of choice for young patients with aplastic anemia, particularly those who do not respond to immunosuppression.

3. Inherited disorders

   a. **Hematopoiesis.** This category consists of a variety of rare congenital disorders. Conceptually, this is an important group because it shows that any disease involving an HSC or its progeny can be cured through an allogeneic HSC transplant. These diseases are caused by the developmental absence or abnormality of a specific lineage of cells derived from the lymphohematopoietic stem cell.

     (1) **Immunodeficiency diseases**

       (a) Severe combined immunodeficiency is a heterogeneous group of lethal disorders of T and B lymphocytes that predispose the patient to life-threatening infections.

       (b) Wiskott-Aldrich syndrome is an X-linked recessive disorder characterized by T-cell immunodeficiency.

       (c) Osteopetrosis is a rare disease that is a result of dysfunctional osteoclasts (specialized macrophages derived from the marrow stem cell).

     (2) **Hemoglobinopathies**

       (a) This category includes severe disorders of hemoglobin synthesis, such as sickle cell disease and thalassemia.

       (b) In European countries where chronic transfusion support is not readily available, allogeneic HSC transplant is more frequently used for these diseases than in the United States.

   b. **Storage diseases.** This disease category includes a number of rare disorders in which an enzyme deficiency leads to an accumulation of undegraded toxic derivatives leading to a wide range of irreversible neurologic disorders, such as Hurler syndrome, Hunter syndrome, and mucopolysaccharidoses. Transplant provides the deficient enzyme in blood cells that can overcome the target organ's enzyme deficiency. The transplant usually must be completed before the patient becomes symptomatic.

C. Immunologic aspects of allogeneic stem cell transplantation

  1. Human leukocyte antigen system

   a. A donor for the transplant is determined by the matching of HLA proteins. HLA proteins are transmembrane proteins that function normally in antigen recognition of foreign agents (e.g., viruses, bacteria) and are important in immunologic recognition of foreign tissues. They bind to protein fragments and present these fragments (antigens) to T cells, which results in T-cell activation via the T-cell receptor (TCR).

b. HLA proteins are encoded by genes of the major histocompatibility complex (MHC) on chromosome 6. A set of three molecules on each chromosome (A, B, and DR) defines a haplotype. We inherit a separate haplotype from each of our parents, and each haplotype is codominantly expressed on the cell surface.

c. Each HLA antigen is polymorphic, with hundreds of different alleles for each of the three antigens, making the typing process complex.

(1) The A and B antigens, known as the class I antigens, are usually expressed on all cell types except erythrocytes.

(2) The class II antigens, or DR antigens, are usually limited to B cells, monocytes, dendritic cells, and some activated T cells.

2. **Finding a suitable donor**

a. The most desirable source of HSCs is a 6/6 HLA-matched sibling. Each full sibling has a 25% chance of matching. Sometimes other close relatives are matches.

b. If no family members match, there are registries of normal donors who have agreed to donate marrow to patients who need transplants. These unrelated donors are less likely to match for minor H antigens, which can cause immunologic reactions between donor and recipient.

3. **Benefits of donor T cells.** The harvesting of HSCs, either from the peripheral blood or from the marrow, mixes mature WBCs with stem cells and progenitors in the collection bag. Mature T lymphocytes are the principal effectors of cell-mediated immunity; many of the therapeutic benefits and toxicities of allogeneic HSC transplant are derived from immunologic reactions between donor T cells and recipient cells.

a. **Engraftment.** Donor T cells help donor stem cells engraft. These facilitator cells are mostly CD8$^+$, and they eliminate any remaining elements of host immune cells that survive conditioning and might reject the donor graft. These CD8$^+$ cells may also have positive effects on donor stem cells, such as the secretion of cytokines, but that mechanism is controversial. Depletion of donor T cells before allogeneic HSC transplant significantly increases the risk of graft failure.

b. **Graft versus leukemia effect.** Most allogeneic HSC transplants are performed for malignancies that do not respond to conventional doses of chemoradiotherapy. Donor T cells are capable of recognizing and eliminating residual malignant cells in the host. Both CD4$^+$ and CD8$^+$ cells contribute to this graft versus leukemia effect in animal models, although the relative importance of specific subsets in clinical transplantation is not yet clear. Depletion of most T cells increases the risk of relapse, especially for patients with CML. If a patient's disease recurs after HSC transplant, sometimes infusion of additional donor leukocytes can again eradicate the malignancy (CML is the best example).

c. **Immunologic reconstitution.** The thymus involutes with increasing age. Reconstitution of the immune system is slower after allogeneic HSC transplant than after autologous HSC transplant, and T cells are the last of the immune cells to recover. T-cell depletion further retards the pace of T-cell reconstitution, making recipients even more prone to viral infections, cytomegalovirus (CMV) in particular.

4. **Disadvantages of donor T cells.** GVHD is the greatest disadvantage from the presence of donor T cells.
   a. **Overview of graft versus host disease**
      (1) Three conditions are necessary for the development of GVHD:
         (a) An immunocompetent graft (i.e., one containing T cells)
         (b) Histocompatibility (minor or major) differences between donor and recipient
         (c) A recipient who cannot mount an immune response to the graft. This condition is often caused by immunosuppressive drugs given to recipients of solid organ transplants. For example, a recipient of a small bowel transplant can develop GVHD because donor T cells are present in the gut-associated lymphoid tissue of the small bowel.
      (2) The chemoradiotherapy used to condition HSC transplant recipients and the large number of T cells that accompany stem cells combine to make allogeneic HSC transplant the most common setting for acute GVHD. Without additional immunosuppression, more than 90% of allogeneic HSC transplant recipients would develop significant GVHD, even from HLA-identical siblings.
      (3) Other individuals at risk for GVHD (Table 24–3) are recipients of blood transfusions that contain WBCs (including lymphocytes). Normal individuals who are heterozygous for HLA proteins will not reject lymphocytes transfused from a donor who is homozygous for one of the recipient's haplotypes. However, if the donor lymphocytes that are not rejected recognize HLA antigens of the recipient's other haplotype, GVHD may develop. On this basis, GVHD may develop in patients who received directed blood donation but are not otherwise compromised (e.g., transfusion from an HLA-homozygous mother to a heterozygous child). Radiation of blood products prevents lymphocytes from proliferating; therefore, all immunocompromised patients receive irradiated blood products.
      (4) GVHD that occurs before day 100 is termed **acute** GVHD. It affects three primary target organs: skin, gastrointestinal (GI) tract, and liver,

TABLE 24–3 • Procedures Associated with a High Risk of GVHD

Procedure	High-Risk Groups
Bone marrow transplant	Patients receiving no GVHD prophylaxis
	Older patients
	Recipients of HLA-nonidentical bone marrow
	Recipients of bone marrow from allosensitized donors
Solid organ transplant	Recipients of organs containing lymphoid tissue (e.g. small-bowel transplant)
Transfusion of unirradiated blood products	Neonates and fetuses
	Patients with congenital immunodeficiency syndromes
	Patients receiving immunosuppressive chemoradiotherapy
	Patients receiving directed blood donations from partially HLA-identical, HLA-homozygous donors

GVHD, graft versus host disease; HLA, human leukocyte antigen.

often simultaneously. GVHD that occurs after day 100 is termed **chronic GVHD** and can affect the skin, GI tract, liver, eyes, lungs, and joints.

(5) Once established, GVHD is difficult to treat, and severe cases are usually fatal. The mainstay of therapy is high-dose steroids.

b. **Pathophysiology of acute graft versus host disease.** The pathophysiology of acute GVHD can be considered in a framework of three sequential phases.

(1) **Phase one.** The earliest phase of acute GVHD starts before the donor cells are infused. The transplant-conditioning regimen can damage and activate host tissues (e.g., intestinal mucosa, liver). Activated host cells secrete inflammatory cytokines that can up-regulate adhesion molecules and MHC antigens, thereby enhancing the recognition of host allogeneic antigens by mature donor T cells after the cellular component of the graft is infused.

(2) **Phase two.** The second phase of acute GVHD includes antigen presentation, the activation of individual donor T cells, and proliferation and differentiation of these activated T cells. Host antigen-presenting cells are particularly important in graft versus host reactions. When donor and recipient are not MHC identical, donor T cells can recognize host MHC molecules as foreign, and the resultant graft versus host reaction can be dramatic. When the recipient and donor are MHC identical, GVHD occurs through recognition by the T cell and its TCR of different peptides bound to the same MHC. T cells that secrete interleukin-2 and interferon-γ (type 1 cytokines) are critical mediators of acute GVHD.

(3) **Phase three.** Mononuclear phagocytes, which have been primed by cytokines during phase two, have an important role in this phase of acute GVHD. Monocytes receive a second, triggering signal to secrete the inflammatory cytokines tumor necrosis factor-α and interleukin-1. This stimulus may be provided by lipopolysaccharide (endotoxin), which can leak through the intestinal mucosa damaged by the conditioning regimen and subsequently stimulate gut-associated lymphocytes and macrophages. Tumor necrosis factor-α can cause direct tissue damage by inducing either necrosis or apoptosis (programmed cell death) of target cells. Apoptosis is critical to GVHD in the large intestine and skin. Thus, the induction of inflammatory cytokines may synergize with the cellular damage caused by cytotoxic T cells and natural killer cells, resulting in the amplification of local tissue injury.

c. **Prevention of graft versus host disease.** All allogeneic HSC transplant recipients are treated with immunosuppressive agents as prophylaxis against GVHD. Usually at least two drugs are used.

(1) **Tacrolimus (FK-506) or cyclosporine.** Both of these compounds inhibit TCR signaling pathways, so either one (not both) is used. They are very toxic drugs, particularly to the kidneys, which may be weakened by antibiotics. Treatment usually lasts at least 6 months after transplant.

(2) **Methotrexate (MTX).** A dihydrofolate reductase inhibitor, MTX inhibits expansion of all actively dividing cells. MTX is most effective when several doses are given within the first 2 weeks after HSC transplant, the time of maximal donor T-cell response to host antigens. Thus, MTX slows expansion of donor T-cell clones but also that of donor stem cells. Hematopoietic engraftment is often slowed by several days when MTX is used.

(3) **Steroids.** Steroids have many immunosuppressive properties and can lyse lymphocytes. They also inhibit production of inflammatory cytokines that mediate GVHD.

D. Phases of allogeneic stem cell transplantation

1. **Conditioning.** Before the transplant, the patient receives high-dose chemotherapy and/or radiation therapy. The purpose of this conditioning regimen is twofold, and some conditioning agents have both of the activities cited next (e.g., cyclophosphamide).

   a. **Cytoreduction.** Chemotherapy and radiation therapy are used to reduce the tumor cells. It also eliminates the patient's normal or abnormal stem cells. The agents used for this usually have broad antitumor activity. Cytoreduction often relies heavily on alkylating agents and TBI.

   b. **Immunosuppression.** To allow engraftment of the new HSCs, the patient's endogenous lymphocytes must be suppressed so as not to reject the new marrow and stem cells.

2. **Transplant.** The harvested cells are infused into the vein as with a blood transfusion. The stem cells traffic to the appropriate place in the marrow, where they take up residence.

3. **Recovery.** This period of intensive supportive care is similar to the recovery period in autologous HSC transplant. The administration of high-dose chemotherapy and radiation therapy eliminates normal marrow function. It also may cause reversible damage to many organs, including the skin, GI tract, lungs, and liver.

   a. **Aggressive supportive care** is crucial for long-term success because most toxicities are reversible.

      (1) **Transfusion.** There is a mandatory period of aplasia awaiting marrow recovery, during which time patients require RBC and platelet transfusions. Prolonged neutropenia predisposes patients to a multitude of bacterial infections. Granulocyte transfusions are impractical.

      (2) **Cytokine support.** Growth factors (e.g., G-CSF) that hasten neutrophil recovery after HSC transplant are available.

   b. Possible **complications** during recovery include infections and organ toxicities.

      (1) **Infections.** Patients are susceptible to a variety of infections. They lack granulocytes, which help resolve bacterial infections. They also lack a functioning immune system, which helps prevent viral infections and unusual or opportunistic infections. Patients are also taking a number of medications that actually block the new developing immune system to prevent GVHD. In addition to these deficiencies, the normal barriers that prevent entry of these organisms (e.g., skin, GI tract) are now destroyed. However, with prompt administration of various antimicrobials and the judicious use of antiviral and antifungal agents, the risk of these infections has been greatly reduced.

         (a) **Bacterial infections.** Patients get a number of bacterial infections during the period of neutropenia (granulocyte count $< 500/\mu L$), including gram-negative rods (*Pseudomonas* from the GI tract) and gram-positive cocci (usually *Staphylococcus aureus*).

         (b) **Viral infections.** Several viruses (e.g., CMV, HSV, adenovirus, respiratory syncytial virus) can be fatal after HSC transplant. Some of these viral infections, such as CMV and HSV, are preventable through the prophylactic use of antiviral therapy (e.g., ganciclovir, acyclovir). Other viruses are much more difficult to treat. Viral infections occur more frequently after allogeneic HSC transplant than after autologous HSC transplant.

   (c) **Fungal infections.** Candidiasis and aspergillosis are rare but often fatal infections in patients after HSC transplant. Some prophylactic strategies for candidiasis have been beneficial. Use of steroids to prevent or treat GVHD puts these patients at very high risk for fungal infections.

   (2) **GI tract.** Conditioning and GVHD both damage the GI tract. Use of multiple antibiotics during HSC transplant changes bacterial flora (e.g., *Clostridium difficile* colitis). Parenteral nutrition is usually required after allogeneic HSC transplant.

   (3) **Liver.** Both venoocclusive disease (low flow, endothelial damage) and GVHD (acute and chronic) cause liver disease. Venoocclusive disease occurs early after both allogeneic and autologous HSC transplant. Although severe liver disease is usually reversible, it often leads to progressive lung disease.

   (4) **Lungs.** Both autologous and allogeneic HSC transplant damage the lungs. Viral, fungal, and bacterial infections are common (e.g., interstitial pneumonia). Pathogens are identified in only 50% of cases; the remaining cases are probably immunologic. The lungs are a target of both acute and chronic GVHD.

   (5) **Immune system.** Slow reconstitution is caused by added immunosuppressive agents and by GVHD. Active support (e.g., prophylactic IV immunoglobulin, antibiotics) is required after allogeneic HSC transplant for months and sometimes years.

   (6) **Graft versus host disease.** GVHD (see III.C.4.) remains the major complication after allogeneic HSC transplant. It is caused by immunologic activation of the infused donor T cells against the patient's organs. Because this disease is closely linked to the graft versus tumor effect seen in these transplants, it may have a beneficial and detrimental effect.

E. **Outcomes of allogeneic stem cell transplantation.** Outcomes depend on the type of transplant (HLA-identical family member donor versus HLA-nonidentical family member donor versus HLA-identical unrelated donor), underlying disease, and the status of disease at the time of transplant.

   1. In general, the later in the disease course the transplant occurs, the worse the survival rate.

   2. Unrelated transplants generally do worse than sibling transplants because of increased incidence of GVHD and infections.

   3. Relapse can still occur, although at a lower rate than with autologous transplant.

   4. The mortality rate at day 100 is 20%–30%, depending on how closely the donor and recipient are matched. Causes of death include:

      a. Relapse
      b. GVHD
      c. Infection

IV. SUMMARY

HSC transplant is a curative therapy for a number of hematologic disorders, both malignant and nonmalignant. Autologous HSC transplants have fewer immunologic complications but have higher rates of relapse after transplant. Allogeneic HSC transplants have lower rates of relapse but have more immunologic complications, including GVHD, which can be fatal. Advances in HLA typing, supportive care, and newer immunosuppressive agents have significantly improved long-term survival rates after HSC transplant over the last 10 years.

SUGGESTED READING

Ferrara JLM, Deeg HJ, Burakoff SJ, eds. *Graft-vs.-Host Disease*. 2nd ed. New York: Marcel Dekker, 1996: 607–639.

Thomas ED, Blume KG, Forman SJ, eds. *Hematopoietic Cell Transplantation*. Malden, MA: Blackwell Science, 1994:515–560.

Index

Page numbers followed by t indicate tables; those in *italic* indicate figures; those preceded by A indicate Atlas entries.

Hematology for the Medical Student
ATLAS IMAGES

Alvin H. Schmaier, William G. Finn, and Lilli M. Petruzzelli

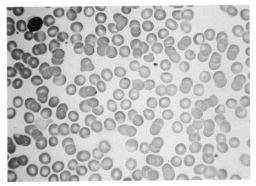

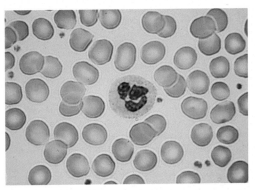

ATLAS FIGURE 1. Medium-power light microscopic view of a normal peripheral blood smear showing normochromic, normocytic red blood cells, a small lymphocyte, and adequate numbers of platelets. The area of central pallor on the red blood cells comprises one third of the diameter of the cell. The diameter of the nucleus of the small lymphocytes is approximately equal to the diameter of the red blood cell. This slide and all other slides in this atlas are stained with Wright-Giemsa stain, the traditional stain for examination of the peripheral blood smear. (Reprinted with permission from the American Society of Hematology Slide Bank CD, prepared by the Center for Educational Resources, University of Washington, 1998.)

ATLAS FIGURE 2. High-power view of a normal polymorphonuclear leukocyte (PMN, neutrophil). The nucleus consists of three lobes, and the cytoplasm has mild granularity that is characteristic of a typical neutrophil. (Reprinted with permission from the American Society of Hematology Slide Bank CD, prepared by the Center for Educational Resources, University of Washington, 1998.)

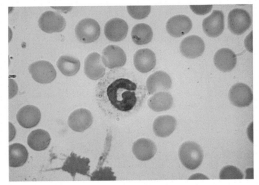

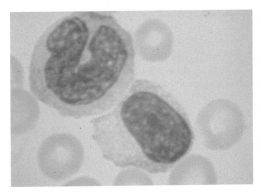

ATLAS FIGURE 3. High-power view of the band form of the neutrophil. The nucleus is not segmented, in contrast to the mature form. The cytoplasm has mild granularity as seen in the mature granulocyte. (Reprinted with permission from the American Society of Hematology Slide Bank CD, prepared by the Center for Educational Resources, University of Washington, 1998.)

ATLAS FIGURE 4. High-powered view of a normal monocyte with a large, lobulated nucleus (on upper left). It is next to a large lymphocyte with abundant agranular cytoplasm (on lower right). (Reprinted with permission from the American Society of Hematology Slide Bank CD, prepared by the Center for Educational Resources, University of Washington, 1998.)

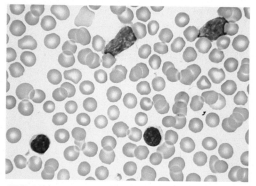

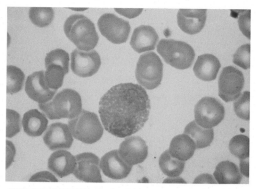

ATLAS FIGURE 5. Medium-power view of two normal small lymphocytes with round nuclei and scant cytoplasm and two large, atypical reactive lymphocytes. Often with reactive lymphocytes, red blood cells make indentations on the lymphocytes' cytoplasm. (This figure is provided by courtesy of Dr. William Finn, Department of Pathology, University of Michigan.)

ATLAS FIGURE 6. High-power view of a normal two-lobed eosinophil. The cytoplasm contains prominent azurophilic granules. (Reprinted with permission from the American Society of Hematology Slide Bank CD, prepared by the Center for Educational Resources, University of Washington, 1998.)

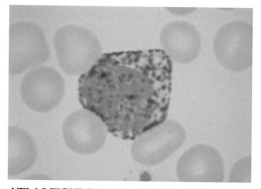

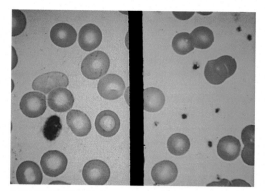

ATLAS FIGURE 7. High-power view of a normal basophil with prominent basophilic cytoplasmic granules that obscure the nucleus. (Reprinted with permission from the American Society of Hematology Slide Bank CD, prepared by the Center for Educational Resources, University of Washington, 1998.)

ATLAS FIGURE 8. High-power view of a large platelet on the left and normal-sized platelets on the right. Large platelets contain basophilic granular cytoplasm. (Reprinted with permission from the American Society of Hematology Slide Bank CD, prepared by the Center for Educational Resources, University of Washington, 1998.)

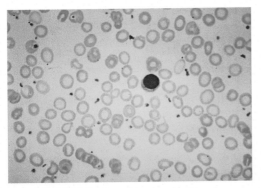

ATLAS FIGURE 9. Medium-power view of hypochromic, microcytic red blood cells. The area of central pallor is greater than a third of the diameter of the cell. This fact is the definition of hypochromia. The diameter of the erythrocytes is smaller than the diameter of the nucleus of the small lymphocyte pictured in this figure, reflecting low red cell volume (microcytosis). The platelet count on this smear is normal or increased. This smear is characteristic of iron deficiency anemia. (Reprinted with permission from the American Society of Hematology Slide Bank CD, prepared by the Center for Educational Resources, University of Washington, 1998.)

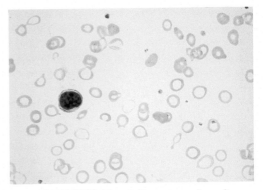

ATLAS FIGURE 10. Medium-power view of markedly hypochromic and microcytic red blood cells. As the patient becomes more anemic, the peripheral blood smear will show increased variation in size (anisocytosis) and shape (poikilocytosis). The pronounced area of central pallor is also noted. (Reprinted with permission from the American Society of Hematology Slide Bank CD, prepared by the Center for Educational Resources, University of Washington, 1998.)

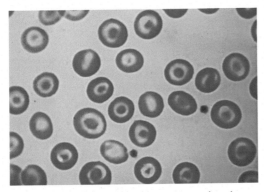

ATLAS FIGURE 11. High-power view of erythrocytes with target cells that are cells with a central appearance of membrane. Target cells arise under conditions of reduced intracellular hemoglobin (e.g. thalassemia or hemoglobin C trait or disease) or when there is excessive red blood cell membrane in relation to the contents of the cells (e.g., liver disease). (Reprinted with permission from the American Society of Hematology Slide Bank CD, prepared by the Center for Educational Resources, University of Washington, 1998.)

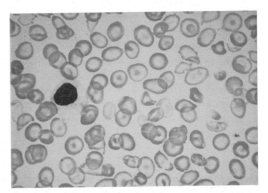

ATLAS FIGURE 12. Medium-power view of targeted hypochromic, microcytic red blood cells that are scattered throughout the smear. Most of the red blood cells have a cell diameter smaller than the nucleus of the lymphocyte. This smear is characteristic of some of the thalassemias. (Reprinted with permission from the American Society of Hematology Slide Bank CD, prepared by the Center for Educational Resources, University of Washington, 1998.)

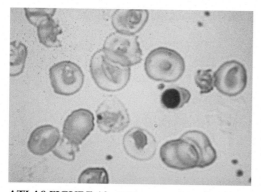

ATLAS FIGURE 13. High-power view of severely hypochromic targeted red blood cells with a nucleated red blood cell. This smear is characteristic of homozygous β-thalassemia or Cooley's anemia. (Courtesy of Dr. William Finn, Department of Pathology, University of Michigan.)

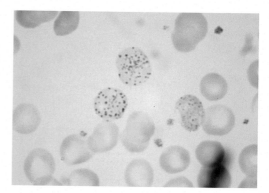

ATLAS FIGURE 14. High-power view of red blood cells showing prominent dark stained deposits with a stippled appearance in their cytoplasm. This feature, called basophilic stippling, indicates pathologic aggregates of ribosomes seen in disorders of hemoglobin synthesis such as thalassemia, hemoglobinopathy, lead poisoning, and myelodysplastic syndromes. (Reprinted with permission from the American Society of Hematology Slide Bank CD, prepared by the Center for Educational Resources, University of Washington, 1998.)

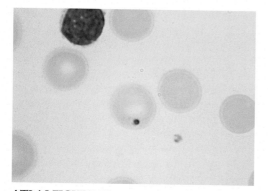

ATLAS FIGURE 15. The dark dot of material seen in the lower portion of the central red blood cell is a Howell-Jolly body, a small remnant of the red blood cell nucleus. It is characteristically seen post splenectomy or when a patient may have developed functional asplenia. (Reprinted with permission from the American Society of Hematology Slide Bank CD, prepared by the Center for Educational Resources, University of Washington, 1998.)

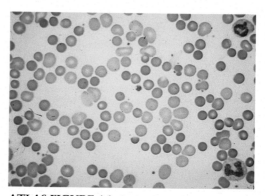

ATLAS FIGURE 16. Low-power view of red blood cells with loss of the area of central pallor. These cells, called spherocytes, can arise from defects in the proteins that constitute red blood cell membranes or when the red blood cells are coated with immunoglobulin or complement and remodeled after traversing the spleen. (Reprinted with permission from the American Society of Hematology Slide Bank CD, prepared by the Center for Educational Resources, University of Washington, 1998.)

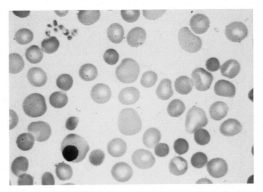

ATLAS FIGURE 17. Medium-power view of spherocytes of varying sizes and a nucleated red blood cell. This smear is characteristic of that seen in a warm (immunoglobulin G) antibody-mediated hemolytic anemia. (Reprinted with permission from the American Society of Hematology Slide Bank CD, prepared by the Center for Educational Resources, University of Washington, 1998.)

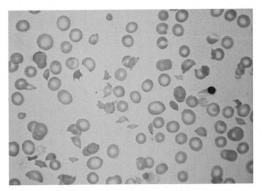

ATLAS FIGURE 18. Low-power view of a peripheral blood smear showing variation in the size (anisocytosis) and shape (poikilocytosis) of red blood cells. Some of the red blood cells appear broken apart and fragmented (schistocytes). The crescent-shaped fragmented cells are called helmet cells. This smear is characteristic of intravascular destruction of red blood cells as is seen in microangiopathic hemolytic anemia of any cause. (Reprinted with permission from the American Society of Hematology Slide Bank CD, prepared by the Center for Educational Resources, University of Washington, 1998.)

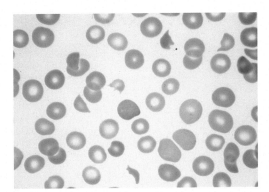

ATLAS FIGURE 19. Medium-power view of fragmented red blood cells with helmet cells and schistocytes. Some of the red blood cells have a different shade of color (polychromasia). Polychromasia indicates younger red blood cells that have remnant ribosomes in their cytoplasm. Its presence indicates that bone marrow is producing and releasing young red blood cells to compensate for peripheral destruction or loss as seen in severe hemolytic anemias (i.e. anemias with shortened red blood cell survival) or brisk hemorrhage. (Courtesy of Dr. William Finn, Department of Pathology, University of Michigan.)

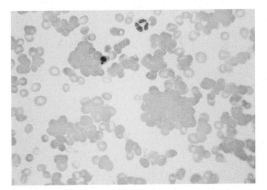

ATLAS FIGURE 20. Low-power view of clumps of red blood cells as seen with immunoglobulin M (IgM antibody) agglutinin disease. Cells agglutinate, or form clumps, on the peripheral blood smear as result of exposure to cool peripheral temperatures. The agglutinated red blood cells can appear as a large smudge on the peripheral blood smear. (Reprinted with permission from the American Society of Hematology Slide Bank CD, prepared by the Center for Educational Resources, University of Washington, 1998.)

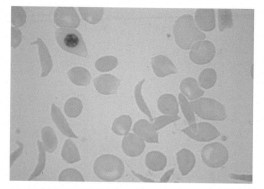

ATLAS FIGURE 21. High-power view of crescent-shaped sickle cells that are characteristic of sickle cell disease. A nucleated red blood cell also appears in the peripheral blood smear. (Reprinted with permission from the American Society of Hematology Slide Bank CD, prepared by the Center for Educational Resources, University of Washington, 1998.)

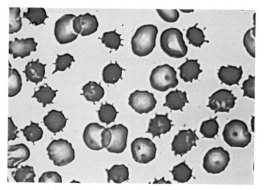

ATLAS FIGURE 22. Medium-power view of spiculated spherocytes (acanthocytes) seen in spur cell anemia associated with liver disease or in abetalipoproteinemia. Acanthocytes indicate abnormal lipid ratios in the red blood cell membrane and are formed as a result of conditioning a less fluid red cell membrane as it transverses a functioning spleen. (Reprinted with permission from the American Society of Hematology Slide Bank CD, prepared by the Center for Educational Resources, University of Washington, 1998.)

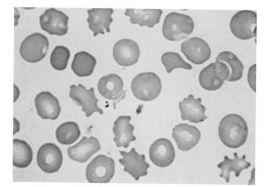

ATLAS FIGURE 23. High-power view of misshapen red blood cells (poikilocytosis). Cells with these bizarre shapes are seen in various metabolic states such as hypothyroidism, hypoparathyroidism, liver disease, and membrane protein abnormalities. (Reprinted with permission from the American Society of Hematology Slide Bank CD, prepared by the Center for Educational Resources, University of Washington, 1998.)

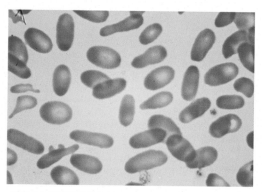

ATLAS FIGURE 24. High-power view of ovalocytosis that results from a defect in the membrane proteins of the cell as seen in hereditary disorders such as hereditary ovalocytosis. (Reprinted with permission from the American Society of Hematology Slide Bank CD, prepared by the Center for Educational Resources, University of Washington, 1998.)

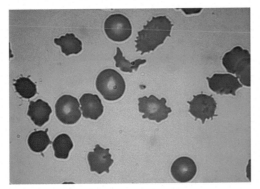

ATLAS FIGURE 25. High-power view of red blood cells from a patient with renal failure. The central red blood cell with crenated edges is called a burr cell. The smear also shows other red blood cells that are spiculated acanthocytes and a spiculated fragmented cell. (Reprinted with permission from the American Society of Hematology Slide Bank CD, prepared by the Center for Educational Resources, University of Washington, 1998.)

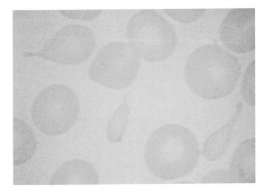

ATLAS FIGURE 26. High-power view of a misshapen red blood cell that looks like a teardrop (dacrocyte). Teardrop cells are seen in patients with myeloproliferative disorders or other causes of marrow fibrosis or extramedullary hematopoiesis. (Reprinted with permission from the American Society of Hematology Slide Bank CD, prepared by the Center for Educational Resources, University of Washington, 1998.)

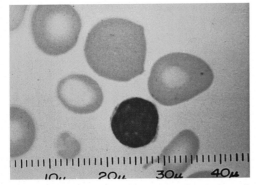

ATLAS FIGURE 27. High-power view of enlarged red blood cells that have a mean diameter greater than the nucleus of the small lymphocyte. These red blood cells are macroovalocytes that can be seen in B_{12} or folate deficiency. (Reprinted with permission from the American Society of Hematology Slide Bank CD, prepared by the Center for Educational Resources, University of Washington, 1998.)

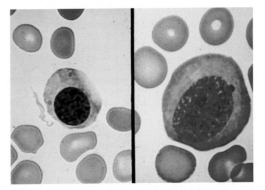

ATLAS FIGURE 28. High-power view of megaloblastic nucleated red blood cells as seen in B_{12} or folate deficiency. These cells are not normally seen in the peripheral blood. The larger cell is an early polychromatophilic normoblast; the smaller cell is an orthochromatophilic normoblast. In both cells, the nuclear chromatin pattern is more open than the tightly packed chromatin in equivalent staged normoblasts in normal individuals. (Reprinted with permission from the American Society of Hematology Slide Bank CD, prepared by the Center for Educational Resources, University of Washington, 1998.)

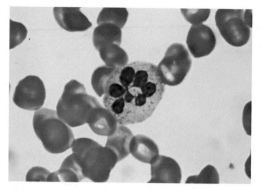

ATLAS FIGURE 29. Medium-power view of a megaloblastic, hypersegmented polymorphonuclear leukocyte. This cell with at least five nuclear lobes is characteristic of B_{12} or folate deficiency. (Reprinted with permission from the American Society of Hematology Slide Bank CD, prepared by the Center for Educational Resources, University of Washington, 1998.)

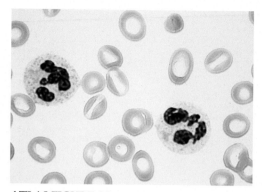

ATLAS FIGURE 30. Medium-power view of two polymorphonuclear leukocytes with bluish bodies in their cytoplasm. These bluish inclusion bodies are called Döhle bodies and are aggregates of rough endoplasmic reticulum in individuals who have had a recent microbial infection or other acute inflammatory condition. (Reprinted with permission from the American Society of Hematology Slide Bank CD, prepared by the Center for Educational Resources, University of Washington, 1998.)

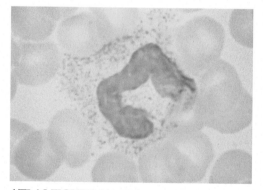

ATLAS FIGURE 31. High-power view of a band form of a polymorphonuclear leukocyte with prominent granules in its cytoplasm. These granules, called toxic granulation, are seen during infections. (Reprinted with permission from the American Society of Hematology Slide Bank CD, prepared by the Center for Educational Resources, University of Washington, 1998.)

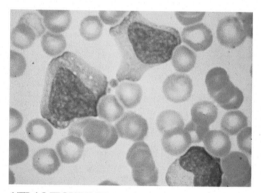

ATLAS FIGURE 32. High-power view of two large lymphocytes in an individual with a recent viral infection or infectious mononucleosis. In large lymphocytes, the cytoplasm of the cell is often indented by adjacent red blood cells. The single leukocyte on the edge of the figure is a monocyte. (Reprinted with permission from the American Society of Hematology Slide Bank CD, prepared by the Center for Educational Resources, University of Washington, 1998.)

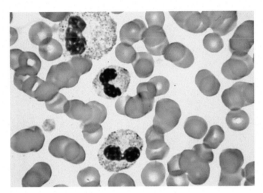

ATLAS FIGURE 33. Medium-power view of three two-lobed polymorphonuclear leukocytes. These cells have the Pelger-Huët anomaly. This entity can be seen as a benign congenital abnormality (the true Pelger-Huët anomaly) or can arise secondarily in reactive conditions (e.g. mycoplasma infection, drug effects) or neoplastic conditions (e.g. myelodysplastic or myeloproliferative syndromes or acute leukemia). Such acquired Pelger-Huët-like changes are called pseudo-Pelger-Huët. (Courtesy of Dr. William Finn, Department of Pathology, University of Michigan.)

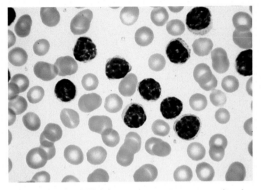

ATLAS FIGURE 34. Medium-power view of multiple small lymphocytes. Cells like this in the peripheral blood are characteristic of chronic lymphocytic leukemia. (Courtesy of Dr. William Finn, Department of Pathology, University of Michigan.)

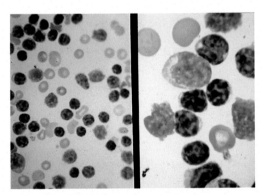

ATLAS FIGURE 35. On one side is a low-power view of small and large lymphocytes seen in chronic lymphocytic leukemia. On the other side is a high-power view of the same cells. In certain instances, an outline of a degenerated cell is seen on the smear. These degenerated cells are called smudge cells and are characteristic of but not specific for chronic lymphocytic leukemia. (Reprinted with permission from the American Society of Hematology Slide Bank CD, prepared by the Center for Educational Resources, University of Washington, 1998.)

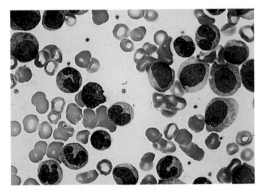

ATLAS FIGURE 36. Medium-power view showing an array of granulocytic precursors in the peripheral blood. The smear shows polymorphonuclear leukocytes, bands, metamyelocytes, myelocytes, and a promyelocyte. It also may have an increase in basophils. This smear is characteristic of chronic myelogenous leukemia. (Courtesy of Dr. William Finn, Department of Pathology, University of Michigan.)

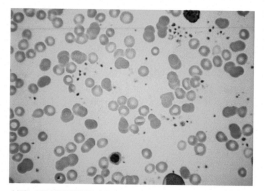

ATLAS FIGURE 37. Low-power view of peripheral blood showing an increase in platelets in clumps, a nucleated red blood cell, and myeloblast. This smear is from a patient with essential thrombocythemia. (Reprinted with permission from the American Society of Hematology Slide Bank CD, prepared by the Center for Educational Resources, University of Washington, 1998.)

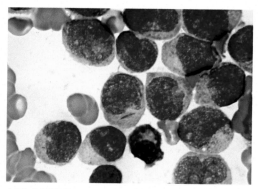

ATLAS FIGURE 38. A high-power view of myeloblasts with prominent nucleoli. One of the myeloblasts contains an Auer rod (a stick-like structure in the cytoplasm); others have granular cytoplasm. This smear is characteristic of acute myelogenous leukemia (M1 morphology). (Courtesy of Dr. William Finn, Department of Pathology, University of Michigan.)

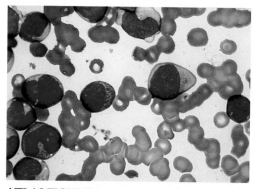

ATLAS FIGURE 39. A medium-power view of homogeneous myeloblasts with prominent nucleoli. Some of the nuclei are folded. This smear is characteristic of acute monocytic leukemia (M4/M5 morphology). (Courtesy of Dr. William Finn, Department of Pathology, University of Michigan.)

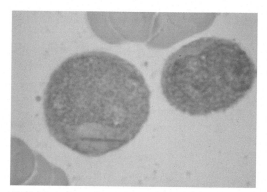

ATLAS FIGURE 40. A high-power view of bone marrow from a patient with acute myeloid leukemia showing two large primitive myeloblasts with very prominent granules and an Auer rod. Auer rods are seen only in malignant proliferation of myeloid cells. (Reprinted with permission from the American Society of Hematology Slide Bank CD, prepared by the Center for Educational Resources, University of Washington, 1998.)

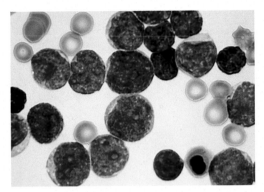

ATLAS FIGURE 41. A high-power view of primitive cells in the peripheral blood. Many of these cells have nucleoli. The large ratio of nucleus to cytoplasm of the blasts is characteristic of acute lymphocytic leukemia. (Reprinted with permission from the American Society of Hematology Slide Bank CD, prepared by the Center for Educational Resources, University of Washington, 1998.)

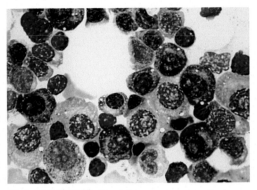

ATLAS FIGURE 42. A bone marrow specimen showing a syncytium of plasma cells with an eccentric nucleus, clumped chromatin in the nucleus, prominent nucleoli and perinuclear Golgi apparatus. This smear is characteristic of multiple myeloma. (Courtesy of Dr. William Finn, Department of Pathology, University of Michigan.)

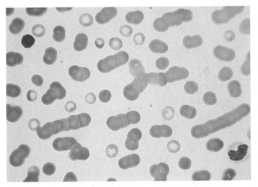

ATLAS FIGURE 43. A low-power peripheral blood smear showing a stacking of red blood cells. This entity called rouleaux is characteristic of hypergammaglobulinemic states such as multiple myeloma. (Reprinted with permission from the American Society of Hematology Slide Bank CD, prepared by the Center for Educational Resources, University of Washington, 1998.)

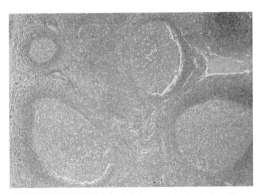

ATLAS FIGURE 44. A low-power view of well-formed germinal centers of a hyperplastic lymph node cross-section. The follicular architecture is intact. (Courtesy of Dr. William Finn, Department of Pathology, University of Michigan.)

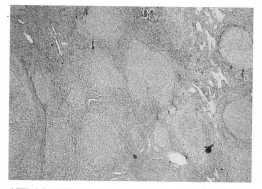

ATLAS FIGURE 45. A low-power view of a follicular lymphoma showing increased number of follicles with crowding of the germinal centers. (Courtesy of Dr. William Finn, Department of Pathology, University of Michigan.)

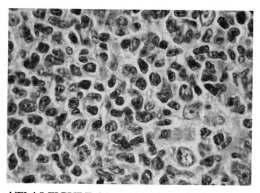

ATLAS FIGURE 46. A high-power view of a neoplastic follicle in follicular lymphoma showing a monotonous population of small cleaved lymphocytes. (Courtesy of Dr. William Finn, Department of Pathology, University of Michigan.)

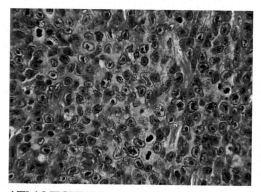

ATLAS FIGURE 47. A medium-power view of diffuse large B-cell lymphoma. (Courtesy of Dr. William Finn, Department of Pathology, University of Michigan.)

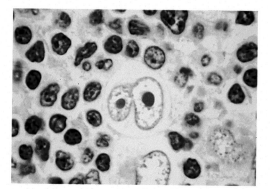

ATLAS FIGURE 48. A high-power view of a Reed-Sternberg cell from a lymph node involved with Hodgkin disease. Note the characteristic bilobed nucleus with prominent nucleoli. (Courtesy of Dr. William Finn, Department of Pathology, University of Michigan.)